Register Now for Online Access to Your Book

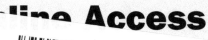

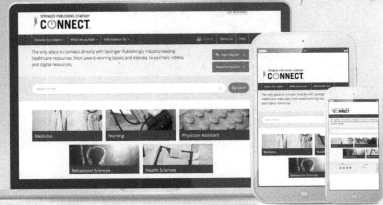

Your print purchase of *Evidence-Based Practice in Nursing,* **includes online access to the contents of your book**—increasing accessibility, portability, and searchability!

Access today at:

**http://connect.springerpub.com/content/book/978-0-8261-2759-4
or scan the QR code at the right with your smartphone
and enter the access code below.**

NADDR4G2

*Scan here for
quick access.*

If you are experiencing problems accessing the digital component of this product, please contact our customer service department at cs@springerpub.com

The online access with your print purchase is available at the publisher's discretion and may be removed at any time without notice.

Publisher's Note: New and used products purchased from third-party sellers are not guaranteed for quality, authenticity, or access to any included digital components.

LS

SPRINGER PUBLISHING COMPANY
View all our products at springerpub.com

EVIDENCE-BASED PRACTICE
IN NURSING

Thomas L. Christenbery, PhD, RN, CNE, is professor and director of program evaluation at Vanderbilt University School of Nursing in Nashville, Tennessee. He is responsible for evaluation and improvement of program outcomes. Dr. Christenbery has 30 years of teaching experience and has held an academic appointment at Vanderbilt University since 2000. He teaches courses in pre-licensure, MSN, DNP, and PhD programs. In each of these programs, Dr. Christenbery has designed and coordinated evidence-based practice courses. For 17 years, he has led faculty across programs in educating learners to effectively engage in interprofessional collaboration that uses evidence-based practice to provide patient-centered care and improve quality of healthcare outcomes. Dr. Christenbery has a publication and research record focused on evidence-based practice. Prior to academia, he was a staff nurse in pediatrics and a nurse manager.

EVIDENCE-BASED PRACTICE IN NURSING

Foundations, Skills, and Roles

Thomas L. Christenbery, PhD, RN, CNE

Editor

SPRINGER PUBLISHING COMPANY

Springer Publishing Company, LLC
11 West 42nd Street
New York, NY 10036
www.springerpub.com

Acquisitions Editor: Joseph Morita
Senior Production Editor: Kris Parrish
Compositor: diacriTech, Chennai

ISBN: 978-0-8261-2742-6
ebook ISBN: 978-0-8261-2759-4
Instructor's Manual ISBN: 978-0-8261-2787-7
Instructor's PowerPoints ISBN: 978-0-8261-2819-5
Instructor's Test Bank ISBN: 978-0-8261-2674-0

Instructor's Materials: Qualified instructors may request supplements by emailing textbook@springerpub.com.

17 18 19 20 / 5 4 3 2 1

The author and the publisher of this Work have made every effort to use sources believed to be reliable to provide information that is accurate and compatible with the standards generally accepted at the time of publication. Because medical science is continually advancing, our knowledge base continues to expand. Therefore, as new information becomes available, changes in procedures become necessary. We recommend that the reader always consult current research and specific institutional policies before performing any clinical procedure. The author and publisher shall not be liable for any special, consequential, or exemplary damages resulting, in whole or in part, from the readers' use of, or reliance on, the information contained in this book. The publisher has no responsibility for the persistence or accuracy of URLs for external or third-party Internet websites referred to in this publication and does not guarantee that any content on such websites is, or will remain, accurate or appropriate.

Library of Congress Cataloging-in-Publication Data
Names: Christenbery, Thomas Lee, editor.
Title: Evidence-based practice in nursing : foundations, skills, and roles /
    [edited by] Thomas L. Christenbery.
Description: New York, NY : Springer Publishing Company, LLC, [2018] |
    Includes bibliographical references and index.
Identifiers: LCCN 2017044828| ISBN 9780826127426 | ISBN 9780826127594 (eISBN)
Subjects: | MESH: Evidence-Based Nursing | Translational Medical Research
Classification: LCC RT42 | NLM WY 100.7 | DDC 610.73—dc23 LC record available at https://lccn.loc.gov/2017044828

Contact us to receive discount rates on bulk purchases.
We can also customize our books to meet your needs.
For more information please contact: sales@springerpub.com

Printed in the United States of America by Bradford & Bigelow.

This book is dedicated to nursing students who continually deepen their understandings of evidence-based practice through critical attitudes of their own nursing practices and development of evidence. Without these bright minds, healthcare organizations would be hard pressed to provide "best evidence."

Contents

Contributors

Molly Bradshaw, DNP, APN, FNP-BC, WHNP-BC   Instructor, Specialty Director: Family Nurse Practitioner Program, Rutgers University, School of Nursing, New Brunswick, New Jersey

Elizabeth Borg Card, MSN, APRN, FNP-BC, CPAN, CCRP   Nursing Research Consultant, Vanderbilt University, Nashville, Tennessee

Thomas L. Christenbery, PhD, RN, CNE   Professor, Director of Program Evaluation, Vanderbilt University, Nashville, Tennessee

Joanne R. Duffy, PhD, RN, FAAN   Executive Vice President and Senior Consultant, Qualicare; Adjunct Professor, Indiana University, Indianapolis, Indiana

Alison H. Edie, DNP, FNP-BC   Assistant Professor, Duke University, Durham, North Carolina

Lianne Jeffs, PhD, RN   Associate Professor, Lawrence S. Bloomberg Faculty of Nursing, University of Toronto; Director, Nursing/Clinical Research, Nursing Administration, St. Michael's Hospital, Toronto, Ontario, Canada

Elaine Kauschinger, PhD, ARNP, FNP-BC   Assistant Professor, Duke University, Durham, North Carolina

Susie Leming-Lee, DNP, MSN, RN, CPHQ   Assistant Professor, Vanderbilt University, Nashville, Tennessee

Rene Love, PhD, DNP, PMHNP-BC, FNAP, FAANP   DNP Director, Clinical Associate Professor, University of Arizona, Tucson, Arizona

Donna Behler McArthur, PhD, FNP-BC, FAANP, FNAP   Clinical Professor of Nursing, University of Arizona, Tucson, Arizona

Mary N. Meyer, PhD, APRN   Associate Professor, University of Missouri Kansas City, Kansas City, Missouri

Lydia D. Rotondo, DNP, RN, CNS   Associate Professor of Clinical Nursing, Associate Dean for Education and Student Affairs, DNP Program Director, University of Rochester, Rochester, New York

Marianne Saragosa, RN, MN   St. Michael's Hospital, Toronto, Ontario, Canada

Philip D. Walker, MLIS, MSHI   Interim Director, Annette and Irwin Eskind Biomedical Library, Vanderbilt University, Nashville, Tennessee

Richard Watters, PhD, RN   Associate Professor of Nursing, Vanderbilt University, Nashville, Tennessee

Nancy Wells, DNSc, RN, FAAN   Research Professor, Vanderbilt University School of Nursing, and Director of Nursing Research, Vanderbilt University Hospitals and Clinics, Vanderbilt University, Nashville, Tennessee

Michelle Zahradnik   Research Coordinator III, St. Michael's Hospital, Toronto, Ontario, Canada

Foreword

Over the years there has been growing acceptance of the need for sound evidence on which to base clinical decisions. By reviewing the evidence, nurses can select the best interventions and approaches for their patients, considering also patient preferences and the nurses' own judgments. In evidence-based practice (EBP), nurses and other healthcare providers identify questions about patient care, search for and critique relevant evidence to help answer those questions, and use that evidence as a basis for decisions. EBP also enables healthcare providers to keep current with the best scientific evidence available, allowing them to provide quality and safe care to patients.

Evidence-based practice is not only important to clinicians: we need evidence to guide educational practices and make sound decisions about the best teaching approaches and assessment methods to use with students. Evidence also should be used to guide policy, management, and other decisions in healthcare and community systems, and as a basis for changing practice.

We cannot have EBP in nursing without preparing nurses who understand the process and can implement it in their own practice. Tom Christenbery has assembled a book to educate nursing students about EBP, enable them to meet the relevant EBP competencies for their program level, and prepare them to develop and implement evidence-based decisions in their clinical practice as students and later as providers. While other books may have a chapter on EBP, the strength of this book is its inclusiveness: The book provides EBP core knowledge for students across each level of nursing education from bachelor of science in nursing (BSN) to master of science in nursing (MSN) and doctor of nursing practice (DNP). I also think the book is relevant to students in associate degree nursing programs. Chapters in the book enable learners to develop competencies to engage in EBP appropriate for their level of education.

The beginning of the book provides readers with foundational knowledge about EBP. Chapters in Part I are particularly relevant to prelicensure nursing students, but many graduate students and nurses have not been prepared in EBP. For that reason, students in MSN and DNP programs and clinicians will find these chapters of value in learning about EBP. Chapter 1 compares EBP with research and quality improvement (QI). These differences are important to understand not only as students but also as healthcare providers. Other chapters address levels of evidence, literature search techniques, and other core concepts of EBP.

Readers need more than a foundational knowledge of EBP. All too often that is all students get. To use EBP in clinical practice, students need to know how to develop, implement, and evaluate EBP projects. In Part II of this book, chapters describe various examples of EBP projects, beginning with developing PICOT (patient population, intervention, comparison, outcome, time frame) questions. It is difficult to implement EBP without understanding change theories, which are addressed in one of the chapters.

Faculty teaching graduate-level courses will find the chapters in Part III to be critical readings for their students. Students will learn about translational research and QI and how these relate to the implementation and evaluation of EBP. I think all students in advanced practice and DNP programs should read these chapters as well as nurses and other health care providers.

The last set of chapters in the book (Part IV) address the importance of developing an organizational culture that promotes EBP. The role of nurse leader, resources for EBP in the work setting, mentoring, and strategies that empower nurses are presented to readers. Empowering nurses to engage in EBP and providing resources and support will lead to improved patient outcomes and higher quality care. Who can argue with that?

This is a must-read book for students across all levels of nursing programs, for faculty and nurse educators in other roles, and for clinicians. The book will be an excellent textbook for students: Chapters include scenarios, case studies, and examples that help students *apply* the concepts they are learning; templates to develop EBP implementation plans; tables and figures that highlight key learnings; and other tools that students can use for learning and later in their own practice. What I like best about this book is its continuity in the development of key EBP concepts and competencies across varied program levels, from prelicensure through DNP programs and into practice.

Marilyn H. Oermann, PhD, RN, ANEF, FAAN
Thelma M. Ingles Professor of Nursing
Director of Evaluation and Educational Research
Duke University School of Nursing
Editor, Nurse Educator and Journal of Nursing Care Quality
Durham, North Carolina

Preface

Evidence-based practice (EBP) is transforming the way healthcare providers, and the public, view healthcare delivery and associated health outcomes. EBP supports healthcare providers to expand beyond insular discipline-specific views of healthcare. Implementation of EBP enables healthcare providers to use, collaboratively, the best scientific evidence, clinical expertise, and patient and population values to deliver quality healthcare. Nurses are present at the point of patient care; therefore, they are at the vanguard of designing and implementing optimal patient-centered care decisions with EBP.

Intellectual curiosity and ingenuity are expected of nursing students as they develop and implement EBP patient-centered care decisions throughout their educational experiences and lifelong careers. As nursing students progress throughout their educational trajectories (e.g., baccalaureate [BSN], master's [MSN], and doctoral [DNP]), it is anticipated they will master degree-appropriate EBP essentials. In addition, nursing students need understanding, skillsets, and integration of critical knowledge about implementation of EBP. Knowledge areas intrinsically woven into successful implementation of EBP include healthcare organizational complexities, interprofessional collaboration, epistemology, philosophy of science, translational science, disruptive innovation, ethics, database algorithms, concept mapping, clinical practice guidelines, continuous quality improvement, and empowerment theory.

GOALS OF THIS BOOK

This book is a response to the need for nursing students to have resources about core EBP knowledge and competencies for each level of nursing practice degrees. Addressing EBP essentials and competencies across BSN, MSN, and DNP levels provides learners an opportunity to develop degree-appropriate skillsets to engage productively in all expected levels of EBP implementation. In addition, while there have been targeted foci to help practitioners appraise and apply appropriate evidence to practice, limited attention has been given to critical knowledge areas that augment successful implementation of EBP.

Importantly, this book acknowledges that EBP involves more than nurses learning about critical evidence appraisal and evidence application exercises. Put another way, this book recognizes that a "one size EBP exercise fits all nurses" approach across their educational and career trajectories is a misrepresentation of real-world EBP clinical practice. Instead, this book addresses critical essentials that nursing students must master as they move from one nursing degree level to the next.

The American Association of Colleges of Nursing (AACN) *Essentials* series for baccalaureate, master's, and doctoral education for advanced practice nursing outlines a stepwise mastery of distinct and increasing complexities of EBP essentials as follows:

BSN:
Essential III: Scholarship for Evidence-Based Practice

MSN:
Essential IV: Translating and Integrating Scholarship Into Practice

DNP:
Essential III: Clinical Scholarship and Analytical Methods for Evidence-Based Practice

Each of the nursing practice degree levels requires specific EBP knowledge, skillsets, and abilities to conceptualize and integrate science, clinical expertise, and patient values and preferences. For example, BSN students must be able to integrate reliable evidence from multiple ways of knowing before they can lead continuous improvement processes based on translational research skills expected at the MSN level. Mastery of translational research skills enables DNP students to practice as specialists/consultants in collaborative knowledge-generating research.

The idea for this book arose from many conversations with nursing students, practitioners, faculty, and researchers about the need for an EBP book in nursing that:

1. Takes an inclusive view of EBP from the perspectives of direct care nurses, advanced registered nurse practitioners, healthcare systems leaders, researchers, and faculty;
2. Aligns EBP content with specific BSN, MSN, and DNP Essentials outlined by the AACN;
3. Addresses leveling EBP process and content across curricula;
4. Uses a theoretical view to describe and explain the empowering impact EBP has on nurses and the patient-centered and population-focused decisions nurses make.

PART I: CONCEPTUAL FOUNDATIONS OF EVIDENCE-BASED PRACTICE

Part I contains five chapters and provides readers with necessary foundational knowledge on which to build clinical decision-making skills based on the best available evidence. Part I, while targeted for BSN students, is relevant for MSN and DNP students. MSN and DNP students may have received their EBP education under an "umbrella effect," which exposes learners only to evidence appraisal and research methodologies, resulting in limited familiarity with critical background information for understanding the development of evidence and science. Chapter 1, "Nursing's Commitment to Best Clinical Decisions," outlines pertinent historical and discipline-specific views of EBP. Because conceptual clarity is needed about evidence and EBP, Chapter 1 distinguishes the similarities and differences among EBP, research, and quality improvement. The chapter highlights scholarly characteristics associated with nurses who engage in EBP activities. Chapter 2, "Using Evidence to Inform and Reform Clinical Practice," describes the state of healthcare quality in the United States and the role of nurses who use EBP in making positive changes in the quality of healthcare. The chapter explores the existence and rationale for facilitators and barriers to EBP. Strategies to capitalize on facilitators and limit barriers are discussed. Chapter 2 helps nursing students identify the breadth and depth of potential EBP projects. Chapter 3, "Integrating Best Evidence Into Practice," outlines levels of evidence, describes how each level is used in practice, identifies strengths and limitations of each level, and provides examples for each level from the literature. The chapter describes literature-search techniques nurses use and provides a detailed illustration of how to access and use an EBP database. The chapter emphasizes the collaborative role of health science librarians and nurses. Chapter 4, "Setting the Boundaries for Nursing Evidence," recognizes the AACN statement that BSN nurses must be able to integrate reliable evidence from *multiple ways of knowing* to inform practice and make clinical judgments. Carper's Ways of Knowing and the nursing metaparadigm serve as frameworks for explaining the origin and boundaries of nursing knowledge. Chapter 5, "Using Nursing Phenomena to Explore Evidence," provides examples of inductive and deductive thinking as approaches to understanding nursing phenomena and examines how concepts and propositions comprise nursing theory. The use of concept mapping, as a tool to clarify meaning and linkages among concepts, illustrates an integral resource for EBP. Criteria for analysis of theory credibility are presented.

PART II: DESIGNING AND IMPLEMENTING EVIDENCE-BASED PRACTICE PROJECTS

Part II contains six chapters that systematically explore the critical elements of conceptualizing, developing, implementing, and evaluating EBP projects. Each chapter focuses on implementation strategies. Content in Part II is appropriate for learners who are beginning to explore EBP, for those who need a refresher in foundations of EBP, and for those who have not covered more advanced areas related to EBP, such as evaluation of clinical practice guidelines. Chapter 6, "Evidence-Based Practice: Success of Practice Change Depends on the Question," demonstrates strategies and rationales for identifying appropriate EBP topics and developing context-specific PICOT (patient population, intervention, comparison, outcome, time frame) questions. Chapter 7, "Change Theories: The Key to Knowledge Translation," guides learners through understanding the important role of change theory in EBP. Facilitators and barriers to change are identified, and strategies to negate barriers are presented. Application and evaluation of change theories used in EBP are covered. Chapter 8, "How to Read and Assess for Quality of Research," presents a concise and thorough prototype for reviewing and analyzing quantitative and qualitative research articles. Chapter 9, "Clinical Practice Guidelines," examines development, application, and evaluation of clinical practice guidelines, which are often central to EBP but frequently absent from EBP books. Chapter 10, "Identifying Significant Evidence-Based Practice Problems Within Complex Health Environments," describes unique methods to align EBP endeavors with healthcare organizational goals. In addition, the chapter explores roles of key stakeholders and interdisciplinary teams for successful implementation of EBP. Chapter 11, "Organizing an Evidence-Based Practice Implementation Plan," sets forth the elements and application of developing effective EBP implementation plans, including analyses and syntheses of knowledge, rollout plan, and SWOT (strengths, weaknesses, opportunities, threats) analysis.

PART III: SCIENCE-BASED DECISIONS AND EVIDENCE-BASED PRACTICE

Part III contains three chapters that emphasize the importance of translational research and quality improvement for the implementation and evaluation of EBP. Topics for each chapter are central to advanced practice registered nurses and DNP students. Chapter 12, "Translational Research," reviews the evolution of translation search. The role of EBP in filling the gap in the translation of knowledge into practice is described. Chapter 13, "Translational Science: Bridging the Gap Between Science and Application," is a valuable resource that depicts nursing's role in translational research and provides a review of translational models for real-world application and evaluation. Chapter 14, "Quality Improvement Processes and Evidence-Based Practice," articulates clearly the important relationship between quality improvement processes and EBP. Chapter 14 compares quality improvement models as a resource for selecting appropriate quality improvement methods.

PART IV: EVIDENCE-BASED PRACTICE: EMPOWERING NURSES

Part IV contains six chapters that address the importance of an EBP culture and structural empowerment strategies required to achieve and sustain a culture that fosters EBP. Chapter 15, "Evidence-Based Practice: A Culture of Organizational Empowerment," defines structural empowerment (e.g., support, resources, information, opportunity) and provides examples of the structural empowerment elements. The chapter outlines the linkages between an empowering work environment and desired healthcare organizational outcomes. Chapter 16, "Nursing Leadership: The Fulcrum of Evidence-Based Practice Culture," underscores the multifaceted role of leadership in *supporting* a flourishing culture of EBP. Chapter 17, "A Prosperous Evidence-Based Culture: Nourishing Resources," reviews organizational *resources* needed to foster an EBP infrastructure. Chapter 18, "Advancing Evidence-Based Practice Through Mentoring and Interprofessional

Collaboration," provides a realistic depiction of mentorship and interprofessional collaboration as a means to access *information and knowledge* to support an EBP culture. Chapter 19, "Evidence-Based Practice: Sequential Layering of BSN, MSN, and DNP Competencies and Opportunities," using a crosswalk of AACN EBP Essentials, illustrates *opportunities* for nurses to engage in EBP at each practice degree level. Chapter 20, "Evidence-Based Practice: Empowering Nurses," recounts the positive outcomes of healthcare organizations that empower nurses to engage in EBP. The chapters in Part IV provide guidance and strategies for using structural empowerment to foster a culture of EBP.

CONCLUSION

Whether you are a new student in a BSN program, in the process of achieving your MSN, or completing your DNP, the editor and contributors believe you will find the content and examples in this book practical and useful. All students of nursing are on a lifelong learning trajectory. The aim of this book is to support your understandings and applications of EBP and critical related content, wherever you may be on the scholarly journey in the quest to provide high-quality patient care.

KEY FEATURES

- Chapter objectives align with AACN Essentials.
- Opening scenarios for each chapter demonstrate negative and positive examples of EBP applications. Each chapter provides content and examples of how to avoid negative EBP outcomes and how to strategize for positive EBP outcomes.
- Key words and concepts are italicized and defined.
- The strong focus on EBP case examples helps readers understand the various contexts in which they will engage in EBP endeavors.
- Practical design templates enable readers to develop EBP implementation plans with critical guideposts.
- Broad coverage of relevant and current examples of ethics, interprofessional collaboration, quality improvement, translational science, and clinical practice guidelines within discussions of EBP context appear throughout the book.
- Continuity in the development of key concepts and skills facilitates a seamless transition for learners between different levels of nursing degree expectations.
- Liberal use of interesting and relevant illustrative tables, boxes, and figures reinforces learning of important concepts.
- EBP hierarchies for quantitative and qualitative research are compared. A quality improvement tool kit is included.

Qualified instructors may obtain access to ancillary materials, including an instructor's manual, PowerPoints, and test bank, by emailing textbook@springerpub.com.

Thomas L. Christenbery

Acknowledgments

I would like to thank Springer Publishing Company and my editor, Joseph Morita, for their faith in this book and their support with editing, designing, and marketing. I am gratefully indebted to my primary mentor, Larry E. Lancaster, for his time, honest critique, and constant encouragement. Many thanks to Betsy Kennedy for her wisdom and guidance throughout the writing process. I want to thank Mia S. Wells for her patience with my unending questions about format and style. A very special thanks to Keith Douglas Wood for his expertise in designing graphics for the book. Last, but certainly not least, thanks to David Beckett Frese, whose support kept me well-balanced throughout the process.

PART I

Conceptual Foundations of Evidence-Based Practice

CHAPTER 1

Nursing's Commitment to Best Clinical Decisions

Thomas L. Christenbery

Objectives

After reading this chapter, learners should be able to:

1. Draw conclusions about the effectiveness of evidence-based practice (EBP) in a variety of clinical situations among various patient populations
2. Outline historical and discipline-specific viewpoints on EBP
3. Distinguish the similarities and differences among EBP, research, and quality improvement as used in clinical environments

EVIDENCE-BASED PRACTICE (EBP) SCENARIOS

Scenario 1

Pediatric clinic nurses in a medically underserved area were concerned when they discovered their patients' rate of tooth decay, prior to starting kindergarten, surpassed the national average of 40%. To alleviate the tooth decay problem, the nurses contacted a major oral healthcare product distributor and subsequently received a large supply of toothbrushes and toothpaste. At the end of each clinic visit, nurses gave each family a toothbrush and toothpaste for each child. Despite these efforts, the clinic continued to report excessive rates of tooth decay in their pediatric population.

Scenario 2

Pediatric clinic nurses in a medically underserved area were concerned when they discovered their patients' rate of tooth decay, prior to starting kindergarten, surpassed the national average of 40%. Nurses observed that the American Academy of Pediatric Dentistry (AAPD) Oral Health Risk Assessment guidelines to assess and manage early childhood dental caries were underused by the clinic's practitioners. In fact, a methodical review of the electronic health records (EHRs) indicated that clinic practitioners were following AAPD assessment and management guidelines 10% of the time. The nurses' concern led them to inquire, "In patients, between ages 2 and 5 years, would an EHR reminder promote practitioner adherence to AAPD guidelines compared with no use of an EHR reminder?" The nurses reviewed relevant research literature about the efficacy of EHR reminders for clinic populations and found strong evidence supporting the use of EHR reminders. At a monthly team meeting with clinic practitioners, the nurses discussed implementing EHR AAPD guideline reminders for all 2- to 5-year-olds. Clinic practitioners noted that patients' parents expressed concern about the tooth decay problem, and they agreed on the value of trying the EHR reminder. Thus, the EHR reminder was implemented at the clinic. A chart review, conducted 6 months postimplementation, found AAPD guidelines were incorporated by practitioners into the clinic visits of children 2 to 5 years of age 90% of the time.

Discussion

The preceding scenarios are emblematic of today's healthcare service. Unfortunately, Scenario 1 dominates as an example of the more practiced method of healthcare service. In Scenario 2, nurses are actively engaged in the process of EBP by demonstrating standardization of best evidence in practice and reducing illogical variation in care (Stevens, 2013). Since 2001, the Institute of Medicine (IOM) has repeatedly recommended EBP as the preferred course to close the gap between what healthcare providers know to be effective healthcare practices and what is actually practiced (Committee on the Robert Wood Johnson Foundation Initiative on the Future of Nursing, 2011; IOM, 2001, 2003, 2008a, 2008b). Scenario 2 focuses on the IOM recommendation that nurses lead interprofessional teams to improve both patient care and healthcare delivery systems (Committee on the Robert Wood Johnson Foundation Initiative on the Future of Nursing, 2011).

In Scenario 2, the nurses' curiosity related to a client-centered care problem led them to question current practice standards. The nurses collected data associated with an identified problem and then searched the research literature for best evidence and evaluated the merit of the evidence. The nurses intentionally integrated research, clinical expertise, and patient/family values to implement an effective practice change. Importantly, the practice change was followed up using an appropriately focused evaluation.

The nurses in Scenario 1, while meaning well, relied on their best inclinations to inform practice. They failed to question whether best or current practices were being used, and whether those practices could bring about desired health outcomes. Critical thinking was insufficient in Scenario 1; therefore, a systematic approach to the evaluation and resolution of a significant health problem was overlooked. Unlike the nurses in Scenario 2, those in Scenario 1 failed to use a formal process with specified steps to change and evaluate clinical practice concerning an important health problem.

COMMITMENT TO BEST CLINICAL PRACTICES

EBP Defined

EBP is defined as *the conscientious, explicit, and judicious use of the integration of current best evidence, clinical expertise, and patient values into the decision-making process for patient care* (Duke University, 2016; Sackett, Rosenberg, Gray, Haynes, & Richardson, 1996; Sackett, Straus, Richardson, Rosenberg, & Haynes, 2000). The key terms within this definition are permanently at the core of nursing care and therefore worthy of review:

- **Conscientious:** Being cautious and thorough in the selection and review of all evidence.
- **Explicit:** Being open and transparent regarding the detection of flaws and gaps in the evidence.
- **Judicious:** Using logic and sound judgment to build compelling cases for practice changes.
- **Current best evidence:** "Best" implies a ranking. Typically, nurses engaged in EBP use quantitative or qualitative research from the highest order or level, and that possesses the utmost quality as evidence. However, not all phenomena related to nursing care have been researched; therefore, nurses sometimes rely on the best nonresearch evidence, such as opinions from expert panels or case studies.
- **Clinical expertise:** The nurse's cumulative experience in clinical practice, education, administration, and informatics.
- **Patient values:** The patient's preferences, individual concerns, and expectations related to quality care.

Commitment to Best Clinical Decisions

Nursing, as a profession, seeks to ensure the care nurses deliver is scientifically sound, clinically effective, compassionate, and meets each patient's needs. Research evidence alone may not always lead to the highest quality care and best practice outcomes. However, integration of best research evidence, clinical experience, and patient values may better determine the provision of optimal nursing care and enhanced patient outcomes. For example, nurses caring for residents in a rural long-term care facility were concerned about the residents' nighttime restlessness. The nurses reviewed relevant research literature and found evidence to suggest that a daytime social dancing activity decreased nighttime restlessness, and the nurses decided to implement a dance therapy program for residents. After some reflection, the nurses understood dancing would be contraindicated for a number of residents in regard to their religious/cultural heritages. To derive the benefits of movement while respecting all residents' religious/cultural values, the nurses implemented a low-impact step aerobics social, which was acceptable as a cultural norm. Integrating research, clinical background experience, and resident values/preferences, the nurses were able to initiate a program that decreased nighttime restlessness.

Regardless of academic degree or program type (e.g., ADN, BSN, MSN, DNP), all nurses and nursing students, with direct patient care responsibilities, are expected to use EBP (American Association of Colleges of Nursing, 2017). This directive is based on substantive reasons:

- EBP helps ensure patients receive nursing care that best addresses their individual needs and, therefore, leads to improved healthcare outcomes (Wells, Pesaro, & McCaffery, 2008).
- At the point of care, EBP provides sound rationale for clinical decision making and conceptually clarifies the rationale (Scott & McSherry, 2008).
- Because EBP provides a sound basis for individualized care, risk, and harm are minimized for the patient (Barnsteiner, 2011).
- Nurses engaged in EBP become proficient in evaluating research evidence and consequently expose gaps and inconsistencies in healthcare knowledge (Fawcett & Garity, 2009).
- EBP has been associated with lower healthcare-related cost compared with care that remains founded on tradition and dated policies and procedures (Sedwick, Lance-Smith, Reeder, & Nardi, 2012).
- EBP has demonstrated a relationship with greater job satisfaction and enhanced professional collaboration (Hughes, 2008).

Nurses engaged in EBP typically follow a practice change trajectory from initial nurse inquiry to practice recommendation (see Figure 1.1). Depending on academic degree and role expectations, all nurses have designated levels of responsibility to make significant commitments to patient care along an EBP path to practice change. Commitment means going above and beyond normally expected behaviors. Individuals committed to a profession, such as nursing, generally invest considerable personal involvement in the work of the profession and tend to do the work well (Friss, 1983). Because the decisions nurses make have

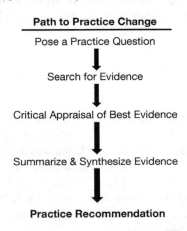

FIGURE 1.1   Evidence-based path to practice change

Source: Courtesy of Nancy Wells.

important patient outcomes, clinical decision making is a hallmark of nursing's professional work (Benner, Hughes, & Sutphen, 2008). Nurses who are deeply committed to making optimal clinical decisions often share a scholarly commitment to the use of EBP.

SCHOLARLY CHARACTERISTICS OF NURSES ENGAGED IN EBP

A scholar is someone with a keen focus who delineates an area of inquiry related to his or her work (Tolk, 2012). Nurses who support their practices using EBP seem to share certain scholarly attributes. For example, nurses who use EBP are *inquisitive* about the current state and standards of patient care and through *questioning* begin to *challenge* the status quo (Christenbery, Williamson, Sandlin, & Wells, 2016). Nurses who seek the best current knowledge, in union with clinical expertise and patient values, display mental integration consistent with *critical thinking* (Profetto-McGrath, Hesketh, Lang, & Estabrooks, 2003). The transference of new knowledge to influence patient care is the essence of *disruptive innovation* (Christensen, Horn, & Johnson, 2011; Nieva et al., 2005). Nurses engaged in EBP use effective *change agent* skillsets to modify practice (Greenhalgh, Robert, Macfarlane, Bate, & Kyriakidou, 2005). The adoption of best evidence into practice is facilitated by nurses who use constructive interpersonal *communication* skills (Berry, 2016). By necessity, nurses who implement EBP are *context oriented* to the patient's environment (DiCenso, Guyatt, & Ciliska, 2002). Nurses who *evaluate* outcomes related to the application of new research findings to practice are engaged in validating *knowledge creation* (Nieva et al., 2005). Importantly, a *collaborative spirit* is needed when nurses share significant EBP findings and outcomes (Titler & Everett, 2001).

In summary, making evidence-based clinical decisions and practice changes requires an assemblage of scholarly strengths and characteristics (see Table 1.1). An important aim of this book is to help you identify, further develop, and apply these scholarly characteristics so that your commitment to making the best clinical decisions and practice changes may be maximized, befitting a nurse engaged in EBP.

EVIDENCE

Evidence, in healthcare, was traditionally thought of as a body of facts indicating whether a belief (e.g., patients desire pain relief) or proposition (e.g., foot elevation decreases pedal edema) was true. In both medicine and nursing, the "body of facts" was typically derived from the scientific method (see Figure 1.2) and applied to healthcare decision making (Claridge & Fabian, 2005). Nightingale used the scientific method (i.e., research) to great effect in exploring differential mortality among population subgroups (Nightingale, 1863) and excess mortality after childbirth (Nightingale, 1871).

The scientific method consists of a systematic set of skills to investigate phenomena for the purpose of acquiring new knowledge or validating and

TABLE 1.1   Scholarly Characteristics of Nurses Engaged in Evidence-Based Practice (EBP)

EBP Scholarly Characteristic	Definition	Demonstrated Behavior
Inquisitive	Having a desire to learn more about patient care and healthcare systems	• The nurse wonders if music CDs at bedtime will promote quality of sleep for patients on a cardiac surgery unit.
Challenger	A query regarding the truth or efficacy of healthcare-related phenomena	• The nurse begins to ask peers if alternative methods of sleep promotion have ever been tried on the unit.
Critical thinker	Actively and skillfully analyzing and synthesizing information from a variety of evidence sources	• The nurse reviews and assesses research literature regarding music therapy relaxation interventions. • Using intake admission forms, the nurse begins chart review to assess patients' preferred bedtime rituals.
Disruptive innovator	Creating or modifying an intervention/procedure that eventually disrupts an old intervention/procedure	• The nurse seeks support from peers, physicians, and managers to pilot music tape relaxation intervention on selected patients.
Change agent	Actively engaged in transforming patient care by altering current patient care standards	• The nurse develops a plan to manage and resolve resistance to change regarding music therapy relaxation.
Communicator	Effective use of communication skills to convey ideas, innovations, and plans regarding evidence-based intervention	• The nurse develops a clear vision of a plan for use of music relaxation tapes and clearly articulates that plan to others.
Context oriented	Aware of the circumstances that form the setting for EBP intervention	• The nurse is aware of and sensitive to the unit's established evening care routines.
Evaluator	An activity to assess the amount or value of EBP implementation	• The nurse creates a plan to evaluate sleep quantity and quality postintervention.
Knowledge creator	Formation of new ideas regarding EBP implementation	• The nurse learns that the music CD relaxation intervention is efficacious.
Collaborative spirit	Working with others to accomplish a desired patient outcome	• The nurse recognizes the contributions of the team effort and shares outcomes with the team and others.

integrating previously gained knowledge. The scientific method of inquiry is empirical and requires a working hypothesis that can be tested through observation or experiment (Goldhaber & Neito, 2010). Not all nursing research questions are a suitable fit for experimental research designs; thus, nursing research uses multiple other forms of inquiry (e.g., qualitative research, descriptive studies) to study its phenomena.

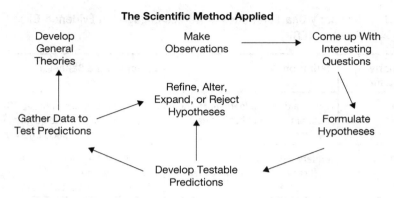

FIGURE 1.2   Representation of the scientific method

Prior to the 1970s, the process by which the scientific method and research were selected and applied in medicine and nursing was highly individualized and subjective. Physicians (DiCenso et al., 2002) and nurses (Beyea & Slattery, 2013) frequently determined independently what research evidence, if any, to consider and how to merge that research with their personal beliefs and contextual factors. There was no formal process in healthcare to determine which research evidence to use, how best to use the research, to what extent to use the research evidence, and on what population. There was an implicit assumption that physicians and nurses would appropriately incorporate research evidence into their practices based on their qualifications as educated, licensed, and altruistic practitioners.

HISTORICAL PERSPECTIVE OF EBP

In 1972, Archibald Cochrane cast doubt on the effectiveness of practitioners independently and arbitrarily applying select scientific knowledge to clinical decision making. Cochrane was especially concerned that practitioners would avoid the results of a single study if the study's results failed to fit the practitioner's preconceived ideas. This concern led Cochrane to advocate rigorous and systematic reviews of research (i.e., randomized controlled trials, cohort studies) to provide exhaustive summaries of science related to specific research questions (Beyea & Slattery, 2013; Claridge & Fabian, 2005). Cochrane's advocacy of systematic reviews of randomized controlled trials led to the development of the Cochrane Library database of systematic reviews (www.cochranelibrary.com). Today, the Cochrane Library is an invaluable resource for nurses and other healthcare providers engaged in EBP.

In 1992, Guyatt introduced the term *evidence-based medicine* (Evidence-Based Medicine Working Group, 1992; Zimerman, 2013). Similar to Cochrane, Guyatt wanted to shift clinical decision making from a position of instinctive, unsystematic clinical experience and pathophysiologic rationale to clinically relevant research. In 1996, Sackett and physician colleagues explained evidence-based clinical decision making as a confluence of systematic research, clinical expertise, and patient preferences (Sackett et al., 1996). Since then, evidence-based clinical decision making has been widely accepted in multiple health disciplines including nursing, social work (Social Work Policy Institute, 2016), and public health (Developing Healthy People 2020, 2010).

Prior to Sackett's definition of evidence-based clinical decision making, nursing as a profession focused its clinical decision making on *research utilization* as a method of translating research into practice (Titler & Everett, 2001). Although research utilization incorporates the critical appraisal and application of research to practice, research utilization did not integrate the nurse's clinical experience or patient's values.

Current nursing leaders, in the area of EBP, include nursing's rich tradition of using meaningful research findings in conjunction with best experiential evidence and patient values to inform clinical decision making as the definition of nursing EBP (Dearholt & Dang, 2012; Melnyk & Fineout-Overholt, 2015; Stevens, 2013). This definition of EBP is specific to nursing and at the same time aligns nursing with medicine and other disciplines engaged in providing care in the patient's best interest.

DIFFERENTIATING EBP, RESEARCH, AND QUALITY IMPROVEMENT

Quality is central to healthcare. The IOM (2001) describes quality as the degree to which healthcare services increase the likelihood of desired health outcomes and are consistent with up-to-date professional knowledge. The Agency for Healthcare Research and Quality (n.d.) explains quality healthcare as doing the right thing, at the right time, in the right way, for the right patient, and having the best possible outcomes. An informed and effective level of quality care is dependent on three key factors: (a) a nursing workforce engaged in EBP, (b) a culture that is amenable to quality improvement practices, and (c) a work environment that supports the use and practice of healthcare-related research. In addition to EBP, this book explores the direct linkages that research and quality improvement (QI) contribute to clinical decision making and, consequently, the richer repertoire of healthcare options and higher quality patient care outcomes.

EBP, *research*, and *QI* are three distinct terms that are essential to quality healthcare, yet are frequently used interchangeably and, therefore, used improperly (Hedges, 2009; Newhouse, 2007; Newhouse, Pettit, Poe, & Rocco, 2006; Shirey et al., 2011). The literature is unquestionable in reporting that much misunderstanding exists in how these terms are used improperly.

Misnomers are often harmless; however, using the terms *EBP*, *research*, and *QI* interchangeably in clinical practice leads to unwarranted outcomes such as disregard for Internal Review Board (IRB) protocol, absence or lack of required project oversight, and most importantly, risks (e.g., absence of full disclosure) to participants or subjects. Misusing these three terms may be related, in part, to the nature of their unique and corresponding relationships (Newhouse, 2007). Nevertheless, nurses and other healthcare providers need to make a deliberate effort to use these three terms appropriately.

To assist in the appropriate use of EBP, research, and QI, it is helpful to consider each term in regard to classifications of *context, methodology,* or *scholarly relevance.* Context consists of circumstances that form the background for EBP, research, and QI and includes (a) history, (b) definition, (c) and purpose. Methodology refers to various functions and entities that put EBP, research, and QI into action and include (a) rigor, (b) data collection and measures, (c) project oversight, (d) population of interest, (e) funding, (f) interconnections, (g) models and methods, and (h) data analysis. Scholarly relevance demonstrates the intellectual contributions to quality that proper use of EBP, research, and QI provide and is composed of (a) generalizability and transferability and (b) dissemination of findings.

Importantly, the summation in Box 1.1 provides a rationale for remaining vigilant in using EBP, research, and QI as separate terms. Table 1.2 depicts each major classification and related dimensions as a means to help clarify confusion and misuse among EBP, research, and QI.

The EBP nursing movement is in its early decades. Both healthcare organizations and schools of nursing have important roles in assisting nurses to clearly differentiate among EBP, research, and QI. When clarity among these three problem-solving processes is achieved, nurses can more easily begin to develop the necessary skills and appropriate activities to more fully engage in and support EBP, research, and QI.

To illustrate the differences among these three processes (i.e., EBP, research, QI), consider the following clinical example. While monitoring (QI) patients on a chronic respiratory unit, nurses found that patient fall rates had increased significantly over the past 6 months. The majority of these falls occurred in patients over 75 years of age and occurred during the night shift. To address this problem, unit nurses conducted an extensive systematic review of the literature related to falls in elderly hospitalized patients (EBP). The systematic literature review found evidence to support the following protocol: Hourly rounds on all high-risk fall patients by direct care staff (to include prompted voiding

---

BOX 1.1   **Summary of Evidence-Based Practice, Research, and Quality Improvement**

Summation:

Evidence-based practice (EBP): This requires practitioners to ask compelling questions, search for best evidence, evaluate the strength and quality of evidence, and implement practice change if warranted. An EBP project is only as good as the "best evidence" related to research, clinical experience, and patient values. Therefore, EBP *is not* synonymous with research or quality improvement (QI).

Research: Quantitative research can possibly establish correlation or causality. Qualitative research can provide new understandings of phenomena. The approach to research should be to discover new knowledge, which *is not* an expected function of EBP or QI.

Quality improvement: This does not establish correlation or causality. Methodologically, QI designs are weak and have poor, if any, internal validity, reliability, and sustainability related to QI projects. Therefore, QI *should not* be misconstrued as EBP or research enterprises. A commonly held, erroneous belief suggests that generation of QI data signifies nurses are actively engaged in research. QI does not, as a rule, meet federally instructed research design requirements or human participant protection rules.

TABLE 1.2   Distinguishing Characteristics of Evidence-Based Practice (EBP), Research, and Quality Improvement (QI)

Context	Evidence-Based Practice	Research	Quality Improvement	Comments
Historical roots	• Originated with Cochrane, 1972 • Founded on criticism of lack of reliable evidence to support commonly used interventions	• Dates to antiquity • Heavily influenced by scientific method beginning in 17th century	• Credited to William Deming, 20th century, as a means to improve product quality	• EBP, research, and QI have three distinct historical origins underscoring the heterogeneity of each term
Definition	• Integration of clinical expertise, patient values, and best research evidence into the decision-making process for patient care (Duke, 2016)	• Systematic inquiry using orderly, disciplined methods to establish facts or achieve new knowledge (Polit & Beck, 2012)	• Data-driven systematic method with individuals collaborating to improve select internal systems, processes, costs, productivity, and quality outcomes (Shirey et al., 2011)	• Not within the realms of EBP or QI to generate new knowledge and should not be credited as reliable (i.e., consistently producing the same results under similar circumstances) methods for generating new knowledge
Purpose	• To rank evidence that will be used to answer clinical or systems questions	• Describe, explain, or predict phenomena to either verify existing knowledge or create new knowledge	• Identify organizational or systems problems to improve safety, efficiency, and quality of healthcare	• EBP and QI use existing knowledge to implement improvement; research creates the knowledge used for EBP and QI

(continued)

TABLE 1.2 Distinguishing Characteristics of Evidence-Based Practice (EBP), Research, and Quality Improvement (QI) *(continued)*

Methodology	Evidence-Based Practice	Research	Quality Improvement	Comments
Rigor	● Rigorous to the extent that certain steps are followed to determine the best evidence for select patient care scenarios	● Whether quantitative or qualitative, must be extremely rigorous to produce the highest levels of evidence	● QI is considered least rigorous and produces the lowest level of evidence	● Level of scientific rigor provides rationale for clear and accurate use of terms ● Research: most rigorous ● EBP: Somewhat rigorous ● QI: Least rigorous
Data collection and measures	● Data collection usually straightforward and efficient	● Uses complex measures, requiring precise administration ● Measurement tools expected to have high estimates of reliability, validity, specificity, and/or sensitivity	● Data collection usually straightforward and efficient	● Depending on the scope of the project, resources and cost usually minimal for EBP and QI ● Research requires well-planned allocation of resources and is often time consuming
Project oversight	● Regulating body is the home organization	● Extensive and includes oversight by Institutional Review Board (mandatory) and at times Office of Human Research Protection, Food and Drug Administration, as well as state and local laws	● Oversight from the home organization ● May be influenced by Joint Commission on Accreditation of Healthcare Organizations and Centers for Medicare and Medicaid Services	● EBP and QI require IRB approval if there is possibility of publishing findings or if patients may possibly be exposed to harm ● IRB approval unquestionably required for qualitative and quantitative research

(continued)

TABLE 1.2 Distinguishing Characteristics of Evidence-Based Practice (EBP), Research, and Quality Improvement (QI) *(continued)*

Population of interest	• Specific unit (e.g., Renal Dialysis Unit) or a patient population (e.g., children with thalassemia) within a healthcare organization	• Persons for whom the findings may be generalized (quantitative) to or transferable (qualitative) to	• Specific unit (e.g., Renal Dialysis Unit) or a patient population (e.g., children with thalassemia) within a healthcare organization	• Population benefit is usually immediate with EBP and QI • Population benefit may be delayed with research populations
Funding	• Usually internal to organization	• May be internal or external (e.g., National Institutes of Health) depending on research question and scope of project	• Usually internal to organization	• EBP and QI frequently do not require funding • Research almost always requires funding
Interconnections	• Provides insight for potential QI projects • May detect gaps in evidence, indicating need for research	• Informs opportunities for both EBP and QI projects • Impetus may be from QI projects that fail to produce quality or gaps found in literature as part of EBP project • Research evidence is often essential for the development of interventions to improve patient outcomes in QI endeavors	• Inform both EBP and research • Research may support need for QI projects	• Corresponding relationships among EBP, research, and QI are beneficial in providing a richer, more informed basis for nursing care

(continued)

TABLE 1.2 Distinguishing Characteristics of Evidence-Based Practice (EBP), Research, and Quality Improvement (QI) *(continued)*

	Evidence-Based Practice	Research	Quality Improvement	Comments
Models and methods used	Examples of frequently used *models* include: • Iowa Model of EBP • Academic Center for EBP Star Model of Knowledge Transformation (ACE Model) • Rosswurm and Larrabee	• Uses scientific method or variation of scientific method if quantitative • Phenomenology, ethnography, grounded theory if qualitative	Examples of frequently used *methods* include • Six Sigma • LEAN Six Sigma • FOCUS-Plan Do Study Act (PDSA) • FOCUS-Plan Do Check Act (PDCA)	Discrete models and methods to achieve results indicate that EBP, research, and QI are not interchangeable terms
Data analysis	• Usually descriptive statistics or bivariate analysis	• Complex inferential statistics are often used with quantitative research, while qualitative analysis requires rich descriptive narrative	• Usually descriptive statistics or statistical process control charts	
Scholarly relevance				
Generalizability or transferability	• Results may be transferable to other similar settings	• Findings may be generalizable (quantitative) or transferable (qualitative) beyond home organization, depending on design and study rigor	• Not generalizable beyond home organization • External organizations may benefit from lessons learned	• Lessons learned from EBP and QI projects are often shared with external organizations • Results from research findings are often generalizable or transferable to other organizations or populations
Dissemination of findings	Dissemination of findings excepted within organization; findings are frequently shared as posters/podiums at nursing conferences	Dissemination of findings expected in poster/podium and literature; expected to reach regional, national, and international audiences	Dissemination of findings excepted within home organization but not necessarily expected beyond home organization	Important to keep in mind at outset of EBP and QI projects, if dissemination of findings is expected, IRB approval will be needed

protocol) between 2400 and 0500 hours. If nurses had detected inconsistencies in the review of literature such as limiting evening fluid intake, the nurses may need to initiate a research study to more fully address prevention of the fall phenomenon (research). If the unit's patients continue to experience an excessive number of falls following implementation of the fall protocol, additional monitoring may be needed to determine if direct care staff are indeed following the protocol (QI). Using the Agency for Healthcare Research and Quality Falls Management Program Self-Assessment Tool may identify a lack of staff adherence to the protocol and provide opportunity for further staff education on the value of the protocol. The nurses in this example monitored both practice and patient outcomes (QI), systematically reviewed the literature, and recommended a practice change (EBP). They were amenable to further scientific investigation (research) if the literature presented gaps or inconsistences related to relevant implementations.

CLINICAL DECISION MAKING AND EBP

Clinical decision making is the contextual, ongoing, and evolving process, whereby nurses gather, interpret, and evaluate data for the purpose of selecting optimal evidence-based courses of action (Tiffen, Corbridge, & Slimmer, 2014). Clinical decision making is a complex process requiring nurses to make choices far beyond limited, categorical options that lead to a defined course of action. Clinical decisions made by nurses occur within active, goal-shifting, and dynamic contexts. Clinical decisions consist of numerous practice-oriented considerations such as assessment, planning, implementation, and evaluation. External influences such as organizational support and allocated resources greatly impact clinical decisions. Internal factors such as the nurse's degree of confidence and perceived controllability of clinical outcomes influence clinical decision making. Effective clinical decision making requires the use of a broad and in-depth knowledge base. Additionally, clinical decisions are almost always encumbered by a degree of uncertainty.

The complexities and ambiguities surrounding clinical decision making are frequently numerous and overwhelming. As nurses become increasingly involved in clinical decision making, it becomes more important for them to use EBP to make the most significant and justifiable decisions in the patient's best interest. Joining the best research evidence, knowledge arising from the nurse's clinical experience, and patient preferences supports an informed evidence-based clinical decision-making process.

SUMMARY

EBP leads to better patient outcomes; therefore, it is an important aspect of nursing care. EBP is widely encouraged at the organizational, state, and federal levels. Understanding essential contextual knowledge about EBP is vital to successfully generating best evidence into practice. This chapter explores background knowledge related to EBP as a foundation for understanding its importance to healthcare and application to a more informed practice of modern nursing.

REFERENCES

Agency for Healthcare Research and Quality. (n.d.). A quick look at quality. Retrieved from http://archive.ahrq.gov/consumer/qnt/qntqlook.htm

American Association of Colleges of Nursing. (2017). AACN essentials. Retrieved from http://www.aacnnursing.org/Education-Resources/AACN-Essentials

Barnsteiner, J. (2011). Teaching the culture of safety. *The Online Journal of Issues in Nursing, 16*(3). doi:10.3912/OJIN.Vol16No03Man05

Benner, P., Hughes, R. G., & Sutphen, M. (2008). Clinical reasoning, decision making and action: Thinking critically and clinically. In R. G. Hughes (Ed.), *Patient and safety quality: An evidence-based handbook for nurses* (Vol. 1, pp. 1–23). Rockville, MD: Agency for Healthcare Research and Quality.

Berry, M.-E. (2016). Better, safer patient care through evidence-based practice and teamwork. *The American Nurse.* Retrieved from http://www.theamericannurse.org/index.php/2014/09/02/better-safer-patient-care-through-evidence-based-practice-and-teamwork

Beyea, S. C., & Slattery, M. J. (2013). Historical perspectives on evidence-based nursing. *Nursing Science Quarterly, 26*(2), 152–155.

Christenbery, T., Williamson, A., Sandlin, V., & Wells, N. (2016). Immersion in evidence-based practice fellowship program. *Journal for Nurses in Professional Development, 32*(1), 15–20.

Christensen, C., Horn, M. B., & Johnson, C. W. (2011). *Disrupting class: How disruptive innovation will change the way the world learns.* New York, NY: McGraw-Hill.

Claridge, J. A., & Fabian, T. C. (2005). History and development of evidence-based medicine. *World Journal of Surgery, 29*, 547–553. doi:10.1007/s00268-005-7910-1

Committee on the Robert Wood Johnson Foundation Initiative on the Future of Nursing. (2011). *The future of nursing: Leading change, advancing health.* Washington, DC: National Academies Press.

Dearholt, S., & Dang, D. (2012). *Johns Hopkins nursing evidence-based practice model and guidelines.* Indianapolis, IN: Sigma Theta Tau International.

Developing Healthy People 2020. (2010). Evidence-based and clinical public health: Generating and applying the evidence. Retrieved from http://www.healthypeople.gov/2010/hp2020/advisory/pdfs/EvidenceBasedClinicalPH2010.pdf

DiCenso, A., Guyatt, G., & Ciliska, D. (2002). *Evidence-based nursing: A guide to clinical practice.* St. Louis, MO: Mosby.

Duke University. (2017). What is evidence-based practice (EBP)? Retrieved from http://guides.mclibrary.duke.edu/c.php?g=158201&p=1036021

Evidence-Based Medicine Working Group. (1992). Evidence-based medicine: A new approach to teaching the practice of medicine. *Journal of the American Medical Association, 268*, 2420–2425.

Fawcett, J., & Garity, J. (2009). *Evaluating research for evidence-based nursing practice.* Philadelphia, PA: F. A. Davis.

Friss, L. (1983). Organizational commitment and job involvement in directors of nursing services. *Nursing Administration Quarterly, 7*(2), 1–10.

Goldhaber, A. S., & Neito, M. M. (2010). Photon and graviton mass limit. *Reviews of Modern Physics, 82*, 39–979. doi:10.1103/RevModPhys.82.939

Greenhalgh, T., Robert, G., Bate, P., Macfarlane, F., & Kyriakidou, O. (2005). *Diffusion of innovations in health service organisations: A systematic literature review.* Malden, MA: Blackwell.

Hedges, C. (2009). Pulling it all together: QI, EBP, and research. *Nursing Management, 40*(4), 10–12. doi:10.1097/01.NUMA.0000349683.16542.e4

Hughes, R. G. (2008). Nurses at the "sharp end" of patient care. In R. G. Hughes (Ed.), *Patient and safety quality: An evidence-based handbook for nurses* (Vol. 1, pp. 1–30). Rockville, MD: Agency for Healthcare Research and Quality.

Institute of Medicine. (2001). *Crossing the quality chasm: A new health system for the 21st century.* Washington, DC: National Academies Press.

Institute of Medicine. (2003). *Health professions education: A bridge to quality* (A. C. Greiner & E. Knebel, Eds.). Washington, DC: National Academies Press.

Institute of Medicine. (2008a). *Knowing what works in health care: A roadmap for the nation.* Washington, DC: National Academies Press.

Institute of Medicine. (2008b). *Training the workforce in quality improvement and quality improvement research.* IOM Forum Workshop. Washington, DC: National Academies Press.

Melnyk, B. M., & Fineout-Overholt, E. (2015). *Evidence-based practice in nursing and healthcare: A guide to best practice.* Philadelphia, PA: Wolters Kluwer.

Newhouse, R. P. (2007). Diffusing confusion among evidence-based practice, quality improvement and research. *Journal of Nursing Administration, 37*(10), 432–435.

Newhouse, R. P., Pettit, J. C., Poe, S., & Rocco, L. (2006). The slippery slope: Differentiating between quality improvement and research. *Journal of Nursing Administration, 36*(4), 211–219.

Nieva, V., Murphy, R., Ridley, N, Donaldson, N., Combes, J., Mitchell, P., … Carpenter, D. (2005). From science to service: A framework for the transfer of patient safety research into practice. In K. Henrickson, J. B. Battles, E. S. Marks, & D. I. Lewin (Eds.), *Advances in patient safety: From research to implementation.* Rockville, MD: Agency for Healthcare Research and Quality.

Nightingale, F. (1863). Sanitary statistics of native colonial schools and hospitals. In *Transactions in the National Association for the Promotion of Social Science* (p. 477). London, UK: London School of Hygiene and Tropical Medicine.

Nightingale, F. (1871). *Introductory notes on lying-in institutions.* London: Longmans, Green.

Polit, D. F., & Beck, C. T. (2012). *Nursing research: Generating and assessing evidence for nursing practice.* Philadelphia, PA: Wolters Kluwer/Lippincott Williams & Wilkins.

Profetto-McGrath, J., Hesketh, K. L., Lang, S., & Estabrooks, C. A. (2003). A study of critical thinking and research utilization among nurses. *Western Journal of Nursing Research, 25*(3), 322–337.

Sackett, D. L., Rosenberg, W. M., Gray, J. A., Haynes, R. B., & Richardson, W. S. (1996). Evidence based medicine: What it is and what it isn't. *British Medical Journal, 13,* 312(7023), 71–72.

Sackett, D. L., Straus, S. E., Richardson, W. S., Rosenberg, W., & Haynes, R. B. (2000). *Evidence-based medicine: How to practice and teach EBM* (2nd ed.). New York, NY: Churchill Livingstone.

Scott, K., & McSherry, R. (2008). Evidence-based nursing: Clarifying the concepts for nurses in practice. *Journal of Clinical Nursing, 18*(8), 1085–1095. doi:10.1111/j.1365-2702.2008.02588.x

Sedwick, M. B., Lance-Smith, M., Reeder, S. J., & Nardi, J. (2012). Using evidence-based practice to prevent ventilator-associated pneumonia. *Critical Care Nurse, 32*(4), 41–51. doi:10.4037/ccn2012964

Shirey, M. R., Hauck, S. L., Embree, J. L., Kinner, T. J., Schaar, G. L., Phillips, L. A., … McCool, I. A. (2011). Showcasing differences between quality improvement evidence-based practice and research. *Journal of Continuing Education in Nursing, 42*(2), 57–68.

Social Work Policy Institute. (2016). EVIDENCE-BASED practice. Retrieved from http://www.socialworkpolicy.org/research/evidence-based-practice.html

Stevens, K. R. (2013). The impact of evidence-based practice in nursing and the next big ideas. *The Online Journal of Nursing, 18*(2), 1–11. doi:10.3912/OJIN.Vol18No02Man04

Tiffen, J., Corbridge, S. J., & Slimmer, L. (2014). Enhancing clinical decision making: Development of a continuous definition and conceptual framework. *Journal of Professional Nursing, 30*(5), 399–405. doi:10.1016/j.profnurs.2014.01.006

Titler, M. G., & Everett, L. Q. (2001). Translating research into practice: Considerations for critical care investigators. *Critical Care Nursing Clinics of North America, 13*(4), 587–604.

Tolk, A. (2012). What are the characteristics of a scholar? *SCS Modeling and Simulation Magazine, 3*(2), 54–58.

Wells, N., Pasero, C., & McCaffery, M. (2008). Improving the quality of care through pain assessment and management. In R. G. Hughes (Ed.), *Patient and safety quality: An evidence-based handbook for nurses* (Vol. 1, pp. 1–29). Rockville, MD: Agency for Healthcare Research and Quality.

Zimerman, A. L. (2013). Evidence-based medicine: A short history of a modern medical movement. *American Medical Association Journal of Ethics, 15*(1), 71–76.

CHAPTER 2

Using Evidence to Inform and Reform Clinical Practice

Thomas L. Christenbery

Objectives

After reading this chapter, learners should be able to:

1. Recognize barriers to implementing evidence-based practice (EBP)
2. Recommend ideas to support and enhance EBP facilitators
3. Describe the state of healthcare quality
4. Understand the role of EBP in improving healthcare quality
5. Identify potential ethical concerns related to the use of EBP

EVIDENCE-BASED PRACTICE (EBP) SCENARIOS

Scenario 1

A new nurse is working in a clinic for an underserved population of HIV-positive adolescents. The nurse notes that most of the clinic's medication adherence programs are male-oriented, non–gender-specific, and counterproductive in the treatment of the clinic's female clients. The nurse searches the literature for evidence about the most effective medication adherence programs for female adolescent clients and discovers the majority of studies consist of male participants. The few studies with female participants are nonempirical and nonrigorous. The nurse sees no ethical concern in using the available male-oriented research to generalize findings to the clinic's female adolescent population. The adolescent female population at the clinic continues to have low adherence to prescribed HIV medication regimens.

Scenario 2

A new nurse is working in a clinic for an underserved population of HIV-positive adolescents. The nurse notes that most of the clinic's medication adherence programs are male-oriented, non–gender-specific, and counterproductive in the treatment of the clinic's female clients. The nurse searches the literature for evidence about the most effective medication adherence programs for female adolescent clients and discovers the majority of studies consist of male participants. The few studies with female participants are nonempirical and nonrigorous. Because the published research failed to provide gender-specific interventions, the nurse was not ethically comfortable continuing to misuse and apply male-oriented treatment recommendations to females. The nurse deferred to the wisdom of experienced colleagues in similar clinics to provide relevant experience-based evidence to help address the disparity between male and female medication regimen adherence. Using the professional expertise of others, over time the nurse began to notice a decline in medication regimen nonadherence in the clinic's female adolescent HIV population.

Discussion

The nurse in Scenario 1 began the process of EBP but was content to proceed with the status quo when the literature provided no recommended alternatives to the current protocol. The nurse in Scenario 2 recognized the critical intersection of EBP and ethics and was not ethically content to proceed with the status quo and misuse current empirical recommendations.

HEALTHCARE QUALITY

A primary goal for healthcare practitioners is to provide health service that optimizes the well-being of patients (McGlynn & Brook, 2001). Healthcare quality is central to achieving this goal. Many patients perceive healthcare quality in the United States as commendable. This perception is understandable, because, at its best, healthcare in the United States is unsurpassed. For example, the United States is at the vanguard in development of both innovative healthcare technologies and pharmaceuticals; many of its medical centers are world renowned for the caliber of care delivered, and its nurses and doctors are recognized as a well-educated and informed workforce. Despite these notable facts, *healthcare quality in the United States is repeatedly reported as suboptimal and of frighteningly poor quality* (Committee on the Robert Wood Johnson Foundation Initiative on the Future of Nursing, 2011; Institute of Medicine [IOM], 2000, 2001, 2003, 2008a, 2008b).

The Institute of Medicine (IOM, 2001) defined healthcare quality as "the degree to which health services for individuals and populations increase the likelihood of desired health outcomes and are consistent with current professional knowledge"

(p. 232). To augment this definition, the IOM (2001) identified six fundamental components central to the definition of healthcare quality:

Safe: For healthcare quality to be safe, there must be avoidance of harm (i.e., freedom from injury) to patients from the care that is meant to help them. Safe care includes (a) an optimal standard of care at all times, including night shifts and weekends; (b) patients only need to disclose healthcare information once to their healthcare providers; and (c) patient information is not misplaced or lost.

Effective: Healthcare quality is considered effective when it is centered on accessible scientific evidence. Healthcare quality is dependent on relevant evidence that is rigorously and systematically obtained to determine which preventive services, diagnostic tests, and interventions (or nonintervention) would produce optimal patient outcomes.

Patient centered: The provision of patient-centered care is respectful of and responsive to individual patient preferences, needs, and values and ensures that patient values guide all decisions. Patient-centered care encompasses the coordination and integration of communication, information, education, physical comfort, emotional support (e.g., lessening fear and anxiety), and involvement of effective support networks.

Timely: Healthcare quality that is timely is demonstrated by reduced waits and harmful delays, which are often anxiety provoking for those who receive care and those who provide care.

Efficient: Efficient healthcare quality is the avoidance of waste, including equipment, supplies, ideas, and energy.

Equitable: Provision of healthcare is equitable when care is delivered without variation in quality because of personal characteristics, such as gender, ethnicity, geographic location, protected veteran status, genetic test status, and socioeconomic status, that are unrelated to the patient's condition or reason for seeking healthcare (IOM, 1990, p. 21).

Suboptimal patient care experiences attributed to poor healthcare quality in the United States are well documented (Lang, Hodge, Olson, Romano, & Kravitz, 2004; Van Den Bos et al., 2011). In fact, two decades ago, the President's Advisory Commission on Consumer Protection and Quality in the Health Care Industry (1998) noted there is *no assurance* that any person will receive high-quality healthcare for any particular health concern. The following data illustrate salient and persistent features of the healthcare quality crisis:

- Medical error (i.e., unintended act of treatment omission or commission or treatment that does not achieve its intended outcome) is the third-leading cause of death in the United States (Makary & Daniel, 2016).
- Almost 75% of those living with chronic health conditions (e.g., congestive heart failure, AIDS, rheumatoid arthritis) report it is difficult to obtain needed care from their healthcare providers (Harris Interactive and ARiA Marketing, 2002).

- It is estimated that 8 million people in the United States living with diabetes remain undiagnosed (American Diabetes Association, 2017).
- Approximately 5,000 Medicare beneficiaries suffer a *never event* (e.g., wrong surgical site) each month (Levinson, 2010).

VARIATIONS IN HEALTHCARE QUALITY

Overuse

Problems associated with healthcare quality generally fall into one of three categories: *overuse, underuse,* and *misuse* (see Table 2.1). Overuse occurs when a healthcare service is provided under conditions in which the service's potential for harm exceeds possible benefit to the patient (Orszag, 2008). More healthcare (i.e., overuse) is not always better healthcare. Allocating more money for treatment does not necessarily translate into better patient outcomes. For example, 97% of emergency physicians indicate that at least some of the imaging procedures they order are medically unnecessary (Kanzaria et al., 2015). Advanced practice registered nurses (APRNs) are expected to order needed tests or procedures for patients, and direct care nurses are responsible for assessing, preparing, educating, and evaluating patients for tests and procedures. It is important for nurses to base the need and subsequent care for diagnostic procedures, as well as treatments, on the best available research, patient preference, and nurse expertise, rather than on unquestioned and outdated standards of practice.

TABLE 2.1   Overuse, Underuse, and Misuse

Service Abuse	Desired Service	Examples of Outcomes Related to Desired Service
Overuse	Patients have a right to treatments that are cost worthy and have beneficial outcomes without complications.	• Acute bronchitis is a lower respiratory tract infection that does not generally warrant antibiotic treatment. • Nevertheless, 71% of patients with acute bronchitis receive antibiotic therapy; this rate continues to rise (Barnett & Linder, 2014). • Indiscriminate use of antibiotics places patients at risk for life-threatening infections such as *Clostridium difficile* infection (CDI). • It is estimated that appropriate use of broad-spectrum antibiotics will reduce the rate of CDI by 26% (Fridkin et al., 2014)

(continued)

TABLE 2.1   Overuse, Underuse, and Misuse *(continued)*

Service Abuse	Desired Service	Examples of Outcomes Related to Desired Service
Underuse	Patients with advanced cancer and poor prognosis have a right to honest conversations with practitioners including chances of remission and possible benefits/discomforts from various treatment options. Too frequently, discussions of advanced directives are not adequately provided to patients.	Patients over 65 with terminal cancer: • One third spent their last days in hospitals/intensive care units, with a significant number receiving advanced life support (e.g., endotracheal intubation, cardiopulmonary resuscitation). • Six percent receive chemotherapy in the last 2 weeks of life. • In 50 academic medical centers, less than half the patients received hospice service, and many cases of hospice service occurred so close to death it is unlikely the service had any benefit (Goodman et al., 2010).
Misuse	Patients have a right to be free from injury during the course of their treatment(s).	• At least one death occurs daily and 1.3 million patients are injured annually related to misuse associated with medications (U.S. Food and Drug Administration, 2009).

Underuse

Underuse, at the opposite end of the range, is failure to provide healthcare service when the service would have the potential to produce favorable patient outcomes (Orszag, 2008). Underuse or neglecting to provide patients with needed care is as detrimental as overuse. Nearly 10,000 deaths from pneumonia could be prevented each year with the pneumococcal vaccine. Yet, only 63 out of 100 patients age 65 and older have received the pneumococcal vaccination (Agency for Healthcare Research and Quality, 2013a). Morbidity and mortality remain high, in part, because patients do not receive adequate evidence-based care for chronic conditions such as hypertension, diabetes, and heart disease (Kochanek, Murphy, Xu, & Tejada-Vera, 2016). Treatment of hypertension, diabetes, and heart disease, and their associated symptoms, is clearly within the domain of nursing practice and requires nurses to keep abreast of the best evidence to treat these highly prevalent conditions.

Misuse

Misuse arises when healthcare service is provided but a *preventable* complication occurs and, consequently, the patient does not receive the full potential benefit of the service (Chassen & Galvin, 1998; IOM, 2001; Orszag, 2008).

The term *misuse* implies a missed opportunity for prevention and is therefore especially troubling because a cornerstone of nursing's foundation is the practice of prevention (American Nurses Association, 2008). Historically, nurses have used a variety of methods to teach patients and populations to prevent illness and enhance overall wellness. Misuse occurs when healthcare providers fail to stop a preventable problem. Preventable problems range from administering the wrong vaccination to failure to teach new parents adequate infant safety. The frequency of misuse or preventable incidents is alarmingly high in healthcare. For example, between 700,000 and 1,000,000 people in the United States fall in hospitals each year (Agency for Healthcare Research and Quality, 2013b). Additionally, nosocomial infections affect 5% to 10% of all hospitalized patients annually in the United States and result in nearly 100,000 deaths (Centers for Disease Control and Prevention, 2009). Regardless of the cause of misuse, nurses have a deeply embedded investment in improving the health of patients and populations through evidence-based preventive health and safety recommendations.

Clearly, there are alarming gaps in the healthcare patients receive and the healthcare they should receive. Gaps, or illogical variations, in care result in both unconscionable morbidity and mortality and unsustainable financial burden (Riley, 2012). Not trying to improve the quality of healthcare is unacceptable. When nurses base patient-centered care decisions on the best existing evidence, they are more likely to provide the right care, to the right patient, and at the right time (American Hospital Association, 2015; Stevens, 2013). Use of EBP reduces the likelihood of overuse, underuse, and misuse in the delivery of patient care (Agency for Healthcare Research and Quality, 2002). Addressing healthcare concerns through EBP helps guarantee a more efficient, equitable, and higher quality of care (Melnyk, 2016). Through the deliberate use of EBP, important improvements can be made that ameliorate care, save lives, and reduce the burden of morbidity in terms of both human suffering and financial cost.

RESEARCH PRACTICE GAP

A great deal of attention is focused on misuse (i.e., error) related to healthcare quality (Andel, Davidow, Hollander, & Moreno, 2012). A larger portion of preventable burden is likely to be related to EBP gaps associated with overuse and underuse of treatments. Research that should be used immediately to change practice is often ignored for extended periods of time. Examples of delay in use of best evidence related to overuse and underuse include imaging overutilization (Rehani, 2011), unnecessary hospitalization (Dartmouth Atlas Project, 2007), crystalloid instead of colloid use for shock (Wilkes & Navicks, 2001), antibiotic use (Wilson, Dahl, & Wells, 2002), and coronary stent placement (Chan et al., 2011).

The research-practice gap is defined as the lag time between the rate at which research results are produced and research results are used in clinical practice (Fraelich-Phillips, 1986). The often immense gap between research and practice is not restricted to nursing but is seen in many of the practice disciplines, including medicine (Morris, Wooding, & Grant, 2011), education (Greenwood & Abbot,

2001), and psychology (DeAngelis, 2011). EBP is an identified bridge between research and practice; however, it is well known that the delay between research findings and clinical implementation remains far too long. It has often been stated that, on average, it takes 17 years for research evidence to reach the point of clinical care (Green, Ottoson, Garcia, & Hiatt, 2009; Westfall, Mold, & Fagnan, 2007).

Delayed implementation of research into practice is a phenomenon that has been well documented for centuries. In 1753, James Lind, a British military surgeon, set up one of the first systematic randomized controlled trials (i.e., research design that randomly assigns participants to an experimental group or control group to assess the outcome variable being studied) to study the effects of various dietary supplements on sailors suffering from scurvy. The treatment group received two oranges and one lemon daily, while the five control groups received dietary supplements that did not contain high doses of vitamin C. Members in the treatment group were able to return to work after 5 days; those in the control groups remained ill. Although the treatment group experienced remarkable recovery, vitamin C dietary supplement did not become a navel military requirement until 40 years later, and another 70 years passed before vitamin C became a requirement for sailors on merchant ships—a 110-year gap from research to practice (Carlisle, 2004).

KNOWLEDGE CREEP

When asked what he thought of Western Civilization, Gandhi replied, "I think it would be a good idea" (Tripathi, 2004). Research utilization in clinical decision making also sounds like a good idea. Conceptually, research utilization in clinical decision making comes with particular sets of concerns. First, research is often underutilized in direct patient care (Israel, Farley, Farris, & Carter, 2013). Only occasionally does research receive both broad attention and application, such as placing infants on their backs to sleep (Hockenberry & Wilson, 2011). Instead, research in healthcare is exercised in more subtle ways than the term *utilization* would imply (Weiss, 1980). Relevant practice ideas that result from rigorous research generally "creep" into clinical practice instead of being immediately and fully utilized (Pape & Richards, 2010).

Well-established research evidence does not automatically spread to the clinical setting. Instead, nurses and other healthcare providers begin to see a need to change practice and often through word of mouth and based on limited research slowly apply certain aspects of relevant research to clinical practice. This phenomenon is often referred to as *knowledge creep*.

The term *decision*, in relation to clinical practice, may also be problematic. Decision implies a brisk and straightforward set of actions (Weiss, 1980). For example, a group of authorized clinicians and researchers may decide to deal with a particular clinical problem, consider the options for dealing with the problem, and select an appropriate decision. Their decision then becomes the gold standard for dealing with the problem and receives broad application. Again, this behavior is infrequently seen in healthcare.

Undoubtedly, knowledge creep does not allow for the articulation of well-defined clinical problems, provision of state-of-the-art science research articles related to the problem, critical appraisal and synthesis of related research, thoughtful and deliberate application of research findings, and dissemination of the findings. EBP accomplishes each of these steps and has been demonstrated repeatedly as an effective method of planned change in closing the gap between available clinical research and clinical practice (Dearholt & Dang, 2012). Underscoring the positive effects of dissemination related to EBP helps to moderate knowledge creep. By sharing results of EBP, nurses build a network of trusting peers and attract more valuable help from colleagues across similar healthcare environments.

BARRIERS TO USING EBP

Effectively integrating evidence into practice requires the judicious use of each component of EBP: best research evidence, practitioner's expertise, and patient values. Studies show that nurses seek clinical information from other nurses, which may indicate they are comfortable using perceived clinical expertise in others as a guide to implement EBP (Pravikoff, Tanner, & Pierce, 2005). The degree to which nurses feel comfortable integrating patient values and preferences as a guide for clinical practice remains unknown. However, many nurses, with or without extensive clinical experience, remain challenged by both personal and organizational barriers when trying to engage in the EBP process.

EBP helps decrease morbidity, mortality, medical errors, and unscientific variation in care (Melnyk, 2012; Stevens, 2013). Despite positive outcomes related to EBP, studies show that nurses do not consistently or equally implement EBP in healthcare organizations nationwide (Melnyk, Fineout-Overholt, Gallagher-Ford, & Kaplan, 2012). Over the past 20 years, multiple studies have consistently identified and similarly ranked barriers to EBP (Atkinson & Turkel, 2008; Linton & Prasun, 2013). A more recent study exploring the state of EBP in the United States has differed somewhat from previous studies (Melnyk, 2012). Among a sample of over 1,000 nurses, two important shifts related to personal barriers to EBP implementation were detected: (a) Nurses are *ready* to use EBP, meaning they want to gain the necessary knowledge and skills to implement EBP, and (b) nurses *value* EBP. Because nurses' attitudes and beliefs are strongly associated with organizational cultures that support EBP, these findings are of particular importance to nurse managers and nurse administrative leaders (see Chapter 16). Nothing is more important to the health and sustainability of EBP than healthcare organizational support (Christenbery, Williamson, Sandlin, & Wells, 2016).

While it is important that nurses welcome and support EBP and agree that EBP skills are necessary for improving healthcare quality, many nurses still avoid engaging in the tasks associated with EBP. The fact that EBP is not routinely implemented by all nurses, despite positive attitudes by most, suggests that barriers to EBP persist, which include both *individual* and *organizational* responsibility. Historically, these barriers have been broadly identified as perceived (a) lack of time, (b) lack of EBP knowledge and skills, (c) notion that EBP is a burden, and (4) impression that organizational cultures do not support EBP (see Table 2.2).

TABLE 2.2 Frequently Encountered Barriers to Evidence-Based Practice (EBP)

Barriers to EBP			
Time	Burden	Knowledge and Skills	Organizational Support
• Feeling guilt devoting time to EBP and not direct patient care • Lack of time to search literature • Lack of time to analyze, synthesize, and integrate research • Insufficient time to implement practice change	• EBP not seen as part of the clinical role • Challenge of implementing changes, too many obstacles • Pressure of clinical workload • Number of research articles is overwhelming • Perceived lack of autonomy and authority to change practice • Consumer demand for non-EBP (e.g., antibiotics for upper respiratory infection)	• Lack of understanding of EBP • Lack of or outdated skills to access relevant research literature • Inability to evaluate quality of research • Lack of confidence that EBP will result in positive change	• EBP seen as low priority by managers and leaders • EBP not valued by peers, physicians, and other key stakeholders • Lack of EBP infrastructure (e.g., computer access, medical librarian) • Absence of collaborative spirit • Lack of qualified EBP mentors • Lack of education related to EBP activities

Time

Several studies indicate that perceived lack of time is the primary reason for the disparity between positive attitudes toward EBP and the systematic application of EBP (Melnyk, 2012; Pravikoff et al., 2005). Conceptually, a great deal of complexity is associated with the term *lack of time*, which is inadequately addressed in the literature. When weighed against provision of direct care, EBP may receive a lower priority score from both direct care providers and managers. Private and federal insurance mandates place heightened emphasis on rapid delivery of healthcare and pressure to discharge patients as early as possible. Clinicians may experience guilt when engaged in an activity, such as EBP, that may not seem to have an immediate and direct impact on the flow of patients through the healthcare organization. This suggests that direct care providers, managers, and leaders may view EBP and clinical care as two distinct entities with competing priorities. Direct care givers engaged in EBP along with nurse managers/leaders have an important responsibility to clearly demonstrate that applying EBP practice to clinical situations may potentially lead to more efficient and effective patient care outcomes, including improved admission-to-discharge times.

Perceived lack of time may also be a convenient default answer. For example, when asked on surveys why any expected work outcome was not achieved, respondents may unthinkingly select "lack of time" as a safe default answer. Further studies that can provide insight and explore reasons into the factors behind the perception of "lack of time" for EBP are needed.

Burden

Translating evidence into practice requires more than knowing the EBP process and understanding the related evidence. To effectively translate evidence into practice requires considerable effort to implement healthcare organizational change. Changing existing nursing practice requires substantial acceptance and agreement from stakeholders (e.g., patients, nurse peers, physicians, administrators, and other health professionals). Approval for change often requires assent from committees, financial investment for resources, and additional training or retraining for those participants engaged in implementing the change. Sixteenth-century theologian Richard Hooker's (cited in Johnson, 1755) maxim that "change is not made without inconvenience, even from worse to better" holds true for EBP. Nurses may feel that, without adequate organizational support, their personal time and work investment associated with EBP change are too great. There may seem to be limited gain when rigorously evaluating research evidence if the possibility of positive change in patient care is unlikely to occur related to inadequate organizational support (see Chapter 16).

Knowledge and Skills

Lack of EBP knowledge and skills creates an inefficient and ineffective implementation of the EBP process. The ability to effectively search the research literature is an invaluable EBP skillset. Searching the literature for the best and current evidence is a daunting task for some nurses, perhaps especially for those who were educated before the introduction of electronic databases. Sometimes literature search skills taught in collegiate nursing programs are lost if not frequently practiced in the work setting. Inadequate literature search skills can easily lead to nurses' perceptions that they do not have time to engage in EBP. Even if nurses possess up-to-date literature search skills, the amount of information today is overwhelming (see Box 2.1). Nurses need clear and efficient strategies to locate and retrieve new evidence that is most likely to benefit their patients and quality of healthcare (Glasziou & Haynes, 2005).

BOX 2.1   Trends in Scientific Output

- Annually, Medline indexes over 560,000 new articles
- Medline indexes 1,500 new articles per day
- Annually, Medline (nursing journal subset) indexes 23,000 new articles
- Cochrane Central adds 20,000 new randomized controlled trials (55 new trials per day)

Lack of skills to adequately critique, interpret, and integrate evidence-based literature remains problematic for many nurses (Pravikoff et al., 2005). Nurses continue to identify the need to gain more knowledge and skills to better implement EBP (Melnyk et al., 2012). In addition, nurses trust a colleague or manager to provide the most up-to-date evidence over electronic evidence resources (Thompson, 2001). If nurses' literature search and evidence interpretation skills were more robust, they may be inclined to rely more on up-to-date electronic resources than colleagues or managers for relevant and critical patient-centered information or knowledge.

Organizational Resistance

The lack or absence of organizational support for EBP remains a pressing concern. A recent study reported that organizational resistance to EBP is received from peers, physicians, and disturbingly from nurse managers and leaders (Melnyk, 2012). The patient is the primary focus of EBP; thus, EBP is inherently an interdisciplinary endeavor. Historical intradisciplinary and interdisciplinary differences must be overcome for all relevant disciplinary groups to make EBP a collaborative and sustainable component of optimal patient care. In addition, those who lead in healthcare systems must be deeply committed to overcoming organizational barriers to EBP. EBP must be seen as a high organizational priority. Managers and leaders must effectively plan for the challenges of fostering effective EBP teamwork and supporting both innovation and implementation of change. Difficulties in accessing relevant evidence and inadequate systems for disseminating EBP findings need to be effectively addressed by healthcare leadership. Significant organizational barriers to EBP (e.g., lack of information technology support, interprofessional challenges, inaccessible databases) require knowledgeable actions on the part of managers and leaders to successfully manage EBP barriers and foster a culture of EBP.

FACILITATORS OF EBP

Specific facilitators have been identified that are essential for EBP to be embedded into the essence of patient-centered nursing care (Melnyk & Fineout-Overholt, 2015). The adoption of EBP occurs in several steps from learning about the fundamentals of EBP (e.g., how to write a PICOT [patient population, intervention, comparison, outcome, time frame] question) to practice implementation (Pagoto et al., 2007). Several facilitating factors have been identified that support each step (see Table 2.3).

TABLE 2.3   Evidence-Based Practice (EBP) Facilitators

Facilitator Category	Examples
Management and leadership commitment	Managers and leaders must • Demonstrate a deep understanding of EBP (e.g., use the language of EBP in organizational communications) • Use evidence in managerial and leadership roles • Identify barriers to EBP and demonstrate resolve to manage barriers • Align EBP competencies that directly reflect caregiver's role (e.g., job description, performance appraisal) • Publicly recognize organizational values of EBP

(continued)

TABLE 2.3   Evidence-Based Practice (EBP) Facilitators *(continued)*

Facilitator Category	Examples
Time allocation	⦿ Availability of time for retrieval of evidence, analysis, synthesis, and interpretation of evidence, and application of EBP implementation plan
Infrastructure	Nurses must have access to ⦿ Relevant electronic databases and evidence ⦿ Library services and medical librarian ⦿ EBP champions or mentors ⦿ Dedicated nurse researcher to oversee project ⦿ Opportunities to disseminate EBP outcomes at local, regional, and national conferences ⦿ EBP website ⦿ EBP rounds

EBP AND HEALTHCARE QUALITY: LINKING RESEARCH TO PRACTICE

At the core of nursing's heritage lies an incredible determination to provide quality care to all patients and populations. Evidence surrounding the value nurses place on quality related to patient safety (Arnold et al., 2006; Cronenwett, 2001; Maddox, Wakefield, & Bull, 2001), standards of practice (American Nurses Association, 2010), and accreditation (American Association of Colleges of Nursing, 2008) are legendary. Nurses, as both healthcare leaders and direct care providers, have important roles to fulfill to ensure that EBP is used effectively to support and maintain the delivery of healthcare quality.

Nurse participation is critical to safeguarding high-quality care at each step of the EBP process:

1. Pose a practice question
2. Search for evidence
3. Critically appraise best evidence
4. Synthesize and summarize best evidence
5. Make practice recommendations

First, as frontline participants in patient care, nurses are qualified to question the rationale and approaches to "routine care" that may result in unintentional negative outcomes for patients. Second, nurses have database search skills specific to their areas of clinical practice and collaborative relationships with health science librarians to locate the best evidence related to both clinical practice and clinical guidelines. Third, once appropriate evidence is located, nurses have the requisite knowledge to determine the level, quality, and relevance of the scientific merit associated with the evidence. Fourth, nurses have the knowledge and expertise to discriminate between sources of valid and invalid evidence for the purpose of modifying clinical practice. Fifth, nurses are central to forming interprofessional collaborative relationships with the clinical workforce and structure the healthcare environment to facilitate best evidence into new standards of practice.

Additionally, nurses must understand that EBP involves more than scientific evidence. Patient preferences and values along with the nurse's clinical expertise are critical for understanding when it is appropriate to diverge from current standards of practice to deliver a higher form of quality, patient-centered care.

FOSTERING AN ETHICAL EBP

Ethical dilemmas arise out of uncertainty, and evidence is one method to help manage uncertainty. The process of EBP encourages lifelong learning strategies in which knowledge is used to diminish areas of uncertainty. How evidence and ethics interrelate is often a neglected or overlooked dimension of EBP (Upshur, 2013).

Integrating ethics and evidence is essential to avoid biased or arbitrary clinical decisions. For example, at the point of clinical decision, there may not be ample or appropriate evidence or there may be conflicting interpretations of the evidence on which to base a clinical decision. EBP is not necessarily structured to mediate conflicting values or interests of healthcare providers about the application or dissemination of evidence. Thus, ethical frameworks may be needed to help mediate conflicting interpretations of evidence (Chabon, Morris, & Lemoncello, 2011).

It is widely agreed that all healthcare should be informed or centered on evidence. Such a mandate may give the false impression that EBP is inherently morally neutral. Gupta (2003) has pointed out that there is no moral imperative within the steps of EBP. For instance, the nurse's personal values that direct the formation of a PICOT question and the way those values can influence the interpretation of related evidence are seldom given thoughtful consideration in the EBP process literature.

Another area of ethical concern related to EBP steps is the literature review. A value-free view of EBP would consider research literature to be an accumulation of unbiased facts. Beginning nursing students understand that even the most sophisticated published research contains some degree of bias. Given the wide range of influences on published literature, it is doubtful that any research literature appraisal tool would capture or detect all biases in a manuscript. While the word *values* is part of the definition of EBP, values seem to pertain only to the patient and not the published evidence or nurse expertise.

Clearly, the relationship between EBP and ethics is complex and problematic. There is much to be gained from further scholarly exploration of the relationship between EBP and ethics. In the meantime, it is important for nurse managers and leaders to assume the responsibility of integrating sound ethical frameworks or models for clinical decision making in areas where EBP is used to inform patient-centered care (Parker, 2007).

SUMMARY

Healthcare quality in the United States is improving in some areas, such as the percentage of children receiving recommended doses of childhood vaccinations.

However, comparable countries continue to outperform the United States on any number of indicators related to quality healthcare, including life expectancy at birth, cost-related barriers to healthcare access, and burden of disease. This chapter explored deficiencies associated with healthcare quality as a result of overuse, underuse, and/or misuse of healthcare services. EBP as a method by which many of these gaps in services can be effectively and ethically diminished was described.

REFERENCES

Agency for Healthcare Research and Quality. (2002). Improving healthcare quality: Fact sheet. Retrieved from http://archive.ahrq.gov/research/findings/factsheets/errors-safety/improving-quality/improving-health-care-quality.html

Agency for Healthcare Research and Quality. (2013a). National health care quality report. Retrieved from http://www.ahrq.gov/research/findings/nhqrdr/nhqr13/chap2c.html#respiratory

Agency for Healthcare Research and Quality. (2013b). Preventing falls in hospitals: A toolkit for improving quality of care. Retrieved from http://www.ahrq.gov/professionals/systems/hospital/fallpxtoolkit/index.html

American Association of Colleges of Nursing. (2008). *The essentials of baccalaureate education for professional nursing practice*. Washington, DC: Author.

American Diabetes Association. (2017). Statistics about diabetes. Retrieved from http://www.diabetes.org/diabetes-basics/statistics/?referrer=https://www.google.com/

American Hospital Association. (2015). Connecting the dots along the health care continuum. Retrieved from http://www.aha.org/content/15/15carecontinuum.pdf

American Nurses Association. (2008). *ANA's health system reform agenda*. Silver Spring, MD: Author.

American Nurses Association. (2010). *Scope and standards of practice*. Silver Spring, MD: Author.

Andel, C., Davidow, S. L., Hollander, M., & Moreno, D. A. (2012). The economics of health care quality and medical errors. *Journal of Health Care Finance, 39*(1), 39–50.

Arnold, L., Campbell, A., Dubree, M., Fuchs, M. A., Davis, N., Hertzler, B., … Wessman J. (2006). Priorities and challenges of health system chief nurse executives: Insights for nursing educators. *Journal of Professional Nursing, 22*, 213–220.

Atkinson, M., & Turkel, M. (2008). Overcoming barriers to research in a Magnet community hospital. *Journal of Nursing Care Quality, 23*, 362–368.

Barnett, M. L., & Linder, J. A. (2014). Antibiotic prescribing for adults with acute bronchitis in the United States, 1996–2010. *Journal of the American Medical Association, 311*(19), 2020–2022.

Carlisle, R. (2004). *Scientific American inventions and discoverers*. Hoboken, NJ: Wiley.

Centers for Disease Control and Prevention. (2009). The direct medical costs of healthcare-associated infections in US hospitals and the benefits of prevention. Retrieved from https://www.cdc.gov/HAI/pdfs/hai/Scott_CostPaper.pdf

Chabon, S., Morris, J., & Lemoncello, R. (2011). Ethical deliberation: A foundation for evidence-based practice. *Seminars in Speech and Language, 32*(4), 298–308.

Chan, P. S., Patel, M. R., Kline, L. W., Krone, R. J., Dehmer, G. J., Kennedy, K., … Spertus, J. A. (2011). Appropriateness of percutaneous coronary intervention. *Journal of the American Medical Association, 306*(1), 53–61. doi:10.1001/jama.2001.916

Chassen, M. R., & Galvin, R. S. (1998). The urgent need to improve health care quality. *Journal of the American Medical Association, 280*(11), 1000–1005.

Christenbery, T., Williamson, A., Sandlin, V., & Wells, N. (2016). Immersion in evidence-based practice fellowship program. *Journal for Nurses in Professional Development, 32*(1), 15–20.

Committee on the Robert Wood Johnson Foundation Initiative on the Future of Nursing. (2011). *The future of nursing: Leading change, advancing health.* Washington, DC: National Academies Press.

Cronenwett, L. (2001). Educating health professional heroes of the future: The challenge for nursing. *Frontiers of Health Services Management, 18,* 15–21.

Dartmouth Atlas Project. (2007). Effective care: A Dartmouth Atlas topic brief (pdf). Retrieved from http://www.dartmouthatlas.org/downloads/reports/supply_sensitive.pdf

DeAngelis, T. (2011). Closing the gap between practice and research: Two efforts are addressing the reasons practitioners may not always use research findings. *American Psychological Association, 41*(6), 42.

Dearholt, S., & Dang, D. (2012). *Johns Hopkins nursing evidence-based practice model and guidelines.* Indianapolis, IN: Sigma Theta Tau International.

Fraelich-Phillips, L. R. (1986). *A clinician's guide to the critique and utilization of nursing research.* Norwalk, CT: Appleton-Croft.

Fridkin, S., Baggs, J., Fagin, R., Magill, S., Pollack, L. A., Malpiedi, P., & Srinivasan, A. (2014). Vital signs: Improving antibiotic use among hospitalized patients. *Morbidity and Mortality Weekly Report, 63*(9), 194–200.

Glasziou, P., & Haynes, B. (2005). The paths from research to improved health outcomes. *Evidence-Based Nursing, 8,* 36–38.

Goodman, D. C., Fisher, E. S., Chang, C. H., Modern, N. E., Jacobson, J. O., Murray, K., & Miesfeldt, S. (2010). Quality of end-of-life cancer care for medicare beneficiaries regional and hospital-specific analysis. In K. K. Bronner (Ed.), *A report of the Dartmouth Atlas Project.* Retrieved from http://www.dartmouthatlas.org/downloads/reports/Cancer_report_11_16_10.pdf

Green, L., Ottoson, J., Garcia, C., & Hiatt, R. (2009). Diffusion theory and knowledge dissemination utilization and integration in public health. *Annual Review of Public Health, 30,* 151–174.

Greenwood, C. R., & Abbot, M. (2001). The research to practice gap in special education. *Teacher Education and Special Education, 24*(4), 276–289.

Gupta, M. A. (2003). A critical appraisal of evidence-based medicine: Some ethical considerations. *Journal of Evaluation in Clinical Practice, 9*(2), 111–121.

Harris Interactive and ARiA Marketing. (2002). Healthcare satisfaction study-final report. Retrieved from http:/www.harrisinteractive.com/news/downloads/Harris AriaHCSatRpt.PDF

Hockenberry, M. J., & Wilson, D. (2011). *Wong's nursing care of infants and children.* St. Louis, MO: Elsevier Mosby.

Institute of Medicine. (1990). *Medicare: A strategy for quality assurance* (K. N. Lohr, Ed.; Vol. 1). Washington, DC: National Academies Press.

Institute of Medicine. (2000). *To err is human: Building a safer health system* (L. T. Kohn, J. M. Corrigan, & M. S. Donaldson, Eds.). Washington, DC: National Academies Press.

Institute of Medicine. (2001). *Crossing the quality chasm: A new health system for the 21st century.* Washington, DC: National Academies Press.

Institute of Medicine. (2003). *Health professions education: A bridge to quality* (A. C. Greiner & E. Knebel, Eds.). Washington, DC: National Academies Press.

Institute of Medicine. (2008a). *Knowing what works in health care: A roadmap for the nation.* Washington, DC: National Academies Press.

Institute of Medicine. (2008b). *Training the workforce in quality improvement and quality improvement research.* IOM Forum Workshop. Washington, DC: National Academies Press.

Israel, E. N., Farley, T. M., Farris, K. B., & Carter, B. L. (2013). Underutilization of cardiovascular medications: Effect of a continuity-of-care program. *American Journal of Health-System Pharmacy, 70*(18), 1592–1600.

Johnson, S. (1755). A dictionary of English usage. Retrieved from http://johnsonsdictionaryonline.com

Kanzaria, H. K., Hoffman, J. R., Probst, M. A., Caloyears, J. P., Berry, S. H., & Brook, R. H. (2015). Emergency physician perceptions of medically unnecessary advanced diagnostic imaging. *Academic Emergency Medicine, 22*(4), 390–398.

Kochanek, K. D., Murphy, S. L., Xu, J., & Tejada-Vera, B. (2016). Deaths: Final for 2014. *National Vital Statistics Reports, 65*(4), 1–122.

Lang, T. A., Hodge, M., Olson, V., Romano, P. S., & Kravitz, R. L. (2004). Nurse patient ratios: A systematic review on the effects of nurse staffing on patient nurse employee and hospital outcomes. *Journal of Nursing Administration, 34*(7–8), 326–337.

Levinson, D. R. (2010). *Adverse events in hospitals: National incidence among medicare beneficiaries.* Office of Inspector General, Department of Health and Human Services. Retrieved from https://oig.hhs.gov/oei/reports/oei-06-09-00090.pdf

Linton, M. J., & Prasun, M. A. (2013). Evidence-based practice: Collaboration between education and nursing management. *Journal of Nursing Management, 21,* 5–16.

Maddox, P. J., Wakefield, M., & Bull, J. (2001). Patient safety and the need for professional and educational change. *Nursing Outlook, 49,* 8–13.

Makary, M. A., & Daniel, M. (2016). Medical error: The third leading cause of death in the United States. *British Medical Journal, 353,* i2139. doi:10.1136/bmj.i2139

McGlynn, E. A., & Brook, R. H. (2001). Evaluating the quality of care. In R. M. Anderson, T. H. Rice, & G. F. Kominski (Eds.), *Changing the U. S. health care system.* San Francisco, CA: Jossey-Bass.

Melnyk, B. M. (2012). Achieving a high-reliability organization through implementation of the ARCC model for systemwide sustainability of evidence-based practice. *Nursing Administration Quarterly, 36*(2), 127–135. doi:10.1097/NAQ.0b013e318249fb6a

Melnyk, B. M. (2016). Improving healthcare, quality patient outcomes and costs with evidence-based practice. *Reflections on nursing leadership Sigma Theta Tau International.* Retrieved from http://www.reflectionsonnursingleadership.org/features/more-features/Vol42_3_ improving-healthcare-quality-patient-outcomes-and-costs-with-evidence-based-practice

Melnyk, B. M., & Fineout-Overholt, E. (2015). *Evidence-based practice in nursing and healthcare: A guide to best practice.* Philadelphia, PA: Wolters Kluwer.

Melnyk, B. M., Fineout-Overholt, E., Gallagher-Ford, L., & Kaplan, L. (2012). The state of evidence-based practice in US nurses: Critical implications for nurse leaders and educators. *Journal of Nursing Administration, 42*(9), 410–417.

Morris, Z. S., Wooding, S., & Grant, J. (2011). The answer is 17 years what is the question: Understanding time lags in translational research. *Journal of the Royal Society of Medicine, 104*(12), 510–520.

Orszag, P. R. (2008). *The overuse underuse and misuse of health care before the committee on finance United States Senate.* Washington, DC: Congressional Budget Office.

Pagoto, S. L., Spring, B., Coups, E. J., Mulvaney, S., Coutu, M. F., & Ozakinci, G. (2007). Barriers and facilitators of evidence-based practice perceived by behavioral science health professionals. *Journal of Clinical Psychology, 63*(7), 695–705.

Pape, T., & Richards, B. (2010). Stop knowledge creep. *Nursing Management, 41*(2), 8–11.

Parker, F. M. (2007). Ethics: The power of one. *The Online Journal of Issues I Nursing, 13*(1). doi:10:3912/OJIN.Vol13No01EthCol01

Pravikoff, D. S., Tanner, A. B., & Pierce, S. T. (2005). Readiness of U.S. nurses for evidence-based practice. *American Journal of Nursing, 105*(9), 40–47.

President's Advisory Commission on Consumer Protection and Quality in the Health Care Industry. (1998). Appendix A: Consumer bill of rights and responsibilities. Retrieved from http://archive.ahrq.gov/hcqual/final/append_a.html

Rehani, B. (2011). Imaging overutilization: Is enough being done globally? *Biomedical Imaging and Intervention Journal, 7*(1), e6. doi:10.2349/biij.7.1e6

Riley, W. J. (2012). Health disparities: Gaps in access quality and affordability of medical care. *Transactions of the American Clinical and Climatological Association, 123,* 167–174.

Stevens, K. R. (2013). The impact of evidence-based practice in nursing and the next big ideas. *The Online Journal of Nursing, 18*(2), 1–11. doi:10.3912/OJIN.Vol18No02Man04

Thompson, C. (2001). Research information in nurses' clinical decision making. *Journal of Advanced Nursing, 36*(3), 376–388.

Tripathi, S. (2004, January 21). Meanwhile: Gandhi, for one, would have found it funny. *The New York Times*. Retrieved from http://www.nytimes.com/2004/01/21/opinion/meanwhile-gandhi-for-one-would-have-found-it-funny.html?_r=0

Upshur, R. E. G. (2013). A call to integrate ethics and evidence-based practice. *American Medical Association Journal of Ethics, 15*(1), 86–89.

U.S. Food and Drug Administration. (2009). Medication error reports. Retrieved from http://www.fda.gov/Drugs/DrugSafety/MedicationErrors/ucm080629.htm

Van Den Bos, J., Rustagi, K., Gray, T., Halford, M., Ziemkiewicz, E., & Shreve, J. (2011). The $17 billion problem: The annual cost of measurable medical errors. *Journal of Health Affairs, 30*(4), 596–603.

Weiss, C. H. (1980). Knowledge creep and decision accretion. *Knowledge: Creation Diffusion Utilization, 1*(3), 381–404.

Westfall, J., Mold, J., & Fagnan, L. (2007). Practice based research: Blue highways on the NIH roadmap. *Journal of the American Medical Association, 207*, 403–406.

Wilkes, M. M., & Navicks, R. J. (2001). Patient survival after human albumin administration: A mete-analysis of randomized control trials. *Annals of Internal Medicine, 135*, 149–164.

Wilson, S. D., Dahl, B. B., & Wells, R. D. (2002). An evidence-based clinical pathway for bronchiolitis safely reduces antibiotic overuse. *American Journal of Medical Quality, 17*(5), 195–199.

CHAPTER 3

Integrating Best Evidence Into Practice

Philip D. Walker and Thomas L. Christenbery

Objectives

After reading this chapter, learners should be able to:

1. Compare various levels of evidence
2. Assess the quality of scientific studies
3. Use rapid critical appraisal (RCA) for critiquing a scientific study
4. Outline the steps for conducting a literature search for scientific evidence
5. Recognize key contributions of health science librarians for implementing evidence-based practice (EBP)

EVIDENCE-BASED PRACTICE (EBP) SCENARIOS

Scenario 1

A community health nurse was asked by the director of a senior citizens' center to do a 1-hour question-and-answer session for the center's patrons about the use of dietary supplements. To prepare for the session, the nurse performed a Google search for several popular dietary supplements including melatonin, glucosamine chondroitin, and multivitamin/mineral combination. When an elderly patron inquired about the use of a daily multivitamin, the nurse replied, "Half of Americans take vitamins regularly, and the use of very high doses of niacin is being explored as a therapy for high cholesterol. Just be sure you take your vitamins as directed."

Scenario 2

A community health nurse was asked by the director of a senior citizens' center to do a 1-hour question-and-answer session for the center's patrons about the use of dietary supplements. To prepare for the session, the nurse read a systematic review (SR) about multivitamins and also the National Institutes of Health and American Heart Association guidelines on multivitamin use. When an elderly patron inquired about the use of a daily multivitamin, the nurse replied, "If you are a healthy adult with no known nutritional deficiencies, you may save your money and not take multivitamins, since science has found no significant role for one-a-day vitamin supplements in preventing cancer or heart disease. In fact, science suggests that a balanced diet with a variety of foods will be more effective than taking vitamin supplements."

Discussion

The nurses in each scenario are to be commended in preparing for the session at the senior center. The nurse in Scenario 1 relied on a convenient, but potentially weak, source of scientific knowledge regarding the use of multivitamins. The nurse's response was factual but not helpful for the patrons. In Scenario 2, the nurse resorted to the highest source of scientific knowledge, a SR, and also took the time to explore reputable national guidelines to prepare for the session. The nurse in Scenario 2 provided a helpful answer in terms of knowledge related to health promotion, diet, and senior citizens' financial status.

USING EVIDENCE TO INFORM PRACTICE

Defining Evidence

A Google search for "Evidence-Based Practice Nursing" produced over 16,000,000 results in less than 1 second. EBP is undeniably popular in nursing. Although a popular term in nursing, EBP spans interdisciplinary boundaries and assumes different meanings for various disciplines including medicine (Sackett, Rosenberg, Gray, Haynes, & Richardson, 1996), psychology (Chambless et al., 1998), social work (Gambrill, 1999), and public health (Jenicek, 1997). It is important for nurses to understand how nursing, as a discipline, defines evidence, identifies relevant evidence to integrate into nursing practice, and evaluates the merit of evidence.

Evidence, translated from the Latin word *evidentia*, means the *action or process of seeing* (English Living Oxford Dictionary, 2016). Disciplines have differing processes for seeing, perceiving, and measuring evidence. The discipline-specific interpretation of evidence used in nursing may or may not necessarily establish evidence in other disciplines, such as medicine, psychology, social work, and public health. As healthcare disciplines trend toward an *interdisciplinary collaborative* approach to patient-centered care, more consideration will need to be given to how evidence is defined, obtained, and used by various health-related disciplines.

Science

Nurses use evidence derived from various sources of knowledge, both scientific and nonscientific, to answer EBP questions (i.e., patient population, intervention, comparison, outcome, time frame [PICOT] questions). Science is the pursuit of knowledge through systematic study of the physical and behavioral worlds through both observation and testing (Merriam-Webster, 2016). Knowledge is a person's range of information and is central to reasoning and decision making (Higgs & Titchen, 2000). Higher forms of evidence in nursing are considered to be knowledge derived from scientific testing and/or scientific rigor that have been found to be credible (Higgs & Jones, 2008). Nurses select the scientific knowledge they use from two distinct research methodologies: quantitative and qualitative research (Table 3.1). For further discussion of quantitative and qualitative research, see Chapter 8.

TABLE 3.1   Differentiating Quantitative and Qualitative Research

Is It Quantitative or Qualitative?		
Criteria	Quantitative Research	Qualitative Research
Scientific approach	Deductive: Start with a generalization (i.e., theory) and base specific predictions on the theory • Moves from broad to specific	Inductive: Make multiple observations, discern a pattern, and develop a generalization (i.e., theory) • Moves from specific to broad
View of reality	Single truth, highly objective	Multiple truths, highly subjective
Purpose and objectives	Test hypotheses, determine probability of cause-and-effect relationships • Describe • Explain • Predict	Interpret and seek understanding of psychological and social phenomena • Describe • Explore • Discover
Research setting	Controlled to the highest degree possible	Naturalistic as possible, observations are often made in natural setting of phenomenon
Data collection strategies	Based on precise measurements, using instruments that are valid and reliable for the purpose of providing accurate numerical data	Narrative based on lived experiences of participants; collective data composed of words, images, or artifacts; using semistructured or unstructured interviews, focus groups, observations, and documents
Data analysis	Statistical procedures to identify numeric descriptions and relationships among study variables	Holistic interpretation of patterns, categories, and themes to achieve in-depth understanding

(continued)

TABLE 3.1   Differentiating Quantitative and Qualitative Research *(continued)*

Is It Quantitative or Qualitative?		
Dissemination of findings	Numerical report, including descriptive statistics, correlations, and statically significant relationships; purpose is to generalize findings	Narrative report, including rich contextual description, categories, themes, and meaningful quotes; purpose is to provide insight and deeper understanding of phenomena
Research example	Effect of Vibration on Pain Response to Heel Lance (McGinnis, Murray, Cherven, McCracken, & Travers, 2016) Study was based on the premise of Gate Control Theory of Pain and tested vibration as an intervention to decrease behavioral and physiologic response to pain	Exploring the Lived Experience of Women Immediately Following Mastectomy: A Phenomenological Study (Davies et al., 2016) Study provided an in-depth understanding of what women following breast cancer surgery experience upon seeing their mastectomy scars for the first time

Source: Adapted from Johnson & Christensen (2008).

Quantitative researchers focus on both the physical and social worlds and generally view the development of scientific knowledge as orderly, rational, and capable of determining universal laws that make it possible to predict outcomes. Scientists who engage in quantitative research view reality as objective and numerically measurable (Polit & Beck, 2012; Williams, 2007).

In contrast to quantitative researchers, qualitative researchers view phenomena as subjective. Qualitative researchers believe the world is relative and that knowledge will alter with time and place. Qualitative researchers are concerned with deepening the nurse's understanding of phenomena through studying people and events as they exist, without the aid of experimentation (Denzin & Lincoln, 2018; Polit & Beck, 2012).

Appraising Evidence

Nurses care for patients and populations who have multiple and complex layers of illness, recovery, and wellness. The health-related layers of patient/population complexity provide nurses unlimited opportunity to develop relevant, discipline-specific questions. It is seemingly impossible for nursing science to rigorously study every aspect of patient care of interest to nurses; therefore, in addition to knowledge gained from quantitative and qualitative research, nurses use patient-centered care knowledge derived from other credible, yet nonscientific sources such as a panel of experts, quality improvement outcomes, and case studies.

EBP nursing is not about a tension between having scientific evidence and not having scientific evidence, because there is always some form of available evidence; however, EBP nursing is committed to a credible ranking order for all types of available evidence. In general, healthcare disciples have an evidence ranking order to help clarify and determine the selection of evidence they use to inform research and/or practice.

The nursing discipline typically uses a twofold process to help identify and evaluate the worth of evidence: (a) level of evidence and (b) quality of evidence. This process is indispensable in helping nurses determine the best evidence to use in answering PICOT questions and has utility related to ease of use for nurses. First, in this chapter we discuss historical development, logical sequencing, and use of levels of evidence. Second, we explore the assessment of quality of evidence as a means to further select the most sound and relevant evidence to answer PICOT questions and support the implementation of patient-centered care.

Levels of Evidence

A cornerstone of EBP is the ranking system to classify evidence (Burns, Rohrich, & Chung, 2011). Nurses are encouraged to use the highest level of evidence to inform clinical practice (White, Dudley-Brown, & Terhaar, 2016). Levels of evidence ranking, sometimes referred to as hierarchy of evidence, are assigned to studies based on the methodological rigor of a study's design. Various nurse and physician authors have conceptualized levels of evidence in slightly different ways, and in nursing there is no single agreed-upon ranking to use (Dearholt & Dang, 2012; Melnyk & Fineout-Overholt, 2015; Polit & Beck, 2012; Sackett, 1989; Sackett et al., 1996). These slight variations in levels of evidence in nursing do not seem to cause a problem because the authors' intentions for each method of ranking are to identify randomized controlled trials (RCTs) as the highest level of evidence and expert opinion as the lowest level of evidence.

Sackett (1989) first described levels of evidence, as used today, in an article establishing a hierarchy of evidence for research about antithrombotic medications. Sackett ranked research articles according to the degree each study design would prohibit the probability of bias or systematic error (i.e., reproducible inaccuracies that persist throughout the study). RCTs were assigned the highest ranking, because they are designed to limit systematic error and therefore have greater validity. For example, randomly assigning study participants to treatment or control groups randomizes confounding factors (e.g., participants' lack of candor) that may potentially bias study results. Expert opinion is generally biased by the expert's experiences or sentiments; thus, there is no control through randomization of confounding factors.

Nursing journals frequently assign a level of evidence to research articles, and conference presenters often assign a level of evidence to abstracts they submit for research conference proceedings. Readers of journal articles and conference attendees need to be aware that a designated level of evidence does not guarantee the quality of scholarly work or research. For example, level one (i.e., RCT) evidence may not always be the best option for answering a specific research question. For example, a nurse should be doubtful if a study was identified as an RCT, yet the purpose was stated as "to determine the correlation of dyspnea distress and engagement in sports for adolescents with asthma." Because there is no randomization or treatment in this example, an RCT would have been an inappropriate design. Hence, it is imperative that nurses be aware of the various levels of evidence and be capable of independently interpreting and judging a work's claimed level of evidence.

It is important for an individual nurse or an organization to select one method of level of evidence ranking and remain consistent with that selection for the duration of an EBP project. As stated earlier, nurses are encouraged to use the highest level of available evidence to answer PICOT questions. Box 3.1 provides examples of levels of evidence from highest- to lowest-order ranking. In addition to ranking, to help with the selection of best evidence for EBP projects, each type of evidence is provided with a definition, strength and limitation, identified areas of potential risk, type of question that best fits the level of evidence, and real-world examples. The ranking order of evidence for this table is founded on the works of various nurse and physician authors (Dearholt & Dang, 2012; Melnyk & Fineout-Overholt, 2015; Polit & Beck, 2012; Sackett, 1989; Sackett et al., 1996).

BOX 3.1   Levels of Evidence

Level 1: Evidence obtained from meta-analyses and SRs

Meta-analysis defined: A meta-analysis integrates findings of highly controlled studies, such as RCTs, that address similar research questions, hypotheses, or aims. Results from the integrated studies are tabulated to develop a combined conclusion that has greater statistical power and is considered more valid than a single study. The statistical conclusion is referred to as the *effect size*, which is a measure of the strength of the relationship between the integrated studies' key variables. If the integrated studies are all RCTs, a meta-analysis is considered the pinnacle of scientific evidence.

Example in practice: Nurses noted the catheter-associated urinary tract infection (CAUTI) incidence to be higher on their hospital's medical-surgical units than the national CAUTI average. The nurses understood solutions to CAUTI problems had been studied repeatedly. To help find the best solution to the CAUTI incidence, the nurses reviewed research literature for a meta-analysis that pooled data from multiple, credible CAUTI studies to arrive at the best combined RCT answer for reduction in CAUTI. The nurses found appropriate CAUTI reduction meta-analyses in PubMed (MEDLINE), the Cochrane Library, and at ClinicalTrials.gov.

Strengths:

- A meta-analysis provides robust statistical power, or the ability to detect the presence of a true relationship, between independent and dependent variables across similar studies.

- It has greater generalizability to similar populations than a single study.

- It is considered an excellent resource for EBP questions.

Limitations:

- Indiscriminate use of meta-analysis is sometimes seen. Nurses must be certain the meta-analysis is appropriate for answering the specific PICOT question.

Alert for unsuspected risk:

- Studies under review should be of similar type. For example, studies must be all RCTs instead of a mix of RCTs and cohort studies.

(continued)

BOX 3.1   Levels of Evidence *(continued)*

- Meta-analysis should include both published and unpublished studies, including relevant studies that may have had negative outcomes.

Example from research literature: Hervik, J. R., & Stub, T. (2016). Adverse effects of non-hormonal pharmacological interventions in breast cancer survivors, suffering from hot flashes: A systematic review and meta-analysis. *Breast Cancer Research and Treatment, 160*(2), 223–236.

Study conclusion: The odds for experiencing adverse effects were significantly higher in patients randomized to high-dose nonhormonal drugs than those randomized to controls, including placebo, low-dose medication, and acupuncture. These therapies should be considered as potential treatment alternatives.

Systematic review defined: A SR is a comprehensive synthesis of relevant research, often RCTs or cohort studies, focused on a specific health-related research question. Using published and unpublished research, a SR is often conducted by a panel of research and/or content experts. The authors of a SR combine relevant information from the integrated studies to form a summation, which is often used to answer EBP questions. The SR is a highly disciplined and meticulous procedure that heightens the validity of the review process to avoid bias.

Example in practice: A new nursing professor will be teaching psychiatric mental health nurse practitioner (PMHNP) students. The professor wants to better understand PMHNP students' attitudes toward acutely psychotic patients. The professor will conduct a literature search for a SR that collates all relevant and credible empirical studies comparing new student attitudes to experienced nurses' attitudes toward acutely psychotic patients.

Strengths:

- A systematic review provides exhaustive review of current findings and ongoing research.
- It is both cost-effective and time efficient when compared to conducting an individual RCT.
- The study obtains results that can be generalized more broadly than an individual study.
- It is considered an excellent EBP resource.

Limitations:

- This is a meticulous and precise task that is time intensive.
- Biased studies may inadvertently enter the SR and skew the summation of evidence if strict inclusion guidelines are not firmly adhered to.

Alert for unexpected risk:

- Studies in a SR may have varying designs (e.g., RCT, cohort study) but collectively must be studying the same research outcomes. Reviewers need to be certain that variables are an absolute match from study to study. In addition, a SR should never be confused with a *literature review*. Clinical decisions are frequently based on SRs but seldom based on literature reviews.

Example from research literature: LeVasseur, N., Clemons, M., Hutton, B., Shorr, R., & Jacobs, C. (2016). Bone-targeted therapy use in patients with bone metastases for lung cancer: A systematic review of randomized control trials. *Cancer Treatment Reviews, 50*, 183–193.

Study conclusion: Data from included trials suggest benefits of bone-targeted agents in lung cancer for the prevention of skeletal-related events and bone pain. There is a trend toward improvement in overall survival and progression-free survival, although further research is needed. The impact on quality of life and key subgroups for benefit both require future research.

(continued)

BOX 3.1   Levels of Evidence *(continued)*

Level 2: Evidence obtained from at least one well-designed *RCT*

Randomized controlled trials defined: RCTs are studies in which participants are randomly assigned to an experimental group or control group. Participants in the experimental group receive the treatment under investigation, while participants in the control group receive a placebo (i.e., pseudo-intervention) or standard care. Because participants have been randomly assigned to groups, it is expected that there will be equal representation on key variables such as age, gender, ethnicity, and income for each group at the start of the study, thus decreasing potential bias and increasing validity. The only expected difference between the experimental and control group will be the outcome, or dependent variable, being studied.

Example in practice: Direct care nurses on an oncology unit are interested in helping reduce patient anxiety. The nurses have reviewed the literature for possible interventions and have become interested in the potential efficacy of aromatherapy. Working with the medical center's nurse researcher, the nurses set up an RCT in which eligible and willing participants are randomly assigned to a treatment or control group. The treatment and control groups inhale two drops of lavender and normal saline, respectively, for 2 minutes. Salivary cortisol levels are tested before and after the treatments.

Strengths:

- If randomized appropriately, potential bias may be reduced.

- It is possible for both researchers and participants to be blind to who is receiving the treatment, which could further decrease bias.

- Results can be analyzed with sophisticated statistical tests.

- It allows for assignment and administration of treatment in a precise and controlled way.

Limitations:

- Threats to external validity or generalizability of findings remain a concern (i.e., what works in one setting or culture may not work in another).

- Groups often need to be quite large to demonstrate statistical significance.

- Results do not often reflect real-life treatment scenarios related to the RCTs' extremely strict inclusion/exclusion criteria and highly controlled settings.

- RCTs may last for years and are therefore often expensive in terms of time and money.

Alert for unexpected risk:

- Reviewers should be alert to the possibility of confounding variables—variables that inadvertently affect the dependent variables. For example, exercise (independent variable) may be confounded by age (confounding variable) on weight gain (dependent variable).

Example from research literature: Tayyib, N., Coyer, F., & Lewis, P. A. (2015). A two-arm cluster randomized control trial to determine the effectiveness of a pressure ulcer prevention bundle for critically ill patients. *Journal of Nursing Scholarship, 47*(3), 237–247.

Study conclusion: Significant improvements were observed in pressure ulcer-related outcomes with the implementation of the pressure ulcer prevention bundle in the ICU; pressure ulcer incidence, severity, and total number of pressure ulcers per patient were reduced.

(continued)

BOX 3.1   Levels of Evidence (*continued*)

Level 3: Evidence obtained from at least one well-designed quasi-experimental study

The term *quasi* means "being partly or almost." Taken as a group, quasi-experimental designs are more frequently implemented than RCTs. They are extensively used in nursing and social science research because of ease of use in measuring social and psychological variables (e.g., self-efficacy, quality of life, social determinants of health).

Quasi-experimental trial defined: Quasi-experiments are trials with an intervention or treatment, but randomization to treatment and control group is absent. The most commonly used quasi-experimental design is nonequivalent groups (e.g., two separate oncology units), in which there is a pretest and a posttest for treatment and control groups. However, the treatment and control groups are not randomized, thus weakening the study's validity or credibility by allowing the groups to be potentially dissimilar on a number of variables, such as diagnosis, treatments, and length of diagnosis.

Example in practice: Nurses at two separate adolescent asthma clinics wanted to know if adolescents who used a telephone app for an asthma action plan would have fewer asthma exacerbations than adolescents who used the standard paper asthma action plan. Adolescents at clinic A received the asthma action plan telephone app, and adolescents at clinic B received the standard paper asthma action plan. Baseline data were collected for new admissions at each clinic, and the number of reported asthma exacerbations was tabulated after 3 months.

Strengths:

- This is an effective alternative when groups cannot be randomized. For example, the experiment must be conducted in a natural setting as opposed to a controlled setting.

- It saves time, finances, and other resources when compared to RCTs.

- Reactions of study participants may be more genuine because the experiment is not occurring in an artificial laboratory environment.

- Threats to validity (e.g., the effects of taking a test on the outcomes of taking a second test) can be addressed in the research design to minimize their impact on study results.

Limitations:

- The absence of randomization leads to nonequivalent groups, limiting generalizability to larger populations.

- Without randomization, hypotheses about treatment causality are extremely difficult to make.

Alert for unexpected risk:

- Readers of quasi-experimental research need to be aware that results of the study will not stand up to rigorous statistical analysis. For example, a study using two types of diabetic teaching programs may show that one program was more effective than the other. If the researcher did not control for confounding variables, the results will not withstand statistical scrutiny, because one group of patients may have been more motivated learners, may have been better educated, or may have better health support services than the other group.

Example from research literature: Yuan, S.-C., Chou, M.-C., Hwu, L.-J., Chang, Y.-O., Hsu, W.-H., & Kuo, H.-W. (2009). An intervention program to promote health-related physical fitness in nurses. *Journal of Clinical Nursing, 18*, 1404–1411.

Study conclusion: This study demonstrates that the development and implementation of an intervention program can promote and improve the health-related physical fitness of nurses.

(*continued*)

BOX 3.1   Levels of Evidence (*continued*)

Level 4: Designs at level 4, and following, are *nonexperimental*; data are collected without the influence of an experiment or treatment

The terms *nonexperimental* and *observational research* are often used interchangeably. *Case control* and *cohort studies* are two of the most frequently used nonexperimental designs in healthcare.

Case control designs: Case control studies compare participants who have a disease (e.g., lung cancer) or outcome of interest (e.g., lymph edema) with participants who are thought not to have the disease or outcome. The participants serve as the controls. Case control studies look retrospectively to compare how frequently the exposure to a risk factor (i.e., attribute, characteristic, or exposure that increases the probability of disease or injury) is present in each group of participants to determine the presence and degree of a relationship between risk factor and disease or outcome. Case control studies are strictly observational, because there is no intervention or treatment to alter the course of disease.

Example in practice: An advanced practice registered nurse (APRN) works in school health at a large northeast public school system. He understood that some school crossing guards in the school system were applying sunscreen during the winter months because snow can reflect the damaging rays of the sun and cause sunburns, which lead to skin cancer. The APRN contacted researchers, also employed in the school system, to help design a case control study to investigate if sunscreen applied during the winter months was more effective as a skin cancer prevention than not wearing sunscreen in the winter months. The investigation compared a former cohort of crossing guards who developed facial cancer (cases) to a group of crossing guards who did not have facial cancer (controls) and assessed their frequency of sunscreen use in the winter months.

Strengths:

 ● It is efficient for rare diseases (e.g., Huntington's disease) or diseases with a long latency period (e.g., AIDS).

 ● When exposure data are expensive or difficult to obtain, case controls are a less expensive and more time-efficient method for determining risk.

 ● This is ideal for studying dynamic populations (e.g., homeless veterans) in which follow-up is difficult.

 ● Less time is needed to complete the study because the disease or outcome has already occurred.

Limitations:

 ● This design is prone to selection bias.

 ● Recall bias is possible, as this relies on the memory of participants with the condition who may be more motivated to recall risk factors.

 ● Information on exposure may be influenced by observation bias.

Alert for unexpected risk:

 ● It is essential that the cases (e.g., fibromyalgia) be clearly defined at the outset of the study to confirm that all cases have met the same diagnostic criteria.

Example from the literature: Bruderer, S. G., Bodmer, M., Jick, S. S., & Meier, C. R. (2015). Association of hormone therapy and incident gout: Population-based case control study. *Menopause: The Journal of the North American Menopause Society, 22*(12), 1335–1342.

(continued)

BOX 3.1   **Levels of Evidence** *(continued)*

Study conclusion: Current use of oral opposed estrogens, but not unopposed estrogens, is associated with a decreased odds ratio (OR) for incident gout in women without renal failure and is more pronounced in women with hypertension. Use of tibolone is associated with a decreased OR for incident gout. The decreased OR for gout may be related to the progestogen component rather than the estrogen component.

Cohort studies: A cohort consists of a sample of participants who share a common characteristic or event (i.e., risk factors) within a defined period, such as receiving a vaccine or being exposed to polluted water. The cohort is followed prospectively, and receives periodic evaluations, with respect to the development of a specific disease or outcome, to which their exposure to characteristics or events are associated. A statistical correlation determines *absolute risk* (i.e., the proportion of cohort who experienced the disease or outcome) between risk factor and incidence of disease or outcome.

Example in practice: A group of pediatric clinic nurses are interested in targeted specific parent groups who do not follow-up on recommended childhood vaccinations. The nurses want to know if there are differences in childhood vaccination compliance between parents who opt for nurse-midwife care and delivery compared to parents who opt for obstetrician care and delivery. The nurses conduct a prospective cohort study to examine the possible effect of nurse-midwife care and obstetrician care on childhood vaccination compliance over the child's first 5 years of life.

Strengths:

- Participants in a cohort can be well matched, thus limiting the introduction of confounding variables.

- A cohort study is less expensive than a RCT.

- This type of study allows for the identification of temporal sequence; did the exposure to risk precede the disease or outcome?

Limitations:

- Studies may be longitudinal; therefore, large numbers of participants may be followed for lengthy time periods.

- Cohorts can be challenging to identify if there are multiple confounding variables.

Alert for unexpected risk:

- Cohort studies may be either prospective or retrospective. If retrospective, selection bias occurs easily because disease or outcomes have already occurred at the time of participant selection. In addition, because participant records may not have been designed for the study, data may be of poor quality.

Example from the research literature: Milani, A., Mazzocco, K., Gandini, S., Pravettoni, G., Libutti, L., Zencovich, C., . . . Saiani, L. (2017). Incidence and determinants of port occlusions in cancer outpatients: A prospective cohort study. *Cancer Nursing, 40*(2), 102–107

Study conclusion: The use of positive pressure in addition to normal saline reduces the incidence rate of partial occlusions. The type of treatment, blood sample collection, and treatment schedule are determinants of partial occlusion.

(continued)

BOX 3.1   Levels of Evidence (*continued*)

Level 5: Meta-synthesis of *qualitative* studies

Meta-synthesis: A systematic approach to reviewing, interpreting, and integrating findings from qualitative studies. Using qualitative studies, a meta-synthesis analyzes the findings and examines the studies for essential features and themes. The features and themes are combined to deliver a new or broader interpretation of the reviewed research as a whole (Zimmer, 2006). **Note**: *Qualitative research* refers strictly to research that follows a specific qualitative tradition (e.g., phenomenology, ethnography, grounded theory). *Descriptive qualitative* research refers to studies that do not follow a specific qualitative tradition but do engage in content analysis of data to detect themes or patterns for narrative content (Polit & Beck, 2012).

Example in practice: Direct care nurses working in a large adult outpatient oncology clinic noted that some patients seemed resilient when faced with adverse diagnostic or treatment outcomes. The nurses realized they needed a more informed and deeper understanding of resilience and its associated protective factors. The nurses believed increased knowledge of resiliency and its protective factors would provide them with a foundation to be more supportive of patients who resort to resiliency as part of coping. The nurses knew there was an abundance of literature regarding cancer patients and resiliency but did not know which articles would be most helpful. The nurses sought advice from the clinic's nurse researcher. The nurse researcher found a meta-synthesis that provided a coherent analysis and summation of relevant qualitative research articles. The meta-synthesis methodically and succinctly addressed the direct care nurses' inquiry related to resiliency and protective factors in cancer populations.

Strengths:

- This method provides practitioners with a broader and deeper understanding of patients' personal experiences with health and illness.

- It enhances interpretive possibilities of findings.

Limitations:

- It is challenging to determine which articles are similar in terms of substantive phenomena.

Alert for unexpected risk:

- Meta-synthesis should not be confused with meta-analysis. Meta-synthesis is conducted to lead to new interpretations of qualitative research. Meta-analysis is conducted to provide a numeric probability of the effect of one variable on another.

Example from the research literature: Olano-Lizarrag, M., Oroviogoicoechea, C., Errasti-Ibarrondo, B., & Saracíbar-Razquin, M. (2016). The personal experience of living with chronic heart failure: A qualitative meta-synthesis of the literature. *Journal of Clinical Nursing, 25*(17–18), 2413–2429 doi:10.1111/jocn.13285

Study conclusion: Heart failure has a major impact on the entire person, but some areas have not been addressed. By creating new tools to understand and evaluate the impact of this illness and interventions that prevent or improve some situations, we can promote the well-being and the quality of life of this population.

Level 6: Evidence from a well-designed qualitative or descriptive qualitative study

Qualitative research: Exploratory research used to gain a deeper and enriched understanding of participants' perspectives, reasons, and motivations. Helpful in explaining underlying themes, categories, and patterns of relationships of phenomena. May lead to creation of hypotheses and/or theory development.

(*continued*)

BOX 3.1 Levels of Evidence (*continued*)

Example in practice: Nursing faculty at a large BSN program were committed to optimizing all clinical experiences for their students. The faculty had reason to believe that not all male nursing students felt as welcomed into some gynecological and obstetrical clinical settings as female students. The faculty understood this was an important topic that did not lend itself to being measured by observational techniques. The faculty decided that to understand and promote optimal clinical experiences for all students, the topic merited a qualitative research endeavor. Therefore, the faculty developed a research project, using focus groups, to better understand the male students' perceptions of enablers and barriers related to gynecological and obstetrical clinical experiences.

Strengths:

- This system provides in-depth knowledge on a limited number of cases.
- It provides rich detail on phenomena as they occur in a realistic context.
- It allows participants to interpret constructs (e.g., locus of control, self-esteem).

Limitations:

- One is unable to generalize knowledge to a larger population.
- It does not allow for testing of hypotheses or theories.
- One is unable to make quantitative predictions related to probabilities.

Alert for unexpected risk:

- Subjectivity is a trademark of qualitative research but is also an aspect reviewers of qualitative research must be alert to. For example, unwarranted observer bias should be accounted for in the studies to limit misinterpretation of the narrative data.

Example from the research literature: Lemke, M. K., Meissen, G. J., & Apostolopoulos, Y. (2016). Overcoming barriers in unhealthy settings: A phenomenological study of healthy truck drivers. *Global Qualitative Nursing Research, 3*, 1–9. doi:10.1177/2333393616637023

Study conclusion: Seven broad themes were identified: access to health resources, barriers to health behaviors, recommended alternative settings, constituents of health behavior, motivation for health behaviors, attitudes toward health behaviors, and setting approaches to improving health behavior.

Level 7: Evidence from expert opinion without explicit critical appraisal

Expert opinion defined: A person or panel who are considered to have social knowledge or skill, by the practice or scholarly communities, on a particular subject (e.g., pain, dyspnea, motivation, or chest tube removal).

Example in practice: A group of direct patient care dialysis nurses at a large medical center have worked well as a healthcare team for several years. They are interested in learning what changes might be occurring in relation to dialysis as a form of treatment option over the next few years. The nurses would even be interested in working with the medical center's nurse researcher on projects related to possible future concerns and issues for dialysis and patients who receive dialysis. To help identify and describe issues surrounding this topic, the nurses convene a panel of experts for an informal presentation. The panel includes the medical director of the dialysis unit, the chief of nephrology, chief nephrology resident, nurse manager, and clinical nurse specialist for the dialysis unit.

(*continued*)

BOX 3.1   Levels of Evidence (*continued*)

Strengths:

- Evidence may be derived from premier authority in the specialty.

- This can provide evidence that is currently not in print.

- It allows for presentation of differing opinions.

- It can stimulate important discussion and questions.

Limitations:

- Evidence may be sought from individuals who may not be considered authoritative experts by the practice or scholarly communities.

- Strong personalities in the discipline may overshadow the worth of the content presented.

Alert for unexpected risk:

- There is often no formalized method of evaluation once the opinion has been proffered by the expert. If the opinion is widely accepted and later found *not to be credible*, effects of the opinion may be difficult to undo (e.g., vaccinations causing autism).

Example from the research literature: Newhouse, R. P. (2006). Expert opinion: Challenges and opportunities for academic and organizational partnership in evidence-based nursing practice. *Journal of Nursing Administration, 36*(10), 441–445.

Study conclusion: Suggestions included strategies to enhance organizational EBP culture, providing leadership support, using EBP as an opportunity for self-development for nurse leaders, and forming academic-practice collaborative partnerships.

EBP, evidence-based practice; PICOT, patient population, intervention, comparison, outcome, time frame; RCT, randomized controlled trials; SR, systematic review.

Quality Ratings

Because level of evidence provides a single numerical ranking based on a study's design, primary studies (i.e., original research) also must be assessed for their research quality. Research quality refers to the scientific merit encompassing all aspects of the study. In particular, research quality pertains to evaluation regarding the match between methods and research question, participant selection, measurement of outcomes, and systematic and random bias (Lohr, 2004).

Often evaluation of study quality is assessed by use of a comprehensive quality of evidence ranking form, combining aspects of "quality" into three or more categories and assigning an ordinal (i.e., ranking) grade of "A," "B," or "C," and so forth. There are several methodological flaws related to this process of rating evidence quality.

It can be assumed that the authors of the quality of evidence rankings define quality as a *degree of excellence*. It cannot be assumed what the authors are implying by *degree* and *excellence*. It would be challenging to suggest that quality of evidence ratings provide an objective assessment of individual studies or compilations of studies' quality. Instead, the quality of evidence ranking is notably subjective and contextual. In addition to the lack of objectivity, the quality of evidence ranking is flawed for several other reasons. For example, the concept of quality may vary with each study's specific research question. The reader's personal judgments will also alter the perception of quality. Finally, the quality rankings often provide no meaningful quality indices or guide for determining quality (Yarris, Simpson, & Sullivan, 2013).

Many quality assessment ranking scales for research articles are available (Agency for Healthcare Research and Quality, 2009; Dearholt & Dang, 2012). Despite the accessibility of quality of evidence scales, the use of overall ranking scales is becoming less popular (Polit & Beck, 2012). The *Cochrane Handbook* (Higgins & Green, 2008) suggests global scales of quality not be used. Instead, a component approach is recommended in contrast to an overall scale approach. A component approach assesses for individual features of each study and provides an individual or separate score for the study.

HEALTH SCIENCE LIBRARIANS AND EBP IN NURSING

Along with nursing, many healthcare disciplines (e.g., audiology, occupational therapy, physical therapy, medicine) are devoting an increasing amount of attention and resources to developing strategies that foster the use of EBP among their practitioners (Kronenfeld et al., 2007). Since its inception in the late 1990s, the inclusion of EBP into multiple healthcare disciplines has paralleled the swift emergence of the World Wide Web, including freely accessible MEDLINE™, other relevant databases, and full-text electronic healthcare journals. The powerful engagement of EBP and voluminous electronic and digital resources has a significant impact on both access and use of healthcare knowledge (Sieving, 1999). Within the large volume of electronic information is *actionable information*—the information most relevant to clinical decision making (Perry & Kroenenfeld, 2005). Given the unceasing torrent of electronic information, efficient and effective access to evidence-based actionable information is a key concern for all healthcare providers.

Although the steps of EBP are straightforward, the implementation and intellectual process of EBP require nurses to acquire and use a moderately complex set of information management skills (Klem & Weiss, 2005; Sitzia, 2002). Nurses have repeatedly voiced concerns about insufficient preparation and experience related to the use of healthcare information management. For example, nurses report they lack necessary knowledge and skills to effectively search for research literature (Ciliska, Pinelli, DiCenso, & Cullum, 2001; Estabrooks, Chong, Brigidear, & Profetto-McGrath, 2005; Marshall, West, & Aitken, 2011; Profetto-McGrath, Smith, Hugo, Taylor, & El-Haii, 2007). Nurses typically attribute the lack of usage of EBP to limited physical access to information resources and the inability to understand and use accessed information (French, 2005; Marshall et al., 2011; Thompson, McCaughan, Cullum, Sheldon, & Raynor, 2005). Nurses also report that research evidence is not assembled in one location, suggesting another level of complexity in literature searching (McCleary & Brown, 2003; Niderhauser & Kohr, 2005).

In addition to challenges in locating relevant literature, nurses sometimes struggle with critically appraising literature. Between 50% and 70% of nurses indicated they are not confident in their abilities to critically read and evaluate published research and determine its applicability to practice (Johnston &

Fineout-Overholt, 2006; Pravikoff, Tanner, & Pierce, 2005). A series of consensus reports (Institute of Medicine [IOM], 2001, 2008) have set a formal expectation that nurses must use research findings to inform clinical practice; therefore, it is important that nurses find a supportive path to help them identify and determine the highest level and quality of research.

Education has been found to be effective in improving less engaged behaviors related to EBP. Less engaged behaviors include not reading research literature and basing healthcare decisions on information other than research, such as social resources that include opinions of nurse colleagues and previous work experience (Marshall et al., 2011). Research consistently finds strategic training and education to be essential for full participation and implementation of EBP (Christenbery, Williamson, Sandlin, & Wells, 2016; Melnyk & Fineout-Overholt, 2015).

Health science librarians have an important role in advancing and supporting EBP (Kronenfeld et al., 2007), because they hold wide-ranging knowledge and training in information organization and retrieval strategies (Klem & Weiss, 2005). Collaboration between nurses and librarians has consistently demonstrated positive results, including updating accurate advice given to patients, refocusing patient care initiatives, avoiding negative patient care outcomes, and improving efficiency of care (Marshall, Morgan, Klem, Thompson, & Wells, 2014). Nurses report that working with health science librarians and using library resources are valuable activities for improving patient care (Marshall et al., 2014). Nurses who collaborate with health science librarians also report using a wider variety of relevant information resources including Micromedex, PubMed/Medline, and UpToDate. In many cases, nurses are effectively using the same information resources as physicians and other healthcare professionals (Marshall et al., 2014).

Wise nurses collaborate with health science librarians to assist with accessing and evaluating the best evidence to support patient-centered care. Librarians have expertise in using effective search strategies and selecting the best EBP resources, and they are able to help evaluate both the level and quality of selected evidence. Librarians are essential in providing ongoing education activities nurses need to keep pace with the dynamic evolution of electronic resources and other digital data forms associated with EBP. Librarians are noted change agents in helping leaders of heathcare organizations to better understand the need for providing nurses and other healthcare professionals with immediate access to EBP resources (Kronenfeld et al., 2007).

Health science librarians provide a wide range of EBP services and support that enhance clinical care. Nurses, nursing leaders, and other healthcare professionals must understand the roles librarians undertake to provide EBP training and support an optimal EBP culture. In addition, health science librarians have a critical role in supporting nurse educators with integrating critical thinking, information literacy, applied informatics, and research into EBP content as part of associates degree in nursing (ADN), bachelor of science in nursing (BSN), master of science in nursing (MSN), and doctor of nursing practice (DNP) curricular models (Kronenfeld et al., 2007). There is a need to broaden nursing students' knowledge, at each degree level, about the value of information literacy as a

lifelong learning skill for the promotion of EBP with emphasis on locating, evaluating, and using healthcare knowledge and information effectively (Fox, Richter,
& White, 1996; Nayda & Rankin, 2008).

RAPID APPRAISAL OF EVIDENCE

Appraisal of current research evidence is a cornerstone strategy for both direct
care nurses and advanced practice nurses to effectively translate research findings into best clinical practices (Facchiano & Snyder, 2012). Generally, nurses
work in fast-paced, dynamic, and complex healthcare environments. Nurses may
desire to read all research on a given clinical topic, but reality dictates that there
is not enough time to read all relevant evidence (Pravikoff et al., 2005). This is
especially true when evidence may be needed for an immediate patient concern.
Therefore, nurses need to triage evidence—determine research evidence that is
critical to read related to their topic or PICOT question as compared with research
evidence that may be nice to read.

The process for rapidly identifying and selecting the relevant evidence
related to a healthcare topic is referred to as rapid critical appraisal (RCA). The
RCA process is a straightforward progression of three uncomplicated steps that
efficiently and effectively aid nurses in selecting the most appropriate research
literature for answering the EBP question. The three steps of RCA are as follows:

1. Identify the level of evidence.
2. Assess how well the study was conducted.
3. Determine how useful the study is to practice.

Step 1: The first step (Box 3.1), described earlier in this chapter, is to identify
the level of evidence. It is important to remember that the highest level of evidence
indicates the highest level of study validity. Nurses aim for selecting studies that
hold the potential for having the greatest validity. Therefore, depending on the
PICOT question, it is generally wise to select those studies closest to the top of
the level of evidence hierarchy. Level of evidence is almost always indicated in
the study title (e.g., Errors in Preparation of Insulin in Two Northeast Medical
Centers: *An Observational Study*) or abstract (e.g., this study was conducted in
two urban medical centers using *a direct observational method*). Both the title and
abstract indicate this study is Level 4 (nonexperimental observation).

Step 2: The second step helps determine how well the study was conducted.
This step tends to make nurses and other practitioners, such as physicians, pharmacists, and social workers, somewhat anxious. Generally, practitioners do not
view themselves as experienced researchers or statisticians; therefore, they view
themselves as unqualified to determine how well a study was conducted unless
they are using a standard appraisal checklist form to assess the study. Standard
forms have great value for in-depth analysis of a study. Standardized forms are
often lengthy and require additional time to complete. However, at times when it
is not feasible or convenient to complete an in-depth analysis of a study, the use
of a RCA to determine how well a study was conducted can be straightforward

and conducted efficiently by looking at a few specific numbers associated with the study.

First, identify the sample size, commonly referred to as "N" in research articles. A larger sample size is almost always better. Popular news stories frequently make claims such as "one glass of red wine daily will make people live longer." When checking on the original research for such tabloid stories, it is not uncommon to find that the initial study may have had 200 participants. A nurse, or any health practitioner, probably would not make wine-centered healthcare decisions based on a sample of 200 participants; therefore, it is critical to first determine the number of study participants.

Second, identify the frequency and duration of follow-up observations. Adequate follow-up observations need to be conducted to ascertain the effects of any intervention or treatment. The frequency and duration of conducting follow-up observations can vary from a few hours' time span to over many years. In the one glass of wine example, the researchers would have needed to make follow-up observations over several decades. The frequency and duration of follow-up observations are dependent on the study question or study purpose. For example, "*Congestive heart failure as comorbidity in patients admitted to a medical center: A cross-sectional study*" would indicate only one observation point is necessary. However, "*Blood glucose variability in cognitive decline: A longitudinal study*" would indicate frequent observation points over a long time span are required.

Third, it is important to identify the number of participants who withdrew or were removed from the study. Excessive attrition weakens a study's findings. A study's abstract will almost always indicate the number of study participants, but the number of participants who completed the study is often found in the results section of the article. Generally, if a study loses 20% of its participants, the study results become doubtful. High attrition indicates participants were unable or uninclined to complete the study; therefore, patients the nurse is caring for may also find the study intervention undesirable. If the attrition rate is high, over 20%, it is wise to read the article's discussion section to determine if the authors addressed the excessive attrition concern. For example, it is common for smoking cessation studies to have high attrition rates. Many studies provide a flowchart beginning with the original sample size and depicting how many participants made it through to the end of the study (Figure 3.1).

Step 3: The third step involves determining if the study's findings are applicable and useful to the patients for whom the nurse is caring. The demographic and clinical variable table, found in most research articles, provides data indicating how well the study sample matches the population of patients the nurse is caring for related to the EBP question. By examining the variables on demographic and clinical variable tables, nurses can determine the applicability of a study's findings to the population the nurses are caring for. Age, severity of illness, and length of illness are variables frequently identified in demographic tables (Table 3.2).

While not an exhaustive appraisal of the study, the RCA allows nurses to identify research that has the highest level of validity and generalizability to positively influence patient-centered practice changes in their clinical areas.

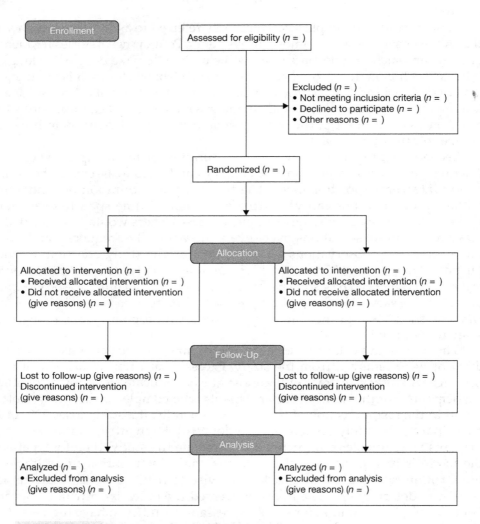

FIGURE 3.1   Flowchart of study design

Source: From Schulz, Altman, and Moher (2010).

TABLE 3.2   Demographic/Clinical Variables (*N* = 79)

Variable	Frequency	Percentage
Gender		
Male	47	60.0%
Female	32	40.0%

(continued)

TABLE 3.2   Demographic/Clinical Variables (*N* = 79) (*continued*)

Variable	Frequency	Percentage
Ethnicity		
White	72	91.1%
African American	7	8.9%
Marital status		
Married/partnered	41	54.4%
Single	11	13.9%
Separated/divorced	13	16.5%
Widowed	12	15.2%
Number in household		
Live alone	21	26.6%
Live with others	58	73.4%
Employment status		
Full time	9	11.4%
Part time	5	6.3%
Retired	37	46.8%
Disabled	28	35.5%
Education		
<High school	8	10.1%
High school	6	7.6%
High school graduate	29	36.7%
College	18	22.8%
College graduate	11	13.9%
Graduate work	7	8.9%
Current smoker	12	15.2%
COPD severity		
Moderate (30%–49% of predicted)*	46	58.2%
Severe (<30% of predicted)*	33	41.8%

COPD, chronic obstructive pulmonary disease.

*Global Initiative for Chronic Obstructive Lung Disease classification.

LOCATING HIGH-QUALITY INFORMATION: AN EASY PROCESS

EBP provides nurses the opportunity to be active seekers of knowledge about critical clinical issues and to build on the knowledge and expertise in their clinical
areas (Newhouse, 2007). Nurses have identified both insufficient literature searching skills and lack of time as significant barriers to implementing EBP (Pravikoff et
al., 2005). Because nurses, on the whole, are not health science librarians or experienced researchers, their literature searching concerns have merit. In addition, not
every healthcare organization provides nurses with immediate electronic access to
healthcare literature. However, the basic technique for conducting healthcare literature searches is straightforward; once demystified, it is usually no longer intimi-
dating. If healthcare organizations do not provide electronic access to healthcare
literature, effective literature searches can be accessed from a mobile phone. This
section of the chapter clarifies the highly manageable steps of conducting a healthcare literature search, attainable from multiple types of electronic devices.

SELECTING THE DATABASE

Basic literature searches regarding any healthcare topic can begin with the Google
search engine. Some information about a healthcare topic will always be found
through an Internet gateway such as Google, and sometimes that information is
useful. However, when using Google, a question of quality and credibility lurks.
Because nurses want the best evidence to use in caring for their patients, it is wise
to move beyond Google to find high-quality evidence in relevant health science
databases specific to healthcare issues and concerns.

A computer database is a large collection of data organized for the purpose of
an efficient search and retrieval. Healthcare databases house massive amounts of
both relevant data and data that may be less relevant for answering an EBP question. For nurses who want to efficiently and effectively retrieve relevant healthcare
data, there are a few uncomplicated and straightforward steps to follow to do so.

Because nurses can select from several databases, the first step is to decide
which electronic bibliographic database would most likely provide the best information (Table 3.3). The bibliographic databases lead nurses to sources of information, typically in journals, that provide the following: (a) citation that includes the

TABLE 3.3   Nursing and Health Databases

Databases Nurses Frequently Use	
Cumulative Index to Nursing and Allied Health Literature (CINAHL)	Available from subscribing library databases. Provides full-text database journals and ebooks on a broad spectrum of nursing and allied health topics. Provides an excellent source of peer-reviewed manuscripts, EBP reports, case studies, systematic reviews, nursing dissertations, nurse practice acts, and standards of professional practice. Includes publications from the American Nurses Association and National League for Nursing. Contains over 900 journals. Primarily bibliographic but provides links to articles when available.

(continued)

TABLE 3.3   Nursing and Health Databases *(continued)*

Databases Nurses Frequently Use	
PubMed (MEDLINE) with full text	A free resource sponsored by the National Library of Medicine. Widely recognized for providing bibliographic and abstract reporting of credible biomedical readings, nursing, medicine, dentistry, and healthcare systems.
ProQuest Nursing and Allied Health Source	Provides credible healthcare information covering nursing, allied health, and alternative and complementary healthcare.

Note: The preceding databases require the reader to analyze the level, quality, and utility of evidence for each article. Cochrane and systematic review databases will provide a combined analysis of the articles for the reader.

EBP Databases	
Cochrane Library	Premier source of systematic reviews and meta-analyses.
Joanna Briggs Institute EBP Database	Sponsored by University of Adelaide. Provides credible EBP resources including evidence summaries, best practice information sheets, and evidence-based recommendations.
National Guideline Clearing House	Public resource for EBP guidelines. Guidelines are searchable by topic or professional organization (e.g., Oncology Nursing Society, American College of Nurse-Midwives).
UpToDate	Designed to immediately answer specific clinical questions at the point of care. Covers a broad array of medical and healthcare topics. Information is concise and practical.

EBP, evidence-based practice.

article's author, title, and source information; (b) name of journal; and (c) volume, issue, and page numbers, and generally an article's abstract.

Nurses generally have the first step completed before even starting the search. The first step is accomplished, in part, by identifying the question the nurse is asking or, more importantly, the well-developed PICOT question (see Chapter 6). A well-developed PICOT will enable the nurse to identify key search terms for the database search. A search term is a word used to electronically retrieve data. For example, "In adults with *COPD*, what is the effect of the *pranayama yoga breathing* technique compared to *pursed lip breathing* on *dyspnea* intensity?" In this example, four key search terms are italicized. Identifying correct search terms is a crucial endeavor. Sometimes lateral thinking or using creative reasoning is helpful in identifying the best search terms. For example, if the nurse is interested in literature focusing on lessening dyspnea intensity, then use of the search term *COPD symptom management* may be a path to relevant evidence.

Using Figures 3.2 through 3.6, we sequentially walk through a MEDLINE (PubMed) search process using the PICOT question: "In adults with *COPD*, what is the effect of the *pranayama yoga breathing* technique compared to *pursed lip breathing* on *dyspnea* intensity?" The basic techniques reviewed in this search can be applied to several databases (see Table 3.3). Please contact your librarian for more advanced searching techniques and additional resources.

The main concepts of the PICOT question comprise the search strategy

(copd OR chronic obstructive pulmonary disease) AND (yoga OR pranayama yoga) AND pursed lip breathing AND dyspnea

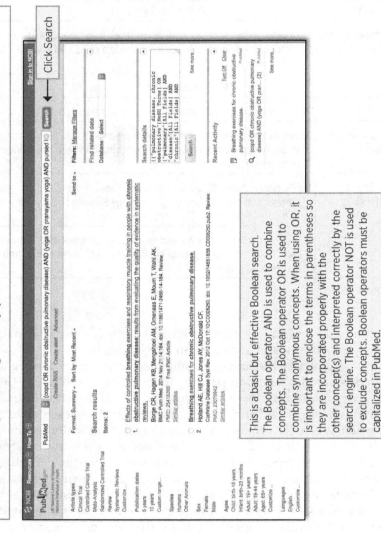

FIGURE 3.2 Searching PubMed.

PICOT, patient population, intervention, comparison, outcome, time frame
Source: National Library of Medicine (n.d.; https://www.ncbi.nlm.nih.gov/pubmed).

- Select appropriate filters to improve relevance.
- EBP content can be quickly identified by using the Article Types filter.

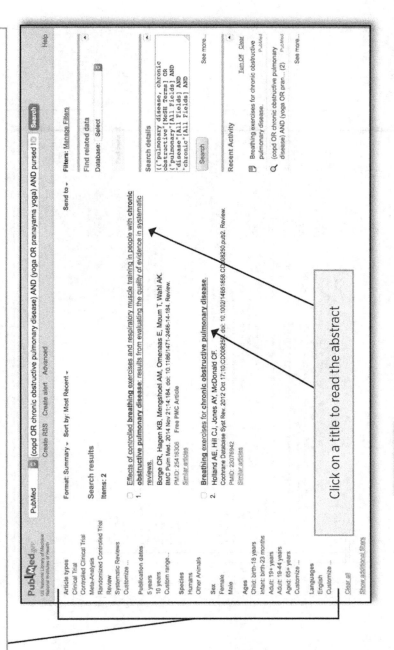

FIGURE 3.3 PubMed filters.

EBP, evidence-based practice.
Source: National Library of Medicine (n.d.; https://www.ncbi.nlm.nih.gov/pubmed).

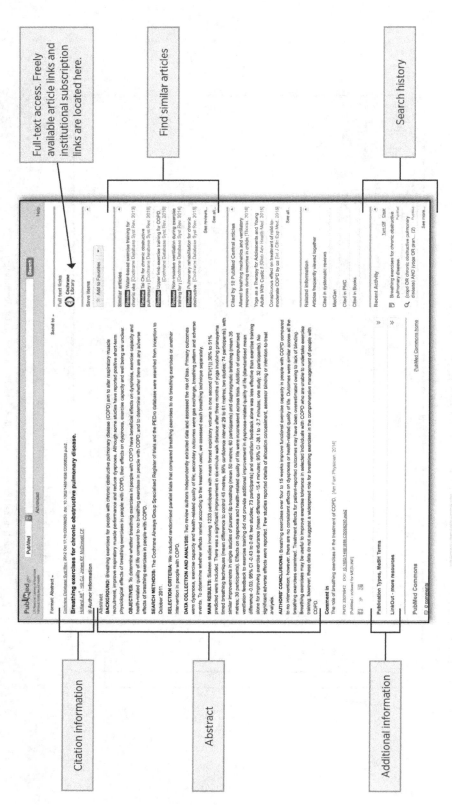

FIGURE 3.4 Abstract and full-text access.

Source: National Library of Medicine (n.d.; https://www.ncbi.nlm.nih.gov/pubmed).

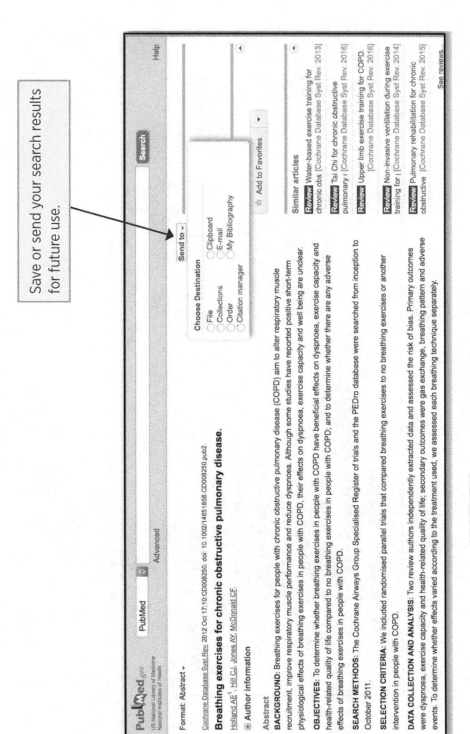

FIGURE 3.5 Exporting results from PubMed.

Source: National Library of Medicine (n.d.; https://www.ncbi.nlm.nih.gov/pubmed).

DATABASE SEARCHING SUMMARY

- Develop a research question using the PICOT Framework.
- Use main concepts from the question to create a search strategy. Incorporate Boolean operators (AND, OR, NOT).
- Search database (PubMed, CINAHL, etc).
- Evaluate results. Revise search if necessary.
- Add filters (study types, dates, ages, gender).
- Read abstract or full-text article.
- Export results for future use.

FIGURE 3.6 Database searching summary.

CINAHL, cumulative index to nursing and allied health literature; PICOT, patient population, intervention, comparison, outcome, time frame.

SUMMARY

Nurses must possess certain essential cognitive and psychomotor skills to be proficient in the process and implementation of EBP. Among the most important of those skills is the ability to use appropriate literature search techniques to find the most pertinent evidence. Once appropriate evidence is located, nurses use essential reasoning skills to determine the strength or level of evidence and the quality of the evidence. This chapter describes efficient and effective research literature techniques that nurses may easily use independently. In addition, the chapter emphasizes the important and growing collaborative role health science librarians and nurses are cultivating to maximize the use of electronic and digital resources to provide the best patient-centered care.

REFERENCES

Agency for Healthcare Research and Quality. (2009). Grading the strength of a body of evidence when comparing medical interventions. Retrieved from https://www.effectivehealthcare.ahrq.gov/repFiles/2009_0805_grading.pdf

Bruderer, S. G., Bodmer, M., Jick, S. S., & Meier, C. R. (2015). Association of hormone therapy and incident gout: Population-based case control study. *Menopause: The Journal of the North American Menopause Society, 22*(12), 1335–1342.

Burns, P. B., Rohrich, R. J., & Chung, K. C. (2011). The levels of evidence and their role in evidence-based medicine. *Plastic and Reconstructive Surgery, 128*(1), 305–310. doi:10.1097/PRS.0b013e318219c171

Chambless, D. L. Baker-Ericzen, M., Baucom, D. H., Beutler, L. E., Calhoun, K. S., Crits-Christoph, P., . . . Woody, S. R. (1998). Update on empirically validated therapies II. *The Clinical Psychologist, 51*(1), 3–16. Retrieved from https://www.researchgate.net/publication/235995889_Update_on_Empirically_Validated_Therapies_II

Christenbery, T., Williamson, A., Sandlin, V., & Wells, N. (2016). Immersion in evidence-based practice fellowship program. *Journal for Nurses in Professional Development, 32*(1), 15–20.

Ciliska, D. K., Pinelli, J., DiCenso, A., & Cullum, N. (2001). Resources to enhance evidence-based nursing practice. *American Association of Critical Care Nurses Clinical Issues, 12*, 520–528.

Davies, C., Brockopp, D., Moe, K., Wheeler, P., Abner, J., & Lengerich, A. (2016). Exploring the lived experiences of women immediately following mastectomy: A phenomenological study. *Cancer Nursing, 40*(5), 361–368. doi:10.1097/NCC.0000000000000413

Dearholt, S., & Dang, D. (2012). *Johns Hopkins nursing evidence-based practice model and guidelines.* Indianapolis, IN: Sigma Theta Tau International.

Denzin, N. K., & Lincoln, Y. S. (2018). Introduction: The discipline and practice of qualitative research. In N. K. Denzin & Y. S. Lincoln (Eds.), *The Sage handbook of qualitative research* (pp. 1–26). Thousand Oaks, CA: Sage Publications.

English Living Oxford Dictionary. (2016). Retrieved from https://en.oxforddictionaries.com/definition/evidence

Estabrooks, C. A., Chong, H., Brigidear, K., & Profetto-McGrath, J. (2005). Profiling Canadian nurses preferred knowledge sources for clinical practice. *Canadian Journal of Nursing Research, 37*(2), 118–140.

Facchiano, L., & Snyder, C. H. (2012). Evidence-based practice for the busy nurse practitioner: Part one: Relevance to clinical practice and clinical inquiry process. *Journal of the American Academy of Nurse Practitioners, 24*(1), 579–586. doi:10.1111/j.1745-7599.2012.00748.x

Fox, L., Richter, J., & White, N. (1996). A multidimensional evaluation of a nursing information literacy program. *Bulletin of the Musical Library Association, 84*(2), 192–190.

French, B. (2005). Contextual factors influencing research use in nursing. *Worldviews on Evidence-Based Nursing, 2*(4), 172–183.

Gambrill, E. D. (1999). Evidence-based practice: An alternative to authority-based practice. *Families in Society, 80,* 341–350.

Hervik, J. R. & Stub, T. (2016). Adverse effects of non-hormonal pharmacological interventions in breast cancer survivors, suffering from from hot flashes: A systematic review and meta-analysis. *Breast Cancer and Research Treatment, 160*(2), 223–236.

Higgs, J., & Jones, M. (2008). Will evidence-based practice take the reasoning out of practice? In J. Higgs & M. Jones (Eds.), *Clinical reasoning in the health professionals.* Amsterdam, the Netherlands: Butterworth Heineman.

Higgs, J., & Titchen, A. (2000). Knowledge and reasoning. In J. Higgs & M. Jones (Eds.), *Clinical reasoning in the health professionals.* Amsterdam, the Netherlands: Butterworth Heineman.

Higgins, J., & Green, S. (2008). *Cochrane handbook for systematic reviews of interventions.* Chichester, England: Wiley-Blackwell.

Institute of Medicine. (2001). *Crossing the quality chasm: A new health system for the 21st century.* Washington, DC: National Academies Press.

Institute of Medicine. (2008). *Knowing what works in health care: A roadmap for the nation.* Washington DC: National Academies Press.

Jenicek, M. (1997). Epidemiology, evidence-based medicine and evidence based public health. *Journal of Epidemiology, 7,* 187–197.

Johnson, B., & Christensen, L. (2008). *Educational research: Quantitative qualitative and mixed approaches.* Thousand Oaks, CA: Sage.

Johnston, L., & Fineout-Overholt, E. (2006). Teaching EBP: The critical step of critically appraising the literature. *Worldviews on Evidence based Nursing, 3*(1), 44–46.

Klem, M. L., & Weiss, P. M. (2005). Evidence-based resources and the role of librarians in developing evidenced-based practice curricula. *Journal of Professional Nursing, 21*(6), 380–387.

Kronenfeld, M., Stephenson, P. L., Nail-Chiwetalu, B., Tweed, E. M., Sauers, E. L. Valovic-McLeod, T. C., . . . Ratner, N. B. (2007). Review for librarians of evidence-based practice in nursing and the allied health professionals in the United States. *Journal of the American Library Association, 95*(4), 394–407. doi:10.3163/1536-5050.95.4.394

Lemke, M. K., Meissen, G. J., & Apostolopoulos, Y. (2016). Overcoming barriers in unhealthy settings: A phenomenological study of healthy truck drivers. *Global Qualitative Nursing Research, 3,* 1–9. doi:10.1177/2333393616637023

LeVasseur, N., Clemons, M., Hutton, B., Shorr, R., & Jacobs, C. (2016). Bone-targeted therapy use in patients with bone metatheses from lung cancer: A systematic review of randomized controlled trials. *Cancer Treatment Reviews, 50,* 183–193.

Lohr, K. N. (2004). Rating the strength of scientific evidence: Relevance for quality improvement programs. *International Journal for Quality in Health Care, 16*(1), 9–18.

Marshall, J. G., Morgan, J. C., Klem, M. L., Thompson, C. A., & Wells, A. L. (2014). The value of library and information services in nursing and patient care. *The Online Journal of Issues in Nursing, 19*(3). doi:10.3912/OJIN.Vol19No03PPT02

Marshall, J. G., West, S. H., & Aitken, L. M. (2011). Preferred information sources for clinical decision making: Critical care nurses' perceptions of information accessibility and usefulness. *Worldviews on Evidence-Based Nursing, 8*(4) 224–235. doi:10.1111/j/1741-6787.2011.00221.x

McCleary, L., & Brown, G. T. (2003). Barriers to pediatric nurses' research utilization. *Journal of Advanced Nursing, 42,* 364–372.

McGinnis, K., Murray, E., Cherven, B., McCracken, C., & Travers, C. (2016). Effect of vibration on pain response to heel lance: A pilot randomized control trial. *Advances in Neonatal Care, 16*(6), 439–448.

Milani, A., Mazzocco, K., Gandini, S., Pravettoni, G., Libutti, L., Zencovich, C., . . .Saiani, L. (2017). Incidence and determinants of port occlusions in cancer outpatients: A prospective cohort study. *Cancer Nursing, 40*(2), 102–107. doi:10.1097/NCC.0000000000000357

Melnyk, B. M., & Fineout-Overholt, E. (2015). *Evidence-based practice in nursing and healthcare: A guide to best practice.* Philadelphia, PA: Wolters Kluwer.

Merriam-Webster. (2016). Science. Retrieved from http://www.merriam-webster.com/dictionary/science

Nayda, R., & Rankin, E. (2008). Information literacy skill development and life long learning: Exploring nursing students' and academics understandings. *Australian Journal of Advanced Nursing, 26*(2), 27–33.

Newhouse, R. P. (2006). Expert opinion: Challenges and opportunities for academic and organizational partnership in evidence-based practice. *Journal of Nursing Administration, 36*(10), 441–445.

Newhouse, R. P. (2007). Crating infrastructure supportive of evidence-based nursing practice: Leadership strategies. *Worldviews on Evidence-Based Nursing, 4*(1), 21–29.

Niderhauser, V. P., & Kohr, L. (2005). Research endeavors among pediatric nurses (REAP) study. *Journal of Pediatric Health Care, 19*, 80–89.

Olano-Lizarrag, M., Oroviogoicoechea, C., Errasti-Ibarrondo, B., & Saracíbar-Razquin, M. (2016). The personal experience of living with chronic heart failure: A qualitative meta-synthesis of the literature. *Journal of Clinical Nursing, 25*(17–18), 2413–2429. doi:10.1111/jocn.13285

Perry, G. J., & Kroenenfeld, M. R. (2005). Evidence-based practice: A new paradigm brings new opportunities for health sciences librarians. *Medical References Services Quarterly, 24*(4), 1–16.

Polit, D. F., & Beck, C. T. (2012). *Nursing research: Generating and assessing evidence for nursing practice*. Philadelphia, PA: Wolters Kluwer/Lippincott Williams & Wilkins.

Pravikoff, D. S., Tanner, A. B., & Pierce, S. T. (2005). Readiness of U.S. nurses for evidence-based practice. *American Journal of Nursing, 105*(9), 40–47.

Profetto-McGrath, J., Smith, K. B., Hugo, K., Taylor, M., & El-Haii, H. (2007). Clinical nurse specialties use of evidence-based practice: A pilot study. *Worldviews of Evidence-Based Nursing, 4*(2), 86–96.

Sackett, D. L. (1989). Rules of evidence and clinical recommendations on the use of anti-thrombotic agents. *Chest, 95*, 2S–3S. doi:10.1378/chest.95.2_Supplement.2S

Sackett, D. L., Rosenberg, W. M., Gray, J. A., Haynes, R. B., & Richardson, W. S. (1996). Evidence based medicine: What it is and what it isn't. *British Medical Journal, 312*(7023), 71–72.

Schulz, K. F., Altman, D. G., & Moher, D. (2010). CONSORT 2010 statement: Updated guidelines for reporting parallel group randomised trials. *British Medical Journal, 340*, c332. doi:10.1136/bmj.c332

Sieving, P. (1999). Factors driving the increase in medical information on the web: One American perspective. *Journal of Medical Internet Research, 1*(1). doi:10.2196/jmir.1.1.e3

Sitzia, J. (2002). Barriers to research utilization: The clinical setting and nurses themselves. *Intensive and Critical Care Nursing, 18*, 230–243.

Tayyib, N., Coyer, F., & Lewis, P. A. (2015). A two-cluster randomized control trial to determine the effectiveness of a pressure ulcer prevention bundle for critically ill patients. *Journal of Nursing Scholarship, 47*(3), 237–247.

Thompson, C., McCaughan, D., Cullum, N., Sheldon, T., & Raynor, P. (2005). Barriers to evidence-based practice in primary care nursing: Why viewing decision-making as context is helpful. *Journal of Advanced Nursing, 52*(4), 432–444.

White, K. M., Dudley-Brown, S., & Terhaar, M. F. (2016). *Translation of evidence into nursing and health care*. New York, NY: Springer Publishing.

Williams, C. (2007). Research methods. *Journal of Business and Economic Research, 5*(3), 65–71.

Yarris, L. M., Simpson, D., & Sullivan, G. M. (2013). How do you define high-quality education research? *Journal of Graduate Medical Education, 5*(2), 180–181.

Yuan, S.-C., Chou, M.-C., Hwu, L.-J., Chang, Y.-O., Hsu, W.-H., & Kuo, H.-W. (2009). An intervention to promote health-related physical fitness in nurses. *Journal of Clinical Nursing, 18*(10), 1404–1111.

Zimmer, L. (2006). Qualitative mete-synthesis: A question of dialoguing with texts. *Journal of Advanced Nursing, 53*(3), 311–318.

CHAPTER 4

Setting the Boundaries for Nursing Evidence

Donna Behler McArthur and Rene Love

Objectives

After reading this chapter, learners should be able to:

1. Describe Carper's patterns of knowing
2. Identify the four metaparadigm concepts of nursing
3. Discuss how each pattern of knowing may inform evidence-based practice (EBP)

EVIDENCE-BASED PRACTICE (EBP) SCENARIOS

Scenario 1

Three community health nurses and a family nurse practitioner identify that a large number of older adults attending the community-based health center have poor nutrition. One of the nurses downloaded a resource on the Internet—*MyPlate for Older Adults*. The other nurses agreed that the tool would be helpful. The nurses made copies of the tool and distributed copies to their patients during clinic visits.

Scenario 2

Three community health nurses and a family nurse practitioner identify that a large number of older adults attending the community-based health center have poor nutrition based on established federal government nutritional guidelines. After reviewing several peer-reviewed articles about nutrition among community-based older adults, they use Pender's Health Promotion Model as a framework for an intervention tailored for individuals. They began by interviewing several patients using a clinical assessment for health promotion based on Pender's model. The nurses were able to identify prior behaviors, personal influences (barriers/benefits, self-efficacy), interpersonal influences, social support, situational influences, and a commitment to a plan of action. By engaging the patient in the decision-making process, individual plans were developed with continued assessments at subsequent visits.

Discussion

The preceding scenarios reflect real-world practice and the overall desire among nurses to influence healthcare outcomes for at-risk populations. Even though both scenarios reflect collaboration among the nurses, the second scenario highlights the engagement of the nurses in reviewing peer-reviewed articles related to their population of interest and identifying potential interventions. In addition, a health promotion model was selected with the behavioral outcome being improved nutrition or eating behaviors of older adults. Pender's Health Promotion Model assisted the nurses in understanding patients' beliefs, which are critical in designing an intervention. The nurses worked collaboratively with the patients to achieve healthier eating behaviors. The nurses assessed evidence and then translated the best evidence to the context of the practice.

In contrast, the well-meaning nurses in the first scenario used a tool (intervention) that was not specific to patients' needs or cognitive capabilities. Feedback from older adults at the health center was not solicited, and outcomes of the Internet resource were not assessed. Using this tool, which has merit because it is based on sound evidence, may be helpful within this community setting and population; however, there are no strategies in place to assess the use.

OVERVIEW OF PROFESSIONAL KNOWLEDGE DEVELOPMENT

The nature of evidence was discussed in Chapter 3. Four types of evidence are needed for healthcare across diverse populations: research, clinical experience, patient experience, and information from the local context (Rycroft-Malone et al., 2004). Historically, empirical evidence has been the gold standard, which requires proof and observation (i.e., research, especially quantitative research) (Sackett, Rosenberg, Gray, Haynes, & Richardson, 1996). The practice of nursing is mediated through relationships between individual practitioners and patients (Kitson, 2002). Hence, evidence-based nursing practice includes knowledge derived from multiple sources.

Other types of knowledge include professional knowledge, which has been explored extensively by Michael Eraut, professor emeritus, University of Sussex, United Kingdom. Eraut (2000) contrasts nonformal learning and tacit knowledge. Further, knowledge is categorized as *propositional* (codified) and *nonpropositional* (personal). The relationship between the two is dynamic (Rycroft-Malone et al., 2004). Propositional knowledge, derived from research and scholarship, is concerned with generalizability, whereas nonpropositional knowledge is informal and derived largely from practice. Tacit knowledge refers to skills, ideas, and experiences that people have in their minds, which are difficult to access because tacit knowledge is often uncodified and not easily expressed. Tacit knowledge is discovered through practice within a particular context and transmitted through social networks (Chugh, 2015). An individual can acquire tacit knowledge without language; for example, a newly graduated master's-educated nurse works with experienced nurses and is mentored by them through observation, imitation, and practice. Shared experience is necessary to acquire tacit knowledge, which is the application of knowledge "know-how" rather than knowing facts.

CARPER'S PATTERNS OF KNOWING

Carper (1978) noted that theorists emphasized objective (empirical) scientific knowledge for nursing practice. Consequently, through her dissertation work, Carper identified fundamental patterns of knowing from an analysis of conceptual and syntactical structure of nursing knowledge. The four domains of knowledge required for nursing practice as posited by Carper are *empirics, esthetics, personal knowledge,* and *ethics.* Carper's pivotal work expanded knowledge necessary for nursing practice to include subjective ways of knowing (personal knowledge and aesthetics) (Thorne & Hayes, 1997). The following provides a brief discussion of each pattern/domain:

- **Empirics** (*the science of nursing*). This is the first fundamental pattern of knowing. Empirical knowing is factual, descriptive, and aimed at developing abstract and theoretical explanations. Publicly verifiable, empirical knowledge is systematically organized into general laws and theories with the goal to describe, explain, and predict phenomena of special interest to the discipline of nursing (Carper, 1978). Some nursing researchers contend that the only valid and reliable source of knowledge is that which is empirical, objectively descriptive, and generalizable.
- **Esthetics** (*the art of nursing*). No one definition works well for this concept. Carper (1978) suggests revisiting the apprentice process in which the apprentice imitates the expert role model with the acquisition of knowledge through experiences. The art of nursing is expressive rather than descriptive—it is a creative process. The nurse gains knowledge of another person's singular, particular, felt experience through empathetic acquaintance. Within the context of Benner's (1984) novice to expert model, the expert nurse is skilled at perceiving and empathizing with the lives of others. In summary, the esthetic pattern of knowing, according to Carper (1978), involves the perception of abstracted particulars as distinguished from abstracted universals.
- **Personal knowing**. This pattern is often identified by advanced practice registered nurse practitioners (APRN) and doctor of nursing practice (DNP) students as the most important way of knowing in understanding patients' health. Personal knowledge is concerned with knowing, encountering, and actualizing the concrete, actual self (Carper, 1978). The pattern speaks to therapeutic use of self in the patient relationship, which is an authentic personal relationship between two persons (e.g., engagement).
- **Ethics**. While standards of practice that include ethical codes of the discipline are inherent in this domain, knowledge of morality in nursing is

extended to capture voluntary actions that are deliberate and subject to the judgment of right and wrong. Once again, this pattern is context specific (e.g., moral choices made in terms of specific actions taken in specific concrete situations) (Carper, 1978, p. 20).

Understanding the four patterns of knowing is essential for nursing students and graduates and reiterates the complexity and diversity of nursing knowledge. While each pattern is mastered within the novice to expert trajectory, the patterns are not mutually exclusive. In summary, nursing depends on the scientific knowledge of human behavior in health and illness, the esthetic perception of significant human experiences, a personal understanding of the unique individuality of the self, and the capacity to make choices within concrete situations involving particular moral judgments (Carper, 1978).

One characteristic of a discipline is its distinct body of knowledge. Critics of EBP highlight the almost exclusive reliance of empirical knowledge, while failing to consider other patterns of knowledge (National Organization of Nurse Practitioner Faculty [NONPF], 2016; Porter, 2010). In contrast, DiCenso, Ciliska, and Guyatt (2005) suggest that research use and research-based practice are subsets within the broader domain of evidence-based nursing (EBN). As such, Carper's (1978) ways of knowing in nursing (empirical, ethical, personal, and esthetic) are included in the clinical decision-making process (Table 4.1).

METAPARADIGM OF NURSING

A metaparadigm is a global statement that identifies the subject matter of each discipline. The metaparadigm of nursing identifies *person/human being*,

TABLE 4.1   Patterns of Knowing: Description and Examples of Evidence

Pattern of Knowing	Description	Evidence for Practice
Empirics	Factual, descriptive, publicly verifiable, generalizable	Randomized controlled trials; original research; translating findings to practice settings
Esthetics	The art of nursing; gaining knowledge of another person's experience though empathetic acquaintance	Reflective practice along the novice to expert continuum
Personal knowing	Knowing, encountering, and actualizing self	Therapeutic use of self in patient engagement
Ethics	Moral choices regarding voluntary actions within specific contexts	Developing own philosophy of nursing; aligning own beliefs with standards of practice

the *environment, health,* and *nursing* as the subject matters of interest to nurses. The distinctive focus of the discipline of nursing is on nursing actions and processes directed toward human beings, which takes into account the environment in which humans reside and in which nursing practice occurs. Within the context of nursing research, theories, which nurses can use in practice, are tested about the health-related experiences of humans within their environments (Fawcett & Garity, 2009; Lee & Fawcett, 2013).

The metaparadigm of nursing continues to evolve with new concepts emerging (e.g., increased emphasis on holistic care, health promotion, and disease prevention; Fawcett, 1984). Outcomes of nursing actions include quality of life in lieu of health. The definitions of each concept vary as to the theoretical underpinning (e.g., the role of "traditional" nurses compared with advanced practice nurses). Likewise, the addition of the concept of "caring" has been suggested. As the discipline continues to mature, new ways of exploring the concepts within the metaparadigm of nursing will evolve. As noted, the concepts are specific to the theoretical underpinnings; hence, the definitions will vary. The preceding definitions are generic. Specific definitions related to Pender's Health Promotion Model and Parse's Theory of Nursing are provided as exemplars (Figure 4.1 and Table 4.2).

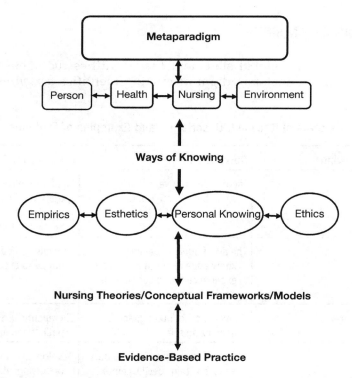

FIGURE 4.1   Relationship among metaparadigm of nursing, patterns of knowing, conceptual models/theories, and evidence-based practice

TABLE 4.2   Metaparadigm of Nursing Concepts: Two Exemplars

Concept	Pender's Health Promotion Model (Pender, 2011)	Parse's Theory of Nursing (Masters, 2017; Parse, 1992)
Person/human being	A biopsychosocial organism partially shaped by the environment that seeks to create an environment in which human potential can be fully expressed. Individual characteristics as well as life experiences shape health behaviors.	An open being; recognized by patterns of relating. Human being freely chooses in situation.
Nursing	Collaboration with individuals, families, and communities to create the most favorable conditions for optimal health and high-level well-being.	A learned discipline; the nurse uses true presence to facilitate the becoming of the person. Goal of nursing is quality of life.
Health	Actualization of individual's inherent and acquired human potential through goal-directed behavior, self-care, and satisfying relationships with others. Health is an evolving life experience.	Process of becoming as experienced and described by person.
Environment	Social, cultural, and physical context in which life unfolds. Can be manipulated by the individual to create positive context and facilitators for health-enhancing behaviors.	Coexists in mutual process with the person.

SUMMARY

Figure 4.1 depicts the relationships among the metaparadigm of nursing, Carper's ways of knowing, theories/conceptual frameworks/models, and evidence-based practice. The relationships are bidirectional, flowing both downstream and upstream.

As a review, evidence-based nursing practice integrates Carper's four domains of knowledge: empirics, esthetics, personal knowledge, and ethics. Nursing practice depends on the scientific knowledge of human behavior in health and illness, the esthetic perception of significant human experiences, a personal understanding of the unique individuality of the self, and the capacity to make choices within concrete situations involving particular moral judgments. Thus, all domains are included in the evidence-based clinical decision-making process.

The metaparadigm of nursing includes the concepts of person/human being, the environment, health, and nursing. The distinctive focus of the discipline of nursing is on nursing actions and processes directed toward human beings that take into account the environment in which human beings reside and in which nursing practice occurs. Understanding the concepts of the metaparadigm and their application within nursing theories helps to inform evidence-based practice within specific settings, thus adding to discipline-specific knowledge.

REFERENCES

Benner, P. (1984). *From novice to expert: Excellence and power in clinical nursing practice.* Menlo Park, CA: Addison-Wesley.

Carper, B. A. (1978). Fundamental patterns of knowing in nursing. *Advances in Nursing Science, 1*(1), 13–23.

Chugh, R. (2015). Do Australian universities encourage tacit knowledge transfer? In A. Fred, D. Aveiro, J. Dietz, J. Filipe, & K. Liu (Eds.), *Proceedings of the 7th International Joint Conference on Knowledge Discovery, Knowledge Engineering and Knowledge Management.* Setúbal, Portugal: SCITEPRESS. 128–135. doi:10.5220/0005585901280135

DiCenso, A., Ciliska, D., & Guyatt, G. (2005). Introduction to evidence-based nursing. In A. DiCenso, G. Guyatt, & D. Ciliska (Eds.), *Evidence-based nursing: A guide to clinical practice* (pp. 3–19). Philadelphia, PA: Elsevier-Mosby.

Eraut, M. (2000). Non-formal learning and tacit knowledge in professional work. *British Journal of Educational Psychology, 70,* 113–136.

Fawcett, J. (1984). The metaparadigm of nursing: Present status and future refinements. *Image: The Journal of Nursing Scholarship, 16*(3), 84–87.

Fawcett, J., & Garity, J. (2009). *Evaluating research for evidence-based nursing practice.* Philadelphia, PA: F. A. Davis.

Kitson, A. (2002). Recognising relationships: Reflections on evidence-based practice. *Nursing Inquiry, 9*(3), 179–186.

Lee, R. C., & Fawcett, J. (2013). The influence of the metaparadigm of nursing on professional identity development among RN-BSN students. *Nursing Science Quarterly, 26*(1), 96–98.

Masters, K. (2017). *Role development in professional nursing practice* (4th ed.). Burlington, MA: Jones & Bartlett.

National Organization of Nurse Practitioner Faculty. (2016). White paper: The doctor of nursing practice nurse practitioner clinical scholar. Retrieved from http://www.nonpf.org/?page=31

Parse, R. (1992). Human becoming: Parse's theory of nursing. *Nursing Science Quarterly, 5*(1), 35–42.

Pender, N. (2011). *The health promotion manual.* Retrieved from https://deepblue.lib.umich.edu/bitstream/handle/2027.42/85350/HEALTH_PROMOTION_MANUAL_Rev_5-2011.pdf

Porter, S. (2010). Fundamental patterns of knowing in nursing: The challenge of evidence-based practice. *Advances in Nursing Science, 33*(1), 3–14.

Rycroft-Malone, J., Seers, K., Titchen, A., Harvey, G., Kitson, A., & McCormack, B. (2004). What counts as evidence in evidence-based practice? *Journal of Advanced Nursing, 47*(1), 81–90.

Sackett, D. L., Rosenberg, W. M., Gray, J. A., Haynes, R. B., & Richardson, W. S. (1996). Evidence based medicine: What it is and what it isn't. *British Medical Journal, 312*(7023), 71–72.

Thorne, S. E., & Hayes, V. E. (1997). *Nursing praxis: Knowledge and action.* Thousand Oaks, CA: Sage.

CHAPTER 5

Using Nursing Phenomena to Explore Evidence

Joanne R. Duffy

Objectives

After reading this chapter, learners should be able to:

1. Describe inductive and deductive models of inquiry
2. Explore relationships among concepts, propositions, and evidence-based practice (EBP)
3. Articulate the value of middle range theory
4. Apply criteria in the analysis of nursing theory

EVIDENCE-BASED PRACTICE (EBP) SCENARIOS

Scenario 1

A group of direct care nurses who represent the cardiac step-down unit at a hospital's Nursing Research Council (NRC) expressed concern about the frequency of clinical alarms in the cardiac step-down unit. Based on policy, each alarm required a nursing response, and the number of alarms was overwhelming. Alarm desensitization often occurred, and nurses tuned out alarms or breached monitoring protocols (e.g., turned off alarms). Consequently, nurses missed important aspects of patient care that led to safety and quality concerns.

The cardiac step-down nurses speculated that nurses on other hospital units might experience a similar alarm frequency phenomenon. Furthermore, the nurses suspected that many alarms were not actionable (i.e., false alarms) and expended nursing time and resources. The nurses were concerned that discounting or turning alarms off, and potentially missing important aspects of care, jeopardized patient safety.

The nurses reviewed relevant literature and found the alarm frequency problem documented and labeled as "nuisance" alarms. However, the literature provided limited evidence about nurses' experiences with nuisance alarms. The nurses thought that if they interviewed nurses on the cardiac step-down unit, a better understanding of nuisance alarms as a phenomenon might emerge. In addition, the nurses hoped to gain insight about how many alarms were actionable compared to nonactionable, and whether nurses perceived if alarm frequency influenced patient care outcomes.

The nurses brought their idea to the hospital's NRC for discussion. The NRC suggested an exploratory qualitative approach to study the phenomenon and to consider how results might provide preliminary evidence about the phenomenon of nuisance alarm frequency. Nurses on the NRC shared concerns about nuisance alarm frequency and offered to support the cardiac step-down nurses in their inquiry, particularly with data collection. The hospital's nurse researcher, who is a standing NRC member, agreed to assist with development of semistructured interview questions and qualitative data analysis. The nurse researcher had experience with evidence exploration, having completed two former studies using *inductive* approaches. The nurses began consulting with the nurse researcher about the exploratory project, and she advised them to seek support from the chief nursing officer (CNO). While meeting with the CNO, the nurses discussed interviewing as a data collection strategy. The CNO suggested using a structured questionnaire to achieve faster results, but the nurses explained that the literature was limited and they were interested in learning about nurses' experiences with alarms, particularly nuisance alarms. The nurses explained that respondents' perceptions and interpretations of nuisance alarms might lead to conceptual clarification and meaning. The CNO agreed with the qualitative exploratory approach and offered support to the pursuit of the plan.

Scenario 2

A group of direct care nurses who represent the cardiac step-down unit at a hospital's NRC expressed concern about the frequency of clinical alarms in the cardiac step-down unit. Based on policy, each alarm required a nursing response, and the number of alarms was overwhelming. Alarm desensitization often occurred, and nurses tuned out alarms or breached monitoring protocols (e.g., turned off alarms). Consequently, nurses missed important aspects of patient care that led to safety and quality concerns.

The cardiac step-down nurses speculated that nurses on other hospital units might experience a similar alarm frequency phenomenon. Furthermore, the nurses suspected that many alarms were not actionable (i.e., false alarms) and expended nursing time and resources. The nurses were concerned that discounting or turning alarms off, and potentially missing important aspects of care, jeopardized patient safety. The nurses reviewed relevant literature and found the alarm frequency problem documented and labeled as "nuisance" alarms. However, the literature provided limited evidence about nurses' experiences with nuisance alarms. The nurses were aware of several safety theories that might provide guidance for the project. After reading the theories, the nurses believed that one particular theory might guide their thinking about alarm frequency.

The nurses brought the theory-focused idea to the hospital's NRC and were encouraged to pursue the *deductive* approach. The nurses were further encouraged to develop specific questions about nuisance alarms and to consider measurements that might aid in answering the questions. NRC members shared concerns about nuisance alarm frequency and offered to support the nurses in their inquiry. The nurse researcher, who is a member of the NRC, stated that an electronic survey would be an efficient way to administer questionnaires to busy clinical nurses, and asked if a valid and reliable questionnaire already existed. One nurse remembered reading an article that used a tool to measure nurses' perceptions of alarms, and she offered to share the questionnaire at the next NRC meeting for review. The nurse researcher suggested if the questionnaire seemed reasonable for this project, she would assist with data collection and quantitative analysis. The nurses spoke with the CNO and received her commitment to support the project.

Discussion

The aim in both scenarios was to discover evidence from which to guide or inform practice and ultimately enhance patient-centered care outcomes. Although each scenario depicted parallel clinical concerns, nurses used different philosophies and methodologies to inquire about and gather clinical evidence. The first scenario is *inductive*, open ended, and exploratory, beginning with specific observations and following up by posing tentative premises for further exploration. Using the inductive approach, results may lead to rich description and new meaning about nuisance alarms and nurses' perceptions of patient care. For example, the results might suggest categories of nuisance alarms and provide insights about nurses' interpretations of nuisance alarms.

The second scenario began with theory evaluation, progressed to formulating theory-originated questions and, subsequently, moved to data collection and analysis to test relevant hypotheses. This *deductive* approach was concerned with testing or confirming hypotheses. In the second scenario, using deduction to explore evidence may lead to a better understanding of the extent of nuisance alarms and may point to information about alarm frequency consequences. Both approaches complement each other and provide results that might inform a practice change. One aim of this chapter is to introduce inductive and deductive models of inquiry to better prepare nurses for EBP implementation.

METHODS OF EXPLORING EVIDENCE

Inductive Inquiry

Inductive approaches to exploring evidence move from specific observations to a search for emerging patterns that eventually lead to development of theoretical explanations (Chinn & Kramer, 2011; Sternberg, 2004). An inductive approach to inquiry involves perceptually synthesizing observations and pieces of information to identify broad generalizations or abstract themes and is associated with qualitative research (Gustason, 1994). Inductive approaches begin with collecting data that are relevant to a topic of nursing interest, such as patient pain perception. Once a substantial amount of data is collected, exploration for patterns begins, with the goal of developing an explanatory theory to clarify patterns. Using an inductive approach progresses from data to theory or from the specific to the general. For example, exploring pain patterns for patients with rheumatoid arthritis may lead to the development of new theoretical understandings of chronic pain self-management strategies.

Deductive Inquiry

While inductive methods move from specific to general, deductive approaches move from general to specific and are aligned with quantitative research. Deductive methods develop specific predictions (e.g., hypotheses) based on general principles or theories (Tarski, 1995). For example, if nurses use a pathophysiologic theory to explain pain occurrence in patients following coronary artery bypass graft (CABG) surgery, then nurses might predict or hypothesize that patients who receive specific CABG preoperative pain management instruction will experience less postoperative pain than patients who do not receive instruction.

Although nurses in both case scenarios did not set out to use a specific philosophical approach, both inductive and deductive strategies are evident in the nurses' respective work. Nurses use inductive and deductive reasoning constantly in clinical practice, although the selection of types of reasoning may not always be conscious (Kaplan, 1964). Applying inductive and deductive approaches to nursing knowledge development helps yield important patient care information that is scientifically grounded and useful to practice. To summarize, quantitative research moves from the abstract to the specific through *deduction*. Qualitative research moves from the specific to the abstract through *induction* (see Figure 5.1).

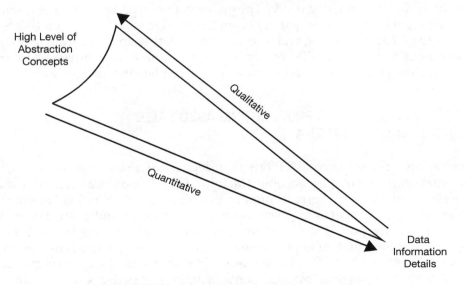

FIGURE 5.1   Information to abstract concepts

Source: Courtesy of Nancy Wells.

NURSING PHENOMENA

Nursing practice is complex and consists of situations, experiences, and perspectives that sometimes generate concerns, requiring improvement in healthcare. Furthermore, nurses work in close contact with patients, families, and communities, which helps generate a holistic view of the healthcare concerns each faces. Nurses are in a unique position to recognize emerging patterns of healthcare concerns or challenges. Processes, occurrences, or events associated with health and illness care are phenomena central to nursing.

Nursing phenomena broadly describes conceptualizations of patient care relevant to nursing practice. Nursing phenomena are areas of concern that influence patients' health and well-being, such as quality-of-life, comfort, and fear. Nurses often think deeply about phenomena central to patient care, which often becomes a focus for further exploration and intervention. For example, while working with recently discharged patients who have heart failure (HF), nurses might observe that many patients with HF have difficulty regularly monitoring cardiac-related signs and symptoms. Limited understanding of symptom importance, lack of motivation, or depression may impede patients with HF from regularly assessing their weight or recording how often they experience fatigue, dyspnea, and coughing. Neglect of symptom self-monitoring is a concern to nursing because such patient oversights frequently lead to illness exacerbation and rehospitalization. Inadequate self-monitoring is a nursing phenomenon that when explored more carefully and methodically may lead to evidence-based interventions to improve health outcomes for patients with HF.

Another example of a nursing phenomenon is the opportunity for patient participation in medication teaching, which is sometimes inadequate in an acute-care environment. The short length of patient stay, coupled with a high task-based nursing workflow, may hinder nurses from adequately attending to patient and family medication teaching needs. The phenomenon of patient teaching is important to nurses because insufficient patient knowledge about medications directly relates to patient well-being and safety. Contemplating and attending to nursing phenomena foster use of EBP by concentrating nurses' inquisitiveness in areas that have the potential to improve patient-centered healthcare outcomes.

THEORY, CONCEPTS, AND PROPOSITIONS ASSOCIATED WITH NURSING PHENOMENA

Theories are abstract generalizations that depict systematic explanations about the relationships among concepts (Meleis, 2012). Theoretical representations describe, explain, and/or predict nursing phenomenon (see Box 5.1). For example, symptom management is a phenomenon closely associated with patient values and nursing care. The Symptom Management Model (see Figure 5.2) is a theoretical representation of phenomena associated with patient symptom experiences (Dodd et al., 2001). The Symptom Management Model is composed of concepts (e.g., symptom management, symptom experience, symptom self-management) with conceptual relationships clearly and logically depicted by the use of arrows and concentric circles. As a theoretical depiction, the Symptom

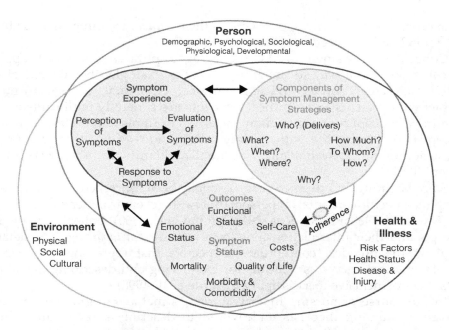

FIGURE 5.2   Symptom Management Model

Source: From Dodd et al. (2001).

BOX 5.1   Uses of Nursing Theory

Nurses use concepts and propositions from theory to:

   Define nursing phenomena

   Formulate compelling PICOT questions

   Retrieve relevant research

   Develop hypotheses

   Measure variables of interest

   Provide evidence on nursing phenomena

PICOT, patient population, intervention, comparison, outcome, time frame.

Management Model provides a means for a clear understanding of symptom experience, guides nurses in selecting targeted symptom interventions, informs research questions, and bridges an array of symptoms associated with disease and illness (Dodd et al., 2001).

   Concepts are mental representations (e.g., symptom management) that allow nurses to draw inferences or propositions (e.g., symptom management influences symptom experience) about phenomena they encounter in daily clinical care. Nurses constantly use concepts in clinical practice to support various mental processes, such as decision making, learning, categorization, making patient-care–related inferences, and memory aids. As abstractions or ideas, concepts describe a portion of reality or vision (Chinn & Kramer, 2014). Concepts label or name processes, occurrences, or events so their clinical meanings may be better understood and conveyed.

Concepts can be single words (e.g., caring) or phrases (e.g., social support). Concepts provide a way to imagine ideas. For example, the concept of caring characterizes various ways (e.g., physical, emotional, and social) nurses interact with patients and families. Concepts are generally multidimensional, meaning a concept represents many ideas. An example of a multidimensional concept is quality of life with reported dimensions of health and functioning, socioeconomic, psychological/spiritual, and family well-being (Ferrans & Powers, 1992).

Since Nightingale, nurses have traditionally been concerned with four broad, discipline-specific concepts: (a) person, (b) health, (c) environment, and (d) nursing (Fawcett & DeSanto-Madeya, 2013; Nightingale, 1860). Collectively, the four concepts and their interrelationships form nursing's *metaparadigm*. A metaparadigm is the broadest conceptual perspective that represents a discipline. A metaparadigm serves as a means for identifying and describing global concepts that are inclusive to a discipline (Thorne et al., 1998).

In the course of nursing history, nursing's metaparadigm concepts have evolved as nursing theorists endeavored to describe, explain, and predict nursing phenomena. For example, concepts such as self-care (Orem, 1985), adaptation (Roy, 1999), and goal attainment (King, 1981) have emerged and formed the source of nursing's *grand theories*. Grand theories are highly abstract and provide an overall explanation of phenomena specific to a discipline (Mills, 1959). Grand theories provide a comprehensive framework that enables nurses to identify primary concepts and principles central to nursing as a discipline.

Subsequent to the development of grand theories, concepts such as comfort (K. Y. Kolcaba, 1994), synergy (Hardin & Kaplow, 2005), and transitions (Meleis & Trangenstein, 1994) have formed a core of nursing middle range theories. According to Merton (1968), a *middle range theory* explains a limited set of phenomena (e.g., symptom management) as compared with grand theories that seek to explain broad, focused phenomena (e.g., unitary human beings).

Currently, nurses work with a broad range of middle range theory concepts to address multifaceted patient care issues. Concepts important to nursing range from the highly abstract (e.g., faith) to profoundly concrete (e.g., sinus mask). Abstract concepts refer to ideas (e.g., comfort, nausea, and fatigue) that have no physical referent. Concrete concepts denote objects or events that can be detected by the senses (e.g., heating pad, ambulate, and nicotine patch). Concepts and conceptual clarity are critical in delineating issues or phenomena in clinical practice and provide the beginning structure for *conceptual propositions* (Walker & Avant, 2005).

Practitioners and researchers alike are seldom interested in a single concept but are instead highly interested in relationships among two or more concepts. For example, the concept "adolescence" evokes images of categories such as young, transitioning, anxious, puberty, and independence. In principle, a concept, such as adolescence, does not exist by itself but is part of a larger propositional system where two or more concepts relate to each other.

Propositional Statements

Propositions are statements about conceptual relationships between two or more concepts (Meleis, 2012). As used in nursing theory, propositions are statements that represent the theorist's view of a concept's properties and how those properties fit together with other concepts and, in most cases, establish how concepts affect one another. If the theorist is concerned with only one concept, the single concept is descriptive or explanatory. For example, Duffy (2013) states, "caring relationships are composed of processes or factors that can be observed" (p. 38). Caring relationship is an example of a single concept depicting a descriptive conceptualization. If the propositional statement is related to two or more concepts, the statement suggests an association among concepts. For example, "caring relationships facilitate growth and change" (p. 38) demonstrates an association between caring relationships, growth, and change.

Concepts and Propositional Statements

Concepts and propositional statements are fundamental to EBP because each helps to translate broad phenomena into more practical components. For example, concepts often identify key words or phrases for literature reviews. Concepts help identify appropriate empirical indicators that measure key EBP outcomes such as the Caring Assessment Tool (CAT) (Duffy, Brewer, & Weaver, 2010) or the Minnesota Living with Heart Failure Questionnaire (MSHFQ) (Rector & Cohn, 1992). Concept and propositional statements form the variables of interest in a PICOT (patient population, intervention, comparison, outcome, time frame) question (Guyatt, Drummond, Meade, & Cook, 2015). *Variables* are concepts that assume variance (e.g., stress, pulse, and level of activity). Propositions form the basis for PICOT questions and suggest the direction of the EBP project. For example, "In adults with osteoarthritis, what is the effect of tai chi as compared with standard stretching exercises, on reports of chronic low-back pain?" EBP draws on concepts and propositions from nursing theory to initiate, hypothesize, measure, and report critical nursing phenomena.

EBP, a widely used term, does not always receive optimal use in healthcare practice environments. Suboptimal application of EBP influences efficiency and effectiveness of patient care. Enabling the full application of EBP in clinical care is a primary goal of nursing and healthcare systems (K. R. Stevens, 2013). One method for further engaging nurses in EBP is *concept mapping*. Concept mapping is a cognitive technique used to facilitate critical thinking about concepts and their connections to other concepts, thus enhancing understanding and applicability to EBP (Kane & Trochim, 2007).

Concept Mapping

Nurses often use concept maps as a learning strategy (Carter-Templeton, Sackett-Fitzgerald, & Carter, 2016). Concept mapping uses a structured and participatory approach to thinking about ideas that result in visual tools or graphical displays to depict clearer conceptual meanings and propositional relationships (Trochim & McLinden, 2016). In EBP, concept mapping is useful for depicting and viewing the interrelatedness of concepts, especially when concepts have various definitions and uses in clinical practice, such as circulatory complication or end-of-life care.

As a communication tool, concept mapping supports EBP by aiding nurses to think critically about nursing phenomena and make important linkages with clinical practice. Concept mapping in clinical areas usually involves nurses working with an experienced facilitator to generate a visual "map" to organize and represent knowledge about a phenomenon of shared concern. Concept map construction enables nurses to understand the meaning of specific concepts and the concept's multifaceted connections. Concept maps help refine PICOT questions, identify key terms for literature searches, and establish priorities for investigation. As concepts become more fully understood, concept mapping aids in targeting key ideas, generating or locating empirical indicators (i.e., measurements), identifying sources of data, deciding how to proceed in terms of clarifying research methods and analytics, developing research models, and guiding practical applications of research.

Concept mapping is a staged process. First, the primary concept is clearly identified, often in conjunction with a preliminary PICOT question followed by identification of secondary concepts. Second, conceptual linkages that logically unite concepts are created. Third, interconnections among concepts are identified and labeled (Daley, Morgan, & Black, 2016). Concept mapping enables nurses to understand the complexities of nursing phenomena and is helpful in conceptualizing EBP projects. Figures 5.3 and 5.4 depict concept maps. In Figure 5.3, the concept map was developed to help clarify the meaning of caring relationships, and in Figure 5.4, a more developed concept map was created to identify possible relationships between caring relationships and patient outcomes in hospitalized older adults (based on propositions in the Quality-Caring Model© [Duffy, 2009, 2013]). Figure 5.4, as a concept map, guided the planning of a performance improvement project aimed at reducing hospital readmissions, reducing the number of falls, and improving patient experiences in hospitalized elderly adults.

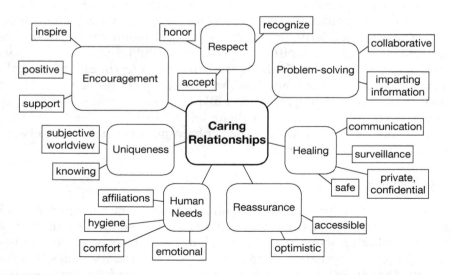

FIGURE 5.3   **Concept map used to describe the meaning of caring relationships**

Source: Courtesy of Joanne Duffy.

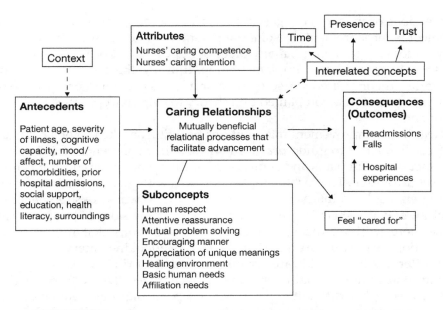

FIGURE 5.4   Concept map derived from the Quality-Caring Model

Source: From Duffy (2013).

From Concept to Middle Range Theoretical Frameworks/Models

Grand theories are broad and far-reaching, while middle range theories address specific nursing phenomena and are directly applicable to a variety of patient populations across many practice settings. Because of their imme- diate applicability to patient-centered care, many middle range theories have emerged and continue to proliferate. Many middle range theories, deduc- tively, originated from grand theories (Peterson & Bredow, 2013). Examples of middle range theories widely used in nursing care include caregiver stress (Tsai, 2003), unpleasant symptoms (Lenz, Pugh, Milligan, Gift, & Suppe, 1997), uncertainty (Mishel, 1997), quality caring (Duffy, 2009, 2013), chronic sorrow (Eakes, 1995), transitions theory (Meleis & Trangenstein, 1994), and comfort theory (K. Kolcaba, 2003).

Nursing, similar to other disciplines, often borrows or shares theory from other disciplines. For example, both researchers and practitioners in multiple disciplines rely heavily on human decision-making theories, which draw from psychology, economics, neuroscience, and nursing (Hall, 2003; Levine, 2001). Examples of borrowed or shared middle range theories that are frequently used in nursing include (a) theory of reasoned action (Ajzen & Fishbein, 1969), (b) adult learning (theory of andragogy) (Knowles, 1984), and (c) social cognitive theory (Bandura, 1986).

Because middle range theories are practical and often conducive to empiri- cal testing, they facilitate EBP by presenting guidance and direction for future research projects. Middle range theories provide the basis for nursing interventions or practice changes and identify and develop empirical indicators for outcome measurement. Despite the potential value of nursing theory, especially middle range theories, many practice improvement projects tend to progress straight from idea to implementation, limiting the critical benefits of an appropriate theory. Often, the source of a problem is present in practice improvement projects but unaccompanied by a theory to help conceptualize and explain a problem.

Healthcare improvement interventions benefit from the use of a change theory (see Chapter 7) to guide practice revisions. In the absence of a theory, outcome measurement plans and significant baseline data required for meaningful analyses are absent. The rush to implementation, without a theoretical underpinning, often results in interventions or improvements whose desired benefits are not clear, and the specific processes required for revision are undocumented. Furthermore, without theory, contextual considerations that might influence intervention evaluation are missing. In fact, overlooking intervention evaluation is often costly to healthcare organizations and a primary reason why many nursing contributions remain insufficiently recognized (Duffy, 2016). Without a guiding theory, it is difficult to demonstrate a particular intervention's effect on patient-centered care.

Theory helps nurses understand the conceptual components of interventions, including how interventions are effective and facilitate clarification of conflicting findings. EBP continually informs and guides practice while simultaneously supporting theory development. Middle range theory, in particular, adds meaning to practice because of frequent application in patient care, research studies, and organizational system changes. To be most effective, theories must be realistic and provide evidence of benefit to patients and families. Selecting theories for application are decisions that require evaluation, including analysis of a theory's value, worth, and significance (Smith & Liehr, 2013).

Analysis of Theoretical Frameworks Guides EBP

As stated earlier, a primary purpose of theory is to provide a framework for identifying and understanding nursing phenomena. Theory has a range of usefulness depending on how well it helps focus, explain, and guide the use of phenomena central to nursing. Therefore, knowing how to evaluate a theory for its usefulness to nursing practice and research is a valuable skillset for nurses to possess. Nurse authors have provided criteria for the analysis of theory.

Johnson (1974), Fawcett (2004), Fitzpatrick and Whall (2004), B. Stevens (1998), Meleis (2012), Fawcett and DeSanto-Madeya (2013), and Smith and Liehr (2013) have developed specific criteria nurses use to analyze the appropriateness of theory for specific practice and research endeavors. *Theory analysis* involves using a set of criteria to examine specific components of a theory. For this chapter, we use the following criteria for theory evaluation: (a) theoretical clarity, (b) logical consistency, and (c) practical usefulness. See Table 5.1 for assessment questions for these three criteria.

TABLE 5.1   Definition Theory Criteria With Examples

Criterion	Assessment Questions
Theoretical Clarity	• Are concepts distinct and unambiguously defined? • Is the theory straightforward and easily understandable? • Does the theory provide sufficient detail to explain the propositional relationship? • Can the theory describe, explain, or predict phenomena? • Do multiple concepts and propositions cloud the theoretical understanding? • Are multiple or lengthy clarifications required to explain the theory?
Logical Consistency	• Is there a diagrammatic representation of the theory? Is there logical agreement between the theory's diagrammatic representation and narrative? • Is the theory consistent with nursing's paradigm (i.e., nurse, patient, health, environment)? • Are propositional statements clearly articulated and logical?
Practical Usefulness	• Is the theory suitable for specific contexts or populations? • Are the concepts and propositional relationships too vague for practical application? • Does the theory have application to clinical settings?

A recent literature review suggests that, with the increased use of middle range theories in nursing, continuing efforts to analyze middle range theories for use in practice, education, and research are necessary to advance the nursing discipline (Im, 2015). Together with articulated values and beliefs about nursing, selecting and using theory to conduct research and ultimately improve practice connects the more abstract (concepts and propositions) with practical data, thus enhancing individual and disciplinary nursing practice. Importantly, theory provides an opportunity to improve patient outcomes.

EXEMPLAR: NURSING PHENOMENA AND EBP

At a Magnet®-designated community hospital in the mid-Atlantic area, elderly adult patients following major surgery are frequently admitted to an intensive care unit (ICU). ICU nurses frequently observed elderly patients fidgeting, intensely focused on the monitors and IVs, and outwardly uncomfortable and apprehensive. Because nurses frequently observed these behaviors among elderly patients, they began to wonder if elderly ICU patients experienced more anxiety surrounding their unstable and high-risk situations than younger patients, and if there was a targeted nursing intervention to reduce elderly patients' anxiety. In addition, ICU nurses were concerned that increased anxiety among elderly ICU patients could negatively affect the patients' illnesses and recovery trajectories.

The nurses brought their concerns about anxiety in elderly ICU patients to the unit's nurse manager. After discussion, the nurses and manager agreed it was a unit concern and perhaps providing a more consistent healing environment— specifically by reorganizing the physical environment around elderly patients' needs; ensuring that family members, when present, were engaged; and providing frequent reassurance from nurses—might reduce elderly patients' anxiety.

One of the nurses remembered from her undergraduate research course the concept of *healing environment* as a nursing phenomenon and asked the group if they were interested in further exploration of the topic of healing environment. The nurses agreed, but remarked they did not know where to start. The nurse manager referred them to a nurse faculty member who had research expertise at the local college of nursing. One of the nurses contacted the faculty member, who agreed to meet with them.

At the meeting, the faculty member seemed eager to help the nurses pursue the topic of healing environment. The group discussed their observations about behaviors of elderly adults in the ICU and their interest in providing a more healing environment for the elderly adult population. The nurses knew that using current and best evidence to guide practice was important, but they admitted they did not know how to proceed. The nurse researcher suggested they look in the literature to see what available evidence existed about the *phenomenon* of healing environment for elderly ICU patients. Although anxious about the process, the nurses were encouraged by the nurse researcher's enthusiasm and decided to pursue the suggested literature search. The nurses used the key search terms "healing environment," "ICU," "anxiety," and "elderly adults." The nurses found many research articles, some that used an *inductive* (e.g., qualitative) approach and others that were more *deductive* (e.g., quantitative), including evaluation of specific interventions, such as music therapy, as a way to reduce anxiety. The nurses could not find any articles that described healing environment in a holistic manner for the ICU setting. The nurses believed that to address the problem of elderly patient anxiety, the definition of healing environment needed to be holistic, addressing concepts such as physical environment, family engagement, and nurse reassurance.

The nurse researcher found the phenomenon of healing environment defined in the literature and provided the nurses with two articles that described the *concepts* associated with healing environment. The nurses were dissatisfied with the definitions and descriptions in the literature, because the definitions were not specific to elderly patients. The nurse researcher suggested the group use *concept mapping* as a technique to help clarify their understandings about healing environments for elderly patients in ICUs to inform the project. The nurse researcher agreed to return and maintain weekly meetings with the nurses until a well-written proposal was ready for approval by the Internal Review Board (IRB). She also promised to send the nurses information about concept mapping for their next meeting.

The nurses went back to their nurse manager to relay information about their meeting with the nurse researcher and seek his support for the project. The nurse manager reminded them of the nursing research policy that specifically stated that the Research Council must approve all nursing research prior to IRB submission. He also referred them to the online research tool kit provided by the Council to help with proposal requirements, and he expressed genuine support of the project.

The nurse researcher sent the nurses three relevant articles on concept mapping and an additional article on fundamentals of the research process. At the next meeting, the nurse researcher and nurses used a whiteboard to diagram thoughts related to the meaning of a healing environment. First, they identified meanings and characteristics of the healing environment such as physical surroundings, including artifacts, spaces, people, sounds, unit culture, and workflow. Second, they thought about the potential benefits (e.g., reduced anxiety, increased comfort, and security) that might result if a healing environment was consistently available to elderly adults. Third, they linked the concepts to the original phenomenon, healing environment. The nurse researcher and nurses reflected on the resulting concept map. There were many terms associated with healing environment, and she helped the nurses see where group agreement existed about the meaning. There were linkages represented in the concept map, and the nurse researcher asked if the nurses could use the map to articulate a PICOT question for the project. The nurses attempted several times to state a PICOT question and finally agreed they needed more reflection and dialogue. The researcher reminded the nurses about the benefits of theory, specifically *middle range theory*, and asked if any theories emerged in their literature review to guide the project. The nurses remembered several theories that considered healing environments, but one theory in particular incorporated their holistic ideas.

Two of the nurses agreed to examine the literature in more detail to identify middle range theories they remembered. They found the Quality-Caring Model (Duffy, 2009, 2013). The nurses located several articles about the Quality-Caring Model and began to read the author's definition of healing environment. Defined as a subconcept in the model, healing environment, together with other subconcepts, contributed to forming a broader concept, "caring relationships." Promotion of healing environments was defined holistically as a caring behavior that nurses use in relationship with patients and families. The definition referred to settings where care takes place and included protecting from harm, providing continuous surveillance, ensuring privacy and confidentiality, preserving comfort, and attending to esthetics. Attentive reassurance (e.g., optimistic, encouraging interactions with nurses) and attention to affiliation needs (e.g., family member engagement) were listed as caring behaviors. Thus, the nurses renamed their phenomenon of interest *caring relationships* and decided to focus on those holistic behaviors they deemed important for the elderly adult in the ICU environment. Furthermore, several propositions listed in the readings provided the nurses opportunities to link caring relationships with other concepts they had discussed (e.g., anxiety).

One of the propositions, "caring relationships influence 'feeling cared for'" (Duffy, 2013, p. 38), seemed intriguing to the nurses. Because the theorist had been a critical care nurse, the nurses decided to contact her for more information about the theory. After discussion, the nurses decided to examine the literature one more time to identify research studies using the model. The review proffered articles that discussed a need for caring relationships, but only one study tested a specific intervention based on the theory; this study examined heart failure patients recently discharged from the hospital. The nurses found two other studies, but only one focused on elderly adults. The study showed an association between caring behaviors and lower anxiety in hospitalized elderly patients. To further clarify whether the theory would be appropriate to guide the proposal, the nurses talked to the nurse researcher who walked them through the process of *analyzing a theory*. After conducting the analysis using specific criteria, the nurses decided the theory fit with their ideas of helping elderly adult ICU patients decrease anxiety. The theory used clear and well-defined concepts, was practical, and offered an empirical indicator (i.e., measurement) for use in the project.

The nurses' work showed a gap in knowledge related to how caring relationships, partially defined as attentive reassurance, healing environments, and affiliation needs, might support elderly adult ICU patients to decrease anxiety in the ICU. A practical middle range theory, an empirical indicator, and possible hypotheses for the project were positive outcomes related to the project. The concept mapping and literature review influenced the nurses to understand that healing environment was part of the broader concept of caring relationships. The nurses hypothesized that when caring relationships are consistently available to older adult ICU patients, the positive emotion, "feeling cared for," may follow, reducing manifestations of patient anxiety the nurses initially observed.

With the help of the Research Council and nurse researcher, the nurses began to develop a proposal for submission to the IRB. The nurse researcher helped the nurses refine a PICOT question to direct the inquiry and operationalize the study variables. The nurses worked with the nurse researcher to adapt a caring-based intervention for care delivery to elderly adults in the ICU. The nurses decided on a deductive approach to evaluate the intervention since empirical indicators already existed. Specifically, the nurses proposed a quasi-experimental study design with pre- and postmeasures of anxiety. The Research Council helped the ICU nurses with the specifics of the proposal and helped them submit the proposal to the IRB. While the nurses were awaiting IRB approval, the nurse researcher found a small critical care grant that the nurses applied for to support data collection and analysis.

The IRB asked for clarification on the consent form, and after some minor editing, the project received approval. The nurses met with peers in the ICU to explain the project and obtain their support for consistently delivering caring relationships via the study protocol for 1 month. The nurses agreed, and the study began 1 year after the nurses first identified the anxiety problem in elderly patients. Following 3 months of consistently delivering the caring intervention to elderly ICU patients, preliminary results showed a statistically significant improvement in anxiety scores for elderly patients.

The ICU staff nurses who first identified and pursued a nursing phenomenon to facilitate better patient outcomes shared their findings at a staff meeting and subsequently at the local critical care nurses' association meeting. In addition, the nurses attended the national American Association of Critical-Care Nurses (AACN) meeting where they presented a poster about their caring intervention. The nurse researcher reminded the nurses of where they started—that is, with the phenomenon of interest. She also reviewed their scholarly learning path, which included inductive and deductive inquiry, concept and proposition identification, concept mapping, use of middle range theory, and theory analysis, to arrive at study findings they could disseminate. The nurses successfully undertook a project to study a phenomenon of interest observed in practice. The nurses were satisfied that elderly ICU patients were now receiving a nursing intervention that led to optimization of patient outcomes. The nurses' persistence and passion made this contribution to the well-being of elderly ICU patients a reality.

SUMMARY

This chapter explored inductive and deductive approaches to understanding nursing phenomena and addressed the concepts and propositions that comprise nursing theory. The use of concept mapping as a tool to clarify meaning and linkages among concepts was illustrated, and middle range theories of particular use to nursing were described as integral to EBP. Criteria for analysis of theory were presented, and a real-world example describing how a nursing phenomenon was initially considered and then used during the research process to advance EBP was described.

REFERENCES

Ajzen, I., & Fishbein, M. (1969). The prediction of behavioral intentions in a choice situation. *Journal of Experimental Social Psychology, 5*(4), 400–416.

Bandura, A. (1986). *Social foundations of thought and action: A social cognitive theory.* Englewood Cliffs, NJ: Prentice Hall.

Carter-Templeton, H., Sackett-Fitzgerald, K., & Carter, M. (2016). Application of concept mapping as a visual thinking strategy in an asynchronous online graduate informatics course. *Computers in Nursing, 34*(8), 331–335.

Chinn, P. L., & Kramer, M. K. (2011). *Integrated knowledge development in nursing* (8th ed.). St. Louis, MO: Mosby.

Chinn, P. L., & Kramer, M. K. (2014). *Knowledge development in nursing: Theory and process* (9th ed.). St. Louis, MO: Elsevier.

Daley, B. J., Morgan, S., & Black, S. B. (2016). Concept maps in nursing education: A historical literature review and research directions. *Journal of Nursing Education, 55*(11), 631–639.

Dodd, M., Janson, S., Facione, N., Faucett, J., Froelicher, E. S., Humphreys, J., . . . Taylor, D. (2001). Advancing the science of symptom management. *Journal of Advanced Nursing, 33*(5), 668–676.

Duffy, J. (2009). *Quality caring in nursing: Applying theory to clinical practice, education, and leadership.* New York, NY: Springer Publishing.

Duffy, J. (2013). *Quality caring in nursing and health systems: Implications for clinical practice, education, and leadership* (2nd ed.). New York, NY: Springer Publishing.

Duffy, J. (2016). *Professional practice models: Successful health system integration.* New York, NY: Springer Publishing.

Duffy, J., Brewer, B., & Weaver, M. (2010). Revision and psychometric properties of the caring assessment tool. *Clinical Nursing Research, 23*, 80–93. doi:10.1177/1054773810369827

Eakes, G. G. (1995). Chronic sorrow: The lived experience of parents of chronically mentally ill individuals. *Archives of Psychiatric Nursing, 9*(2), 77–84.

Fawcett, J. (2004). *Analysis and evaluation of contemporary nursing knowledge.* Philadelphia, PA: F. A. Davis

Fawcett, J., & DeSanto-Madeya, S. (2013). *Contemporary nursing knowledge: Analysis and evaluation of nursing models and theories.* Philadelphia, PA: F. A. Davis.

Ferrans, C., & Powers, M. (1992). Psychometric assessment of the quality of life index. *Research in Nursing and Health, 15*, 29–38.

Fitzpatrick, J., & Whall, A. (2004). *Conceptual models of nursing.* Stamford, CT: Appleton Lange.

Gustason, W. (1994). *Reasoning from evidence: Inductive logic.* New York, NY: Macmillan.

Guyatt, G., Drummond, R., Meade, M., & Cook, D. (2015). *The evidence based medicine working group users' guides to the medical literature* (3rd ed.). Chicago, IL: McGraw-Hill.

Hall, H. (2003). Borrowed theory: Applying exchange theories in information science research. *Library and Information Science Research, 25*(3), 287–306.

Hardin, S. R., & Kaplow, R. (2005). *Synergy for clinical excellence: The AACN synergy model for patient care*. Sudbury, MA: Jones & Bartlett.

Im, E. O. (2015). The current status of theory evaluation in nursing. *Journal of Advanced Nursing, 71*(10), 2268–2278.

Johnson, D. (1974). Development of theory: A requisite for nursing as a primary health profession. *Nursing Research, 23*(5), 372–377.

Kane, M., & Trochim, W. M. K. (2007). *Concept planning for mapping and evaluation*. Thousand Oaks, CA: Sage.

Kaplan, A. (1964). *The conduct of inquiry*. New York, NY: Harper & Row.

King, I. (1981). *A theory of nursing: Systems, concepts, process*. New York, NY: Wiley.

Knowles, M. (1984). *The adult learner: A neglected species* (3rd ed.). Houston, TX: Gulf Publishing.

Kolcaba, K. Y. (1994). A theory of holistic comfort for nursing. *Journal of Advanced Nursing, 19*(6), 1178–1184.

Kolcaba, K. Y. (2003). *Comfort theory and practice: A vision for holistic health care and research*. New York, NY: Springer Publishing.

Lenz, E. R., Pugh, L. C., Milligan, R. A., Gift, A., & Suppe, F. (1997). The middle-range theory of unpleasant symptoms: An update. *Advances of Nursing Science, 19*(3), 14–27.

Levine, D. (2001). In partial defense of softness. *Behavioral and Brain Sciences, 24*, 421–422.

Meleis, A. I. (2012). *Theoretical nursing: Development and progress* (5th ed.). Philadelphia, PA: Wolters Kluwer/Lippincott Williams & Wilkins.

Meleis, A. I., & Trangenstein, P. A. (1994). Facilitating transitions: Re-definition of the nursing mission. *Nursing Outlook, 42*(6), 252–259.

Merton, R. K. (1968). *Social theory and social structure*. New York, NY: US Free Press.

Mills, C. W. (1959). *The sociological imagination*. Oxford, NY: Oxford University Press.

Mishel, M. (1997). Uncertainty in acute illness. *Annual Review of Nursing Research, 15*(1), 57–80.

Nightingale, F. (1860). *Notes of nursing: What it is and what it is not*. New York, NY: D. Appleton.

Orem, D. E. (1985). *Nursing: Concepts of practice* (3rd ed.). New York, NY: McGraw-Hill.

Peterson, S. J., & Bredow, T. S. (2013). *Middle range theories: Application to nursing research* (3rd ed.). Philadelphia, PA: Lippincott Williams & Wilkins.

Rector, T. S., & Cohn, J. N. (1992). Assessment of patient outcome with the Minnesota Living With Heart Failure questionnaire: Reliability and validity during a randomized, double-blind, placebo-controlled trial of pimobendan. *American Heart Journal, 124*(4), 1017–1025.

Roy, C. (1999). *The Roy adaptation model* (2nd ed.). New York, NY: Appleton and Lange.

Smith, M. J., & Liehr, P. R. (2013). *Middle range theory for nursing* (3rd ed.). New York, NY: Springer Publishing.

Sternberg, R. J. (2004). *Cognitive psychology*. Belmont, CA: Wadsworth.

Stevens, B. (1998). *Nursing theory: Analysis, application, and evaluation*. Boston, MA: Little, Brown.

Stevens, K. R. (2013). The impact of evidence-based practice in nursing and the next big ideas. *The Online Journal of Nursing, 18*(2), 1–11. doi:10.3912/OJIN.Vol18No02Man04

Tarski, A. (1995). *Introduction to logic and the methodology of deductive sciences*. New York, NY: Dover.

Thorne, S., Canam, C., Dahinten, S., Hall, W., Henderson, A., & Kirkham, S. R. (1998). Nursing's metaparadigm concepts: Disimpacting the debates. *Journal of Advanced Nursing, 27*(6), 1257–1268.

Trochim, W., & McLinden, D. (2016). Introduction to a special issue on concept mapping. *Evaluation and Program Planning, 60*, 166–175.

Tsai, P. F. (2003). A middle-range theory of caregiver stress. *Nursing Science Quarterly, 16*(2), 137–145.

Walker, L. O., & Avant, K. C. (2005). *Strategies for theory construction in nursing*. Upper Saddle River, NJ: Pearson Prentice Hall.

PART II

Designing and Implementing Evidence-Based Practice Projects

CHAPTER 6

Evidence-Based Practice: Success of Practice Change Depends on the Question

Mary N. Meyer

After reading this chapter, learners should be able to:

1. Express the relationship between well-written clinical questions and the quality of evidence-based interventions
2. Outline the historical development of evidence-based practice (EBP) questions
3. Differentiate between foreground and background clinical questions
4. Develop a clinical question using the PICOT (patient population, intervention, comparison, outcome, time frame) and PICOT-D (PICOT-digital data) formats

EVIDENCE-BASED PRACTICE (EBP) SCENARIOS

Scenario 1

Josh, a registered nurse who works in an orthopedic clinic, knows that continuous passive motion (CPM) therapy is routinely ordered for patients undergoing knee surgery. One of Josh's primary roles in the clinic is preoperative patient education about how to manage mobility restrictions while optimizing long-term joint function. He believed that CPM kept the joint mobile and reduced scar tissue. Recently, Josh learned that some insurance companies have denied payment for CPM for patients undergoing meniscus repair, suggesting CPM was medically unnecessary. Thus, he wondered if evidence might exist to support the practice of recommending CPM therapy for patients undergoing knee surgery. He framed his clinical question as, "Is CPM therapy helpful to patients?"

Josh conducted a Cumulative Index to Nursing and Allied Health Literature (CINAHL) search using the search term "continuous passive motion." The search returned 185 manuscripts. He entered the same search term in PubMed and retrieved 1,643 articles. He did not know how to narrow his search and felt overwhelmed. Before abandoning his inquiry, he contacted the department's clinical nurse leader for assistance.

Scenario 2

Monica, a registered nurse in the adolescent rheumatology clinic, sees over 40 patients a week with juvenile rheumatoid arthritis (JRA). She has noted patients with JRA, as typical of most adolescents, love to lead busy and fulfilled lives to the extent they can. Monitoring and managing patient pain efficiently and effectively is key to helping adolescents with JRA function as well as others in their peer group. Monica noted that many adolescents travel a far distance to the clinic for pain monitoring and management, and she wondered how much time patients could save if pain management was conducted remotely. Monica checked OVID™ for rheumatology pain management and found over 1,500 articles. She remembered that in her BSN (bachelor of science in nursing) program she learned how to construct a PICOT question to effectively manage vast quantities of information. She stated her PICOT question as, "For adolescent patients with JRA, is remote monitoring of arthritic pain as effective as clinic visits for pain management?" Returning to OVID, Monica was able to use the search terms "adolescent" AND "rheumatoid arthritis" AND "pain management." The search produced 12 level one evidence articles that enabled Monica to develop a successful proposal for an EBP project for remote pain monitoring in the JRA clinic. She used a well-built clinical question as an opportunity to make explicit and systematic use of best available evidence.

Discussion

In previous chapters, the importance of using evidence to guide clinical decision making was discussed. This chapter focuses on systematically developing a clinical question so that each component of the question is clear. Clinical questions are the indisputable driving force behind EBP, and without questions EBP would be unnecessary (Davies, 2011). If a question is not stated in a clear, meaningful, and credible way, it is difficult to explore existing knowledge. The mnemonic PICOT is presented, along with several opportunities to explore sample clinical questions that are under development and that are well written. The role of PICOT-D for nurses educated at the DNP (doctor of nursing practice) level is also discussed.

Real-world, clinically focused questions drive EBP. Although it can sometimes be challenging to articulate an answerable question, a well-stated question is the critical first step in retrieving appropriate evidence to guide practice decisions. As described in Scenario 1, when nurses attempt to retrieve applicable literature without first defining important aspects of the question, they may become frustrated and overwhelmed by the amount of data. In a busy clinical setting, nurses do not have time to review hundreds of articles in the process of searching for relevant articles. In fact, time is cited as the number one reason nurses and physicians do not engage in relevant literature searches (Ebell, 1999; Ellsworth et al., 2015; Ely, Osheroff, Chambliss, Ebell, & Rosenbaum, 2005).

This chapter describes how to structure a clinical question to best explore what is known about the topic under investigation. In some cases, a well-stated question will lead a nurse to conclude that a question cannot be answered from the current body of evidence; in that case, the clinical question may serve as a precursor to a needed research question. In fact, in a systematic, retrospective review of published studies, researchers uncovered a correlation between higher-quality research studies and systematically designed research questions (Rios, Ye, & Thabane, 2010).

ORIGINS OF GOOD CLINICAL QUESTIONS

Clinical questions originate from nurses who practice at all nursing degree levels (e.g., ADN, BSN, MSN, DNP). When questions originate at the point of care, there is a higher likelihood that subsequent EBP and/or research initiatives will be relevant to practice. Research closely linked to practice has a high likelihood of benefitting patients. Clinicians often raise important practice-related questions, but they may lack the expertise to develop a question. Similar to the nurse in clinical Scenario 1, when the question fails to guide the exploration of evidence, it becomes unlikely that nurses will be able to use the evidence in practice. Clinical Scenario 2 provides an example of why every clinician needs to be able to properly frame a clinical question.

The methodology used to guide development of clinical questions is known by the mnemonic PICO or PICOT. The letters describe the necessary components of the clinical or research question:

- P: Problem, patient, or population
- I: Intervention, indicator, or independent variable
- C: Comparison
- O: Outcome of interest or dependent variable

In some cases, it is also relevant to explore T: Time frame (Echevarria & Walker, 2014; Elias, Polancich, Jones, & Colvin, 2016). Practice is needed to write answerable PICOT questions. This chapter provides many question examples and opportunities to see how PICOT questions might evolve.

The value of starting an exploration of the evidence with a well-designed clinical PICOT question must not be underestimated. First, a well-stated clinical question provides a nurse with operative search terms to explore literature that considers the important aspects of the healthcare phenomenon. Clearly stating the parameters in the clinical question helps to narrow the literature search so that only relevant studies are included. Unstructured collections of key terms lead to irrelevant literature, which wastes nurses' time and efforts (Davies, 2011).

Following a systematic review of the applicable literature, a nurse can synthesize the literature to determine what is known about the clinical problem and proceed to formulate the next EBP steps.

Before learning how to write a PICOT question, we explore various types of PICOT questions. It is important to understand the types of PICOT questions, because the type of question a nurse is exploring guides the systematic way a question is built. The first step in question development is to determine if a question represents *background* or *foreground* knowledge. The following explores the concepts of both background and foreground clinical questions.

BACKGROUND AND FOREGROUND QUESTIONS

Background Questions

Nurses are sometimes interested in basic information concerning a disease or a healthcare process; therefore, they formulate a background question to arrive at an appropriate answer. A background question explores one or more of the seven Ws: Who, What, for Whom, When, Why, Where, and how Well (Larue, Draus, & Klem, 2009). Specifically, a background question contains a question root with a verb, combined with a diagnosis or other healthcare characteristic (Echevarria & Walker, 2014). The following are examples of background questions: "How often should men over age 65 have a wellness exam?" or "What is the incubation period for mumps?" Background questions are used to gather general knowledge and are often best answered by resources such as textbooks and point-of-care (POC) resources. There are a wide variety of POC resources, such as the Joanna Briggs Institute EBP Database and National Guideline Clearinghouse.

Foreground Questions

General knowledge gained from background questions is indispensable for nurses. Knowing about patients' conditions and appropriate interventions is foundational knowledge that supports nursing practice. As nursing students and nurses accrue background knowledge, their patient-centered clinical expertise begins to necessitate a need to ask more specific and complex questions. Foreground questions enable practitioners to seek answers for more specific and complex questions, and they are formulated to gather specific clinical information relative to a patient or an intervention (Echevarria & Walker, 2014). To find an answer to a foreground question, healthcare databases, such as PubMed, CINAHL, and Cochrane, provide access to current literature. To support the search for best evidence, the PICOT format is used.

HOW TO WRITE A PICOT QUESTION

As mentioned earlier, working through the PICOT acronym provides a complete, yet succinct framework to guide the search for existing evidence. Table 6.1 provides a detailed look at the building blocks needed to construct a PICOT question.

TABLE 6.1 How to Develop Clinical Questions Using PICOT

	Patient, Problem, or Population	Intervention, Indicator, or Independent Variable	Comparison	Outcome or Dependent Variable	Time
Questions to ask yourself	How would I describe a group of patients or a population similar to mine?	What is the main intervention I am considering?	What is the main alternative that I am comparing to the intervention?	What do I hope to accomplish? *or* If my population was exposed to this intervention, what could be expected?	Is there a specific time frame to consider?
Tips for formatting	Balance brevity with precision	Be specific	Be specific	Be specific	Be specific
Example	Newly graduated registered nurses in the United States	First RN employment is in Magnet®-designated hospital	First RN employment is in non-Magnet–designated hospital	Increased job satisfaction	RNs licensed for less than 2 years
Example: Do **newly graduated registered nurses** who have been licensed for less than 2 years report increased job satisfaction when their first job is in a Magnet-designated hospital compared with a non-Magnet hospital?					

PICOT, patient population, intervention, comparison, outcome, time frame.

Types of PICOT Questions

To break down questions into key words, the concept of PICO was initiated and developed by a group of physician colleagues (Richardson, Wilson, Nishikawa, & Hayward, 1995). The PICO acronym enabled physicians and nurses to address these questions:

- **P**—Patient or problem: When identifying the P in PICOT, it is useful to ask the following questions: "Who is the patient?" "What are the most important patient attributes or characteristics?" "What are key demographic and clinical variables (e.g., age, race, ethnicity, gender, current medications, and previous illnesses)?" "What is the primary problem, disease, or coexisting condition?" It is important for nurses to consider if any patient or population characteristics should be considered when conducting the literature search.
- **I**—Intervention: When identifying the intervention, it is important to ask the following questions: "What is the primary intervention being considered?" "What does the nurse plan to do for the patient?" Remember that interventions may be treatments, procedures, tests, medications, or adjunctive therapies.

- **C**—Comparison: When developing the comparison, it is important to ask the following: "What is the primary comparison intervention?" The comparison must be specific and limited to one alternative to simplify the literature search.
- **O**—Outcome: When considering outcome, important questions to consider are as follows: "What measures, improvements, or effects are anticipated?" "What symptoms should be relieved or eliminated?" "What functions will be improved or maintained?"

In considering the questioning behaviors of nurses, Fineout-Overholt and Johnston recommended a five-component arrangement for EBP questions using the acronym PICOT, with the T representing *time frame*. For a clinical question to be directly relevant and able to facilitate searching for a credible answer, the question must be focused and well-articulated for all appropriate components of its anatomy: patient, intervention, comparison, outcome, and time frame.

Clinical or PICOT questions arise from nearly any encounter a practitioner has with patients or populations. Richardson et al. (1995) found that most clinical questions arise from distinct aspects of clinical encounters:

1. **Clinical evidence:** Gathering clinical findings for proper and sound interpretation
2. **Diagnosis:** Selecting and interpreting appropriate tests
3. **Prognosis:** Anticipating a patient's likely course of events
4. **Therapy:** Selecting therapies that are more beneficial than harmful
5. **Prevention:** Screening to reduce risk of disease
6. **Education:** Teaching self, patient, and family what is needed

Based on Richardson and colleagues' suggested grouping of clinical questions within those six categories, five categories are principally used today: *Intervention, Prognosis* or *Prediction, Diagnosis* or *Diagnostic Test, Etiology*, and *Meaning*, as discussed in the following text. Several authors provide templates that clinicians might use to shape the clinical question based on these five categories (Davies, 2011; Dearholt & Dang, 2012; DiCenso, Guyatt, & Ciliska, 2002; Fineout-Overholt & Stillwell, 2015). Table 6.2 reviews the templates for each of the five categories.

Intervention

There are times healthcare workers want to investigate the efficacy of an intervention or compare the effectiveness of two different interventions. For example, "In *postoperative patients* (P), how does *nurse-directed urinary catheter removal* (I) compared to *provider-directed urinary catheter removal* (C) affect *rates of urinary tract infections* (O) *during the first five postoperative days* (T)?"

Prognosis/Prediction

Some questions may be written to explore the course of a problem or disease. A nurse who is interested in predicting a clinical course and perhaps possible complications over time will write a prognosis/prediction question using the PICOT

TABLE 6.2   Types of PICOT Questions

Type of Question	Novice PICOT	Rationale for Rewording	Expert PICOT
Intervention In ____ (P), what is the effect of _____ (I) on _____ (O) compared with _____ (C) within _____ (T)?	Does CPM improve outcomes from total knee replacement?	Similar to Josh's question about CPM after meniscus repair, this clinical question is too vague. The revision is more specific in terms of the intervention and the outcome.	In patients recovering from total knee replacement, does CPM therapy at least 4 hours per day for 4 weeks (I) improve postoperative range of motion (O) at 6 months and 1 year?
Prognosis/prediction Does _____ (I) influence _____ (O) in patients who have _____ (P) over _____ (T)?	If we monitored HgbA1c levels every 3 months, could we decrease the frequency of retinal complications from hyperglycemia in patients with type 2 diabetes mellitus?	Since retinopathy is frequently a result of hyperglycemia over time, specifying the time further improves the quality of the PICOT question. Monitoring the numbers will likely not be an intervention of interest; rather, it is how the information is used.	Do patient coaching phone calls associated with every HgbA1c check (I) influence rates of retinopathy (O) in patients who have type 2 diabetes mellitus (P) for at least 5 years (T)?
Diagnosis/diagnostic test In _____ (P), are/is _____ (I) compared with _____(C) more accurate in diagnosing _____ (O)?	Which test is more accurate for diagnosing type 2 diabetes, serum glucose or HgbA1c?	This clinical question was refined to be more specific by narrowing the results to obese patients.	In obese patients (P), are serum HgbA1cs (I) compared with serum glucose (C) more accurate in diagnosing _____ (O)?
Etiology Are _____ (P) who have _____ (I) at __ (increased/decreased) risk for/of _____ (O) compared with/ without _____ (C) over _____ (T)?	If nurses provided passive range of motion (PROM) at least two times a day (BID) in the intensive care unit (ICU), would deep vein thrombosis (DVT) rates decrease?	Considering the nature of the intervention, the population of interest was further refined, focusing on patients who are not able to ambulate. The nurse is interested in outcomes of care in the ICU, so limiting the scope to include only time in critical care should help target the results.	Are nonambulatory patients (P) who receive PROM at least BID (I) at decreased risk for DVT (O) compared with nonambulatory patients receiving standard care (C) who receive no PROM during their ICU stay (T)?
Meaning (phenomenology) How do ___ (P) with _____ (I) perceive _____ (O) during _____ (T)?	How do people who have been diagnosed with cancer see life differently?	The effects of cancer are quite variable depending on the population and the stage of malignancy. Additionally, what does it mean to "see life differently"? The question was revised to be more specific in all parameters.	How do women (P) who have been diagnosed with stage 1 breast cancer (I) perceive life priorities (O) during the first year after their diagnosis (T)?

CPM, continuous passive motion; PICOT, patient population, intervention, comparison, outcome, time frame.

format. For example, "In *confused patients* (P), how does *physical restraint* (I) compared with *no physical restraint* (C) influence *falls* (O) over the *course of an acute care stay* (T)?"

Diagnosis/Diagnostic Test

To better educate and care for patients, nurses are frequently asked about the comparative accuracy of diagnostic tests. The following is a sample PICO question that guides a diagnostic inquiry: "In *patients with inflammatory bowel disease* (P), is *CT scan of the abdomen* (I) or *endoscopy* (C) more *accurate in diagnosing complications* (O)?"

Etiology

The clinical question may address etiology or cause of a given phenomenon. To better understand causes and/or risk factors for a condition, the nurse may frame a PICOT question to investigate etiology. For example: Are *adolescent boys* (P) *raised in households without fathers* (I) compared with *adolescent boys raised in households with fathers* (C) *more likely to be involved in gun violence* (O)?

Meaning (Phenomenology)

DiCenso, Guyat, and Ciliska (2005) suggested that qualitative questions require two of the PICO components: population and situation (i.e., outcome). In a phenomenological inquiry, the nurse seeks to better understand the significance of an event or incident on a person or group of people. In exploring clinical questions designed to elicit details of an experience, sometimes comparison (C) and time (T) are not appropriate to the question (Echevarria & Walker, 2014). The following is an example of a meaning or phenomenological PICOT question: "How do *spouses of patients with Alzheimer's-type dementia* (P) perceive their own *quality of life* (O)?"

In Scenario 1, Josh's clinical question concerned the use of CPM in postoperative knee surgery patients—that is, *Is CPM therapy helpful to patients?* The clinical nurse leader met with Josh to help him rewrite the question using the PICOT framework. Because Josh was interested in learning if CPM therapy actually helped patients after knee surgery, it seemed appropriate to classify the question as an "Intervention." Table 6.3 demonstrates how the PICOT mnemonic was used to revise the clinical question into a strong foreground PICO question: "In *patients who have undergone knee cartilage repair* (P), how does *CPM for 6 weeks* (I) compared with *no CPM* (C) affect *clinical outcomes* (O)?"

Perseverance is needed to become skilled at writing PICOT questions. Table 6.2 offers a list of sample PICOT questions for each of the five types of questions discussed previously. The first question was written by a novice nurse; the second question was revised by a nurse with experience developing PICOT questions.

TABLE 6.3   Applying the PICOT to a Real-World Scenario

	Patient, Problem, or Population	Intervention, Indicator, or Independent Variable	Comparison	Outcome or Dependent Variable	Time
Questions to ask yourself	How would I describe a group of patients or a population similar to mine?	What is the main intervention that I am considering?	What is the main alternative that I am comparing to the intervention?	What do I hope to accomplish? *or* If my population was exposed to this intervention, what could be expected?	Is there a specific time frame to consider?
Tips for formatting	Balance brevity with precision	Be specific	Be specific	Be specific	Be specific
Example	Patients who have undergone knee cartilage repair	Six weeks of CPM therapy	No CPM	Improved clinical outcomes	A specific timetable was not deemed relevant to the question.
Example: In patients who have undergone knee cartilage repair, how does CPM for 6 weeks, compared with no CPM, affect clinical outcomes?					

CPM, continuous passive motion; PICOT, patient population, intervention, comparison, outcome, time frame.

BENEFITS OF USING THE PICOT FRAMEWORK

Using the PICOT framework can be beneficial to both nurses and patients. To become a skillful PICOT question writer, first the nurse must learn the process. Once equipped with knowledge, a significant amount of practice is required to hone the skill. Investing time and attention to developing the skill of PICOT question writing is beneficial for nurses at all levels of practice as well as for patients.

PICOT Benefits for Nurses

In their work, nurses frequently encounter challenges and questions related to best practices for optimal patient care. Nurses who are able to articulate clinical questions using PICOT format have several advantages. First, prepared with a well-written clinical question, a nurse can more confidently approach the literature search. The nurse understands the scope of inquiry has been appropriately narrowed, and only applicable concepts or variables will be included in the search results. A literature search that targets and identifies only information that is supportive of the clinical question adds to the nurse's efficiency, which is of paramount importance to busy practitioners. PICOT supplies a pathway for nurses to efficiently search a body of evidence and apply the findings to determine if the clinical question can be answered as originally posed.

The systematic process of first writing a PICOT question and then using the question to search the evidence offers a high degree of confidence that the process resulted in a literature search of sufficient breadth and depth. When the search results have been synthesized, the PICOT structure also provides a succinct format for the clinician to share results, ideas, and recommendations with management teams, healthcare leaders, and healthcare providers. It is crucial for nurses to be able to skillfully communicate the findings so that best evidence can be used to guide system change.

To support EBP and to make the search for evidence even more efficient, some academic nurse leaders have proposed an evolution of PICOT to include a plan for how data will be collected, recorded, and analyzed. The process has been identified as PICOT-D. In the same way the PICOT process promotes critical analysis of each aspect of the question, it follows that data may provide answers. In fact, writing PICOT questions to include a data analysis process is particularly well aligned with the scope and goals of the DNP degree. Important components of the PICOT-D are the following: (a) type of data source (e.g., narrative or numeric); (b) form of data (i.e., paper or electronic); (c) location of data (i.e., electronic medical record, system-based records, or paper chart); (d) data steward (i.e., who gives permission for data to be used); and (e) format for extracting data (e.g., Excel spreadsheet) (Elias et al., 2016).

PICOT-D provides nurses the ability to leverage a broader cross section of data to answer clinical questions. For example, a nurse wanted to learn if there was a difference in glucose control between patients who had RN coaching as compared with those with nurse practitioner coaching. If no answer can be found in the literature, PICOT-D would be applicable. In the scenario described, the data might include glucose values downloaded from patients' monitors and HgbA1cs from the electronic health record.

Benefits for Patients

Practicing nurses wish to provide care that makes positive differences in people's lives. Formulating PICOT questions is foundational to EBP. When nurses practice according to the evidence, care is guided by the best research available, and it follows that patients will benefit from use of a scientific approach. Nurses, particularly those at the point of care, must be prepared to write well-designed clinical questions and use the findings to plan and implement care.

This chapter provided many examples of clinical questions that were converted into PICOT questions. Reflecting on the scope of the clinical questions presented as samples in this chapter exemplifies that PICOT can be applied in any nurse–patient interaction to improve patient outcomes. Patients can potentially benefit from direct care nurses being well versed in EBP, and as mentioned earlier, EBP begins with the development of the question. Nurses who are skilled at writing PICOT questions have a positive impact on patient outcomes, such as quality of life, satisfaction, and safety (Black, Balneaves, Garossino, Puyat, & Qian, 2015; Stevens, 2013).

Patients expect nursing care to be consistent and outcome focused. When direct care nurses are able to explore important clinical questions, traditional practices that are not necessarily guided by evidence will be appropriately questioned. When nursing research becomes relevant to nurses at the point of care, evidence will be in the hands of those who have the power to reduce the lag between knowledge discovery and practice integration (Lockwood & Hopp, 2016).

PICOT Benefits for Administrators

The PICOT process supports high-quality patient care and, therefore, aligns with the goals of healthcare administrators. In fact, using the PICOT format to support EBP has the potential to improve efficiency, care quality, and patient and staff satisfaction. PICOT questions identify cost-related variation in healthcare practices (Elias et al., 2016). For example, there may be two therapies available to achieve the same goal. By using the PICOT process, the relative financial value of each therapy can be explored.

PICOT Within the Microsystem of Care

In many healthcare settings, nursing care is provided by teams of nurses who work together regularly to provide care to a defined patient population. These nursing teams are part of a microsystem of care that is usually embedded within a larger macrosystem. Multiple changes concerning healthcare organizations occur at a microsystem level. In fact, the goals of macrosystems are often realized through strategic change initiatives implemented within the microsystem (Institute for Healthcare Improvement, 2017). The microsystem model reinforces the importance of all nurses knowing how to use the PICOT format to frame clinical questions. Nurses working on the front lines of patient care are primarily charged with the responsibility of providing care aligned with current and relevant evidence. The PICOT approach fits appropriately with quality improvement initiatives in contemporary healthcare as described in Chapter 14 (Glascow, Scott-Caziewell, & Kaboli, 2010).

Popular frameworks that guide healthcare quality initiatives include LEAN, Six Sigma, and a combination of the two, referred to as LEAN Six Sigma (Glascow et al., 2010). Using rapid improvement cycles, these approaches focus on workflow processes, error elimination, and outcome measurements with the goal of improving safety outcomes as well as the patient and nurse experience. Involving frontline workers in each step of the process is also a key principle of these quality improvement models. Nurses skilled in PICOT are able to find the best evidence to integrate in ways that are compatible with the quickly evolving quality improvement characteristic of current healthcare environments.

Practitioners are using literature searching skills to locate published evidence. In addition, they are using critical appraisal skills to evaluate the merit and clinical utility of evidence and clinical judgment to determine, along with patients, how best to put evidence into practice. For these essential EBP steps to occur, practitioners must start the fundamental skill for EBP: asking well-designed clinical questions (Richardson et al., 1995). Asking a well-formulated question is a starting point for conducting a quality research project, and for evidence-based clinical practice.

SUMMARY

In the first clinical scenario, the nurse learned that his research question could not be answered by the existing literature. In fact, the existing protocol for ordering CPM on postoperative knee cartilage surgery patients could not be validated as evidence based. More well-designed research was needed, but that would take time. Josh presented his findings to the nursing team. One of the nursing leaders, who had obtained a DNP degree, was familiar with the PICOT-D process. The DNP-educated nurse will be defining a data collection and analysis process to include the amount of time the patient uses the CMP and the joint range of motion measured at each postoperative appointment.

In the meantime, how will the clinic nurse proceed? There was insufficient evidence to support the use of CPM in patients undergoing knee cartilage repair. Should the team consider a change in the protocol based on the lack of evidence? Josh knew that changing practice could be challenging. Even if the interprofessional team wished to adjust the protocol, Josh was not sure of the best way to implement a sustained practice change. The next chapter provides an exploration of change theories to guide the transition of knowledge into practice.

REFERENCES

Black, A. T., Balneaves, L. G., Garossino, C., Puyat, J. H., & Qian, H. (2015). Promoting evidence-based practice through a research training program for point of care clinicians. *Journal of Nursing Administration, 45*(1), 14–20.

Davies, K. S. (2011). Formulating the evidence-based practice question: A review of the frameworks. *Evidence-Based Library and Information Practice, 6*(2), 75–80.

Dearholt, S., & Dang, D. (2012). *Johns Hopkins Nursing Evidence-Based Practice Model and Guidelines.* Indianapolis, IN: Sigma Theta Tau International.

DiCenso, A., Guyatt, G., & Ciliska, D. (2002). *Evidence-based nursing: A guide to clinical practice.* St. Louis, MO: Mosby.

Ebell, M. (1999). Information at the point of care: Answering clinical questions. *Journal of the American Board of Family Practice, 12,* 225–335.

Echevarria, I., & Walker, S. (2014). To make your case, start with a PICOT question. *Nursing 2014, 19,* 18–19.

Elias, B. L., Polancich, S., Jones, C., & Convoy, S. (2016). Evolving the PICOT method for the digital age: The PICOT-D. *Journal of Nursing Education, 54,* 594–599. doi: 10.3928/01484834-20150916-09

Ellsworth, M. A., Homan, J. M., Cimino, J. J., Peters, S. G. Pickering, B. W., & Herasevich, A. (2015). Point-of-care knowledge-based resource needs of clinicians: A survey from a large academic medical center. *Applied Clinical Informatics, 6*(2), 305–317. doi:10.4338/ACI-2014-11-RA-0104

Ely, J. W., Osheroff, J. A., Chambliss, M. L., Ebell, M. H., & Rosenbaum, M. E. (2005). Answering physicians' clinical questions: Obstacles and potential solutions. *Journal of the American Medical Informatics Association, 12*(2), 217–224.

Fineout-Overholt, E., & Johnson, L. (2005). Teaching EBP: Asking searchable, answerable clinical questions. *Worldviews on Evidence-Based Nursing, 2*(3). 157–160. doi:10.1111/j.1741-6787.2005.00032.x

Fineout-Overholt, E., & Stillwell, S. B. (2015). Asking compelling clinical questions. In B. M. Melnyk & E. Fineout-Overholt (Eds.), *Evidence-based practice in nursing: A guide to best practice* (pp. 24–39). Philadelphia, PA: Wolters Kluwer.

Glascow, J., Scott-Caziewell, J., & Kaboli, P. (2010). Guiding inpatient quality improvement: A systematic review of LEAN and Six Sigma. *The Joint Commission Journal on Quality and Patient Safety, 36*, 533–539.

Institute for Healthcare Improvement. (2017). Clinical microsystem assessment tool. Retrieved from http://www.ihi.org/resources/Pages/Tools/ClinicalMicrosystemAssessmentTool.aspx

Larue, E., Draus, P., & Klem, M. L. (2009). A description of a web-based educational tool for understanding the PICO framework in evidence-based practice with a citation ranking system. *CIN: Computers, Informatics, Nursing, 27*, 44–49.

Lockwood, C., & Hopp, L. (2016). Knowledge translation: What it is and the relevance to evidence-based healthcare and nursing. *International Journal of Nursing Practice, 22*(4), 319–321.

Richardson, W. S., Wilson, M. C., Nishikawa, J., & Hayward, S. A. (1995). The well-built clinical question: A key to evidence-based decisions. *American College of Physicians Journal Club, 123*(3), A12.

Rios, L., Ye, C., & Thabane, L. (2010). Association between framing of the research question using the PICOT format and reporting quality of randomized controlled trials. *BMC Medical Research Methodology, 10*. Retrieved from http://bmcmedresmethodol.biomedcentral.com/articles/10.1186/1471-2288-10-11

Stevens, K. R. (2013). The impact of evidence-based practice in nursing and the next big ideas. *The Online Journal of Nursing, 18*(2), 1–11. doi:10.3912/OJIN.Vol18No02Man04

CHAPTER 7

Change Theories: The Key to Knowledge Translation

Lydia D. Rotondo

Objectives

After reading this chapter, learners should be able to:

1. Identify five reasons nurses resist change
2. Explain why the majority of organizational change efforts fail
3. Discuss theoretical approaches to implement planned change
4. Describe the importance of change leadership in planned change initiatives

EVIDENCE-BASED PRACTICE (EBP) SCENARIOS

Scenario 1

At a unit leadership meeting, the unit educator raised the opportunity to develop an interprofessional education (IPE) initiative to maintain pediatric resuscitation skills. For several months, the unit educator worked with nursing and physician leaders, direct care nurses, attending physicians, and residents to develop regularly scheduled simulated pediatric resuscitation sessions. With full endorsement by all stakeholders, the unit educator developed several evidence-based simulation scenarios and created an educational training schedule that best accommodated both unit and participant needs. For five consecutive months, the unit offered well-attended resuscitation simulation sessions that received positive staff reviews. Participants felt the scenario fidelity and subsequent debriefing enhanced their knowledge and skills. Postsimulation evaluations showed improving resuscitation team performance and communication. After the first few simulation sessions, an issue arose when resident rounds started conflicting with the IPE simulation schedule. The resident round change often necessitated nurses coming into work on their days off for rescheduled simulation sessions. In addition to scheduling challenges, financial responsibility for resuscitation teaching supplies became a source of dispute between nursing and medical leadership. The final setback occurred 6 months after program implementation when the nurse educator left the organization.

Within 1 year, the simulation educational sessions ceased. Even though the initiative demonstrated feasibility and positive outcomes, sustainability for the IPE program failed.

Scenario 2

An emergency department (ED) nurse approached the ED leadership team with a proposal about how to promote EBP among the nursing staff. Having spent several years as a direct care nurse, charge nurse, preceptor, and most recently having completed a DNP (doctor of nursing practice) degree, the nurse was acquainted with the unpredictability and frenetic pace of a trauma center. Working with the ED clinical nurse specialist, associate director of nursing, and ED medical director, the DNP nurse proposed development of a practice innovation committee (PIC). The proposal specifically targeted direct care nurses who would meet regularly to design and implement EBP initiatives in the ED under the mentorship of the DNP nurse. The DNP nurse explained that the creation of this work group could facilitate the achievement of several important aims. First, as a Magnet®-designated institution committed to high-quality, evidence-based nursing care, PIC provides an infrastructure to support adoption of evidence-based approaches to nursing practice. In the proposal, the DNP nurse aligned the hospital's nursing department professional practice model with Magnet core principles to create an organizing framework for the committee that integrated with the mission, vision, and values of the healthcare organization.

Second, the PIC provides a means for promoting professional development. With a robust clinical ladder system, nurses could include their EBP projects as part of a professional portfolio needed for clinical advancement. Third, enrollment in the PIC would be open to all nursing staff, including new graduates, licensed practical nurses (LPNs), and registered nurses (RNs) with a range of clinical experience, thereby helping ensure opportunities for full nurse participation.

With endorsement from department leadership, the first committee meeting began with over 40 ED nurses attending. During the first year, direct care nurses implemented six EBP initiatives, and five nurses advanced in the clinical advancement system. The group continued to meet monthly, averaging 15 nurses in attendance each time. The organization's annual practice showcase featured the work of the PIC during National Nurses' Week, and the DNP leader presented the PIC initiative at a national nursing conference.

In the second year, PIC nurses made modifications to the project selection process and committee activities to adapt to changing unit conditions, including the hiring of a large number of graduate nurses. Support for the PIC expanded with the addition of EBP mentors. The mentors are nurses who completed PIC projects and are supporting current unit EBP initiatives. In addition, the nursing department's quality improvement coordinator regularly attends PIC meetings, and EBP project updates are part of the standing agenda for the interdisciplinary unit leadership meetings.

Discussion

Both scenarios describe important change initiatives that have the potential to improve quality and outcomes of patient-centered care. Scenario 1, despite some early success, failed to achieve sustainability. In Scenario 2, adaptive efforts facilitated adoption of new practice initiatives. Both scenarios depict key considerations for EBP initiatives and serve as models throughout the chapter to illustrate principles and consequences of change management.

APPLICATION OF CHANGE MANAGEMENT PRINCIPLES TO EBP

Paradoxically, the one *constant* that has characterized 21st-century U.S. healthcare is *change*. Whether a shift to value-based payment for healthcare services, emergence of population health approaches for chronic condition management, or creation of new practice models to build capacity and increase access to care, change flourishes. Although change can be unpredictable and unsettling, it also provides exciting opportunities for growth and progress (Mitchell, 2013). Successful organizational change is essential for sustaining EBP (Fineout-Overholt, Williamson, Kent, & Hutchinson, 2010).

Organizational change can be emergent or planned. *Emergent change* results as an adaptation to continually changing environmental conditions. Emergent change is often open ended, directed at multiple aims, and occurs as organizational participants respond to needs and opportunities that arise (Burnes, 2005). *Planned change*, on the other hand, begins with an explicit aim and involves intentional actions taken over time. Planned change is participative and directed at disrupting organizational stability to achieve a desired goal (Van der Voet, Groeneveld, & Kuipers, 2014).

Successful implementation of EBP requires a systematic approach to change management that is responsive to the multiple influences in highly complex healthcare systems. Such efforts rely on methodical appraisal of practice environments as well as design and implementation of well-planned, context-sensitive, sustainable change initiatives that have the potential to influence professional nursing practice and positive patient-centered care outcomes.

BARRIERS TO CHANGE: UNDERSTANDING CHANGE RESISTANCE

Resistance to change is complex, multidimensional, and cited as the most common reason for organizational change failure (Erwin & Garman, 2010). Change resistance occurs at individual, group, and organizational levels. At the individual level, nurses may express cognitive, affective, and behavioral dimensions of change disparately (Erwin & Garman, 2010). For example, nurses may have a positive cognitive response to EBP, knowing change will improve patient care, yet feel apprehensive about their abilities to implement EBP, which may lead to resistant behavior. In addition, psychological and personality variables, such as self-concept, resilience, risk tolerance, and flexibility, influence nurse openness or resistance to change (Erwin & Garman, 2010). Given the challenges of translating scientific findings for clinical practice, Eccles, Grimshaw, Walker, Johnston, and Pitts (2005) urge the development of theoretical frameworks to understand the characteristics of nurse clinician behavior related to the adoption of EBP. Theoretical insights offer the potential of reducing change resistance and optimizing integration of best evidence into patient-centered care.

Resistance at group and organizational levels arises from dynamic interrelationships between individuals, group norms, organizational culture (e.g., history, traditions, and values), organizational structure, and leadership (Canning & Found, 2015). Evaluating an organization's level of change readiness is an important consideration in mitigating change resistance. Weiner (2009) describes organizational readiness as the collective state of preparedness attributed to organizational participants' willingness to act (change commitment) and confidence in their ability to implement change (change efficacy) in three key areas: (a) task demands, (b) resource availability, and (c) situational factors. Smith and Donze (2010) emphasize the importance of assessing environmental readiness for successful implementation of EBP. For example, nurses who feel unprepared, as manifested by lack of requisite knowledge and skills to learn the change behavior, may be more likely to resist needed change. Similarly, a scarceness of organizational resources to support EBP and the absence of EPB culture and infrastructure might increase resistance to change and weaken the adoption of EBP (Smith & Donze, 2010).

Resistance to change also can arise from change initiatives. For instance, a poorly designed plan that is incompatible with existing workflow processes may meet resistance. Under these conditions, resistance is not a barrier to overcome but rather an opportunity to reconsider and refine the change plan (Erwin & Garman, 2010). Thoughtful a priori consideration is given as to whether an intended evidence-based initiative has been effectively adapted to a specific practice setting. Understanding the critical interrelationship between change initiative and change context is a major theme in the change theories presented later in the chapter.

WHY NURSES RESIST CHANGE

Potential Threat of Change Outcome(s)

When confronted with a new practice, a nurse may respond to the situation based on perceived benefit(s) and potential threat(s) of the proposed change (Erwin & Garman, 2010). Perceived threats, such as loss of power/expert status, loss of control, or change of habit, increase change resistance (Kanter, 2012; Oreg, 2003). In Scenario 1, the interference of the IPE sessions with residents' new rounding schedule and failure to resolve conflict based on inflexible, entrenched attitudes were potential threats and ultimately endangered project viability.

Concern Over Personal Ability to Accomplish Change

Nurses may believe that they have insufficient knowledge or skill to implement a proposed practice change (Kanter, 2012). In 2015, Black, Balneaves, Garossino,

Puyat, and Qian implemented a research training program for over 150 clinicians who identified unfamiliarity with the research process and inability to critically appraise research evidence as barriers to adopting EBP. Similarly, Melnyk and Fineout-Overholt's (2012) descriptive study of 1,015 nurses found that 76% of respondents reported that they needed additional knowledge and skills to implement EBP. Vanhook (2009) noted that nurses might believe that they do not have the autonomy to initiate EBP based on organizational norms. In addition, lack of infrastructure, such as EBP education programs, contributes to change resistance.

Inadequate Organizational Capacity for Change

Given the multiple stressors and demands that characterize clinical practice environments, nurses may feel too burdened to consider a new EBP approach, even if evidence-based change is potentially beneficial to patients (Kanter, 2012). McMillan and Perron (2013) describe *change fatigue* as an emerging phenomenon in which a constant state of change, characteristic of current healthcare environments, contributes to nurses feeling exhausted and overwhelmed. In addition, the practice setting may be troubled with workflow inefficiencies or lack adequate resources to implement change. In Scenario 1, reliance on nurses to attend the IPE sessions on days off was unsustainable. In addition, the inability of department leaders to consider possible financial solutions to work through managing expenses associated with monthly IPE sessions increased resistance and ultimately undermined project sustainability.

Show Versus Tell Factor (Role Modeling)

Role modeling, in part, involves developing self-awareness of behavior through a process of self-reflection (Karp & Helgø, 2008). Practice colleagues who use EBP offer invaluable observational learning opportunities that exemplify desired practice behavior and reinforce positive change messages (Kotter, 1995). In Melnyk and Fineout-Overholt's (2012) survey of more than 1,000 nurses, only 34.5% of survey respondents' colleagues implemented evidence-based nursing care. Consequently, the limited number of EBP role models slows the diffusion of EBP as well as the opportunity to change resistant organizational behavior. In addition, the lack of demonstrated leadership commitment and understanding to assume responsibility for change and resolve unanticipated consequences, as seen in Scenario 1, may be perceived by nurses as ambivalence to change efforts, which diminishes nurses' commitment and intensifies change resistance (Erwin & Garman, 2010).

The Element of Surprise

It is important to plant seeds of organizational change early and cultivate the seeds with ongoing, clear communication and consensus building (Kanter, 2012). Insufficient knowledge about the impact of EBP change on a nurse's professional practice increases change resistance (Lewis, 2006). Importantly, nurses tend to dislike change imposed on them but instead are inclined to respond positively to preparation for change and the opportunity to offer input (Levasseur, 2010).

WHY ORGANIZATIONAL CHANGE EFFORTS FAIL

Although not empirically validated, it is widely reported that over two-thirds of all change initiatives fail (Burnes, 2011). Kotter (1995), a leading management and organizational change expert and author of the eight-step change model (Table 7.1), identifies the following reasons for organizational change failure.

Failure to Establish a Strong Sense of Urgency Around the Change Initiative

Early in the change process, it is critical to make a convincing case for change. External pressure by regulatory agencies, constraints placed by accrediting bodies, or pressure to comply with professional practice standards can strengthen participant resolve to take action (Smith & Donze, 2010). In Scenario 1, although there was agreement that IPE would be valuable, participants were unable to maintain a sense of urgency once problems arose following implementation. Lack of consistent communication and actions reinforcing the importance of the initiative from department leaders may have undermined interprofessional team readiness for change (Smith & Donze, 2010). It is possible that the original sense of urgency abated because of early success. Although there was demonstrated improvement in team performance early on, connecting the program efforts with improved team performance under real-life conditions could have demonstrated the benefit of the IPE and reinforced the change message.

Failure to Establish a Leadership Coalition to Guide the Change Initiative

Building consensus around the change initiative with leaders and stakeholders is critically important. Establishing an implementation team that includes practice

TABLE 7.1   Kotter's Eight-Step Change Process

Step 1	**CREATE** a sense of urgency around the change opportunity
Step 2	**BUILD** and maintain a guiding coalition for the change effort
Step 3	**FORM** a strategic vision and initiatives to achieve change
Step 4	**ENLIST** engaged stakeholders to support change
Step 5	**ENABLE** change efforts by removing barriers
Step 6	**GENERATE** short-term wins by tracking progress toward achieving change goals
Step 7	**SUSTAIN** success through reinforcement/ modification of change behavior
Step 8	**INSTITUTIONALIZE** change by anchoring in organizational culture

Source: Adapted from Kotter (2014).

and organizational leadership as well as representation from key stakeholders is essential. It is imperative that a change leader actively expand the base of support for the EBP initiative. In Scenario 1, there was early enthusiasm for the IPE project, but the failure to broaden the change coalition contributed to waning interest. In addition, the change agent loss (i.e., unit educator) 6 months after the project launch contributed to abatement of momentum and compromised the unit's ability to address emerging obstacles. Change leadership, an essential part of change initiative, is discussed in a later section of the chapter.

Failure to Connect Change Initiative With Strategic Vision

It is important for nurses to perceive an EBP initiative as part of a larger organizational strategy. Overt organizational commitment to EBP implementation emphasizes organizational recognition that EBP reduces clinical variation in care and focuses on optimal health outcomes. At the organizational level, a hospital's quality and safety agenda or achieving Magnet hospital status are examples of strategic endeavors that support EBP change initiatives (Krugman, 2010). The early appeal of the IPE simulation initiative in Scenario 1 linked the practice change to strategic organizational priorities of high-quality patient-centered care, but the IPE was not integrated into ongoing quality monitoring metrics to monitor and reinforce the importance and benefit of the new practice.

Failure to Communicate the Change Vision

A vital aspect of change management is dissemination of change messages to galvanize support for a change initiative (McClellan, 2014). Active engagement of stakeholders is critical for change success and involves listening to concerns, reiterating the importance of change, and describing how nurses are essential to change efforts (Levasseur, 2010). McClellan (2014) emphasized that effective change communication acknowledges conflicting views and promotes an open conversation among stakeholders to address doubt and support change implementation. Fineout-Overholt et al. (2010) similarly emphasize the importance of active nurse engagement in creating an organizational culture for EBP. In fact, Lewis (2006) reports higher perceptions of information quality about a proposed change lower the resistance to change initiatives. Ongoing communication should emphasize change goals and use carefully constructed verbal and nonverbal messages to build and sustain momentum for change. In Scenario 1, the loss of the change champion and lack of unified leadership to reinforce the importance of the IPE initiative weakened communication and commitment among stakeholders. The waning interest in change led to limited effort for exploring possible resolutions to scheduling conflicts, such as changing program frequency, which might have reinforced program sustainability.

Failure to Remove Obstacles to Proposed Change

Communicating and reinforcing a change vision are necessary but not sufficient to implement and sustain change. Ongoing identification and management of potential barriers that undermine change efforts are crucial. Obstacles to change occur at individual, group, or organizational levels. Development of a systematic approach that mobilizes a broad base of supporters to work through implementation challenges is critical throughout the change process and beyond, as new practices become established within the organizational culture. In Scenario 1, scheduling and financial barriers became seemingly unsurmountable obstacles, contributing to discontinuation of the IPE sessions.

Failure to Create Short-Term Goals to Sustain Change Momentum

A central concept in planned change efforts is the recognition that *change is a process, not an event* (Shirey, 2013). Kotter (1995) noted that a general lesson to be learned from successful change cases is that the change process is a series of phases that, in totality, typically require a considerable length of time. Identifying incremental gains may reinforce the change vision as well as provide important, ongoing feedback about change efforts. For example, setting goals around process measures related to implementation, such as behavioral compliance with new practice guidelines, helps to maintain momentum toward achieving long-term, patient-centered or system outcomes related to EBP. In Scenario 1, the short-term wins achieved improved team performance and communication following the simulation sessions; however, there was no program evaluation of IPE impact on team performance in clinical practice. Program evaluation efforts may have provided additional gains to demonstrate the value of IPE activity and augment sustainability.

Claiming Success Prematurely

Sustainable organizational change is a deliberate, iterative, and multistage process that requires time, persistence, modification, and reinforcement (Kotter, 1995). As stated previously, over two-thirds of all change initiatives fail. Change failure, in part, may be a result of false confidence leading to complacency that sometimes accompanies initial success. With false confidence, enthusiasm for change wanes, previous habits reemerge, preexisting or new obstacles interfere with change adoption, and the permanent organizational structures and processes needed to sustain change do not materialize. Lewin (1951) refers to the *shot in the arm* that accompanies initial change efforts but asserts that achieving *permanency* of change behavior is an ultimate goal. While identified timelines for EBP initiatives are often constructed over weeks or months, the reality is that sustainable change and the creation of an EBP paradigm that is internalized and integrated into standard practice may take years and requires ongoing attention and monitoring (Kotter, 1995). In Scenario 1, there was evidence of early success based on participant feedback and team performance measures, but without ongoing reinforcement and attention to potential program modification to address emerging implementation issues, such as change in resident availability, IPE sustainability was unachievable.

Failure to Integrate Change Into Organizational Culture

Individual and group behavior centers on beliefs, norms, and shared values. For a change initiative to be successfully adopted, the practice must be valued by the group and conform to cultural norms. Kotter (1995) identifies two key elements to promote change adoption. First, change initiative requires assimilation into the practice setting over an extended period. Second, sustained commitment from leadership is critical to minimize the return to former work habits and loss of hard-fought gains throughout the implementation process. Krugman (2010) emphasizes that multiple surveys have confirmed that there is an ongoing lack of long-term administrative support and dedicated resources to support evidence-based nursing practice. Similarly, Smith and Donze (2010) describe the importance of evaluating the environment in three key areas to implement EBP: (a) organizational culture, (b) organizational infrastructure, and (c) organizational resources. In Scenario 1, support for the IPE initiative was rooted in an organizational culture that values high-performing teams, but hierarchical decision making, related to resident scheduling practices, threatened IPE viability. In addition, unit leaders were unable or unwilling to amend organizational processes and find workable alternatives to sustain the new practice.

THEORETICAL APPROACHES TO GUIDE PLANNED CHANGE INITIATIVES

Using change theory to guide systematic implementation of EBP helps bridge the research–practice gap by providing a guiding framework to implement and achieve sustained change (Grol, Bosch, Hulscher, Eccles, & Wensing, 2007). Rossi, Freeman, and Lipsey (1999) divided health change theories into *impact* or *process* categories. *Impact theories* describe assumptions and hypotheses about how specific interventions determine the level of intervention success in improving healthcare. Mechanisms of change in impact theories arise from multiple perspectives and include individual, social, organizational, political, and economic influences. *Process theories* describe specific activities in planning and implementing change and how the target group will use and be influenced by the specific activities. Burnes (2014) stresses that the wide range of available change theories offer a rich opportunity to use several frameworks, either concurrently or sequentially, to guide change efforts. Presented in the following sections are several widely used change theories for consideration to guide EBP change initiatives in nursing.

LEWIN'S THEORY OF PLANNED CHANGE (TPC)

Kurt Lewin was a social scientist whose work focused on social conflict resolution (Burnes, 2004). A pioneer in change management, Lewin introduced the term *planned change* in the 1940s to describe an integrated approach of four interrelated elements of change: *field theory* and *group dynamics* that focus on analyzing group behavior, and the *Three-Step Model of Change* and *action research* that address strategies to change group behavior (Burnes, 2004).

Field Theory, Force Field Analysis (FFA), and Group Dynamics

According to Lewin, social behavior is in a constant state of adaptation. Lewin viewed social behavior as maintained in *quasi-stationary equilibrium* by opposing forces (Lewin, 1951). Lewin developed field theory as a means to explain social behavior within a specific context, and he depicted the nature and strength of opposing forces through *force field analysis* (FFA) (Lewin, 1951). *Driving forces* disrupt the status quo or quasi-stationary equilibrium, and *restraining forces* maintain the current state and/or oppose driving forces (Lewin, 1951). According to Lewin, change occurs because of the introduction of a new force, or a change in the direction and/or strength of existing forces, which destabilize the status quo and create disequilibrium. When nurses plan a practice change, creating a vector map that depicts competing forces within a clinical setting through FFA will help facilitate identification of change strategies that augment driving (helpful) forces and diminish restraining (hindering) forces of change (Lewin, 1951) (Figure 7.1). Clinical change efforts should target group decision making, because nurses are strongly influenced by group norms and socialization processes (Batras, Duff, & Smith, 2014) as outlined in Lewin's work on the principles of group dynamics.

Three-Step Change Model and Action Research

Lewin offers a three-stage model to facilitate planned change efforts (Burnes, 2004).

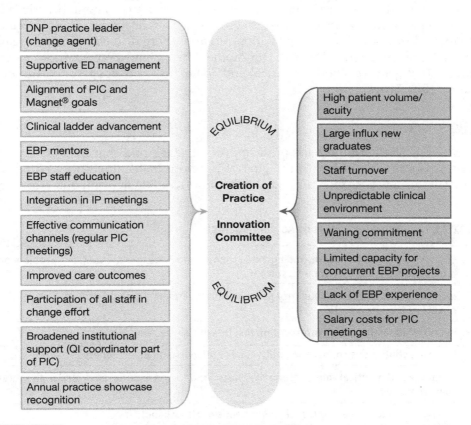

FIGURE 7.1   Force field analysis using Lewin's TPC for implementation of a PIC change initiative

EBP, evidence-based practice; ED, emergency department; PIC, practice innovation committee; QI, quality improvement; TPC, Theory of Planned Change.
Source: From Lewin (1951).

Stage 1: Unfreezing

The unfreezing stage prepares an organization for change. In the unfreezing stage, Lewin theorizes behavior is stabilized (frozen) by the balance of opposing forces. The status quo is destabilized (unfrozen) so new behaviors can be introduced. In the unfreezing stage, it is important to create motivation for change by identifying a change agent(s). The identified change agent must clearly articulate a rationale for change, create a sense of urgency about a proposed change, and build a coalition of support for change initiatives (Shirey, 2013). The change agent helps challenge existing beliefs, values, attitudes, and behaviors that define the current status quo. In addition, Burnes (2004) points out a need for creating psychological safety surrounding change to foster organizational participant openness to new information about the impending change.

Step 2: Moving

During the moving stage, there is maximization of *driving forces* that enhance positive change, and there is minimization of *restraining forces* that create barriers to change. The planned change is trialed and evaluated. Lewin describes the moving stage as an iterative process that requires modification and reinforcement as detailed in his writings about action research (Bargal, 2008). Action research is situational problem solving that combines theory and practice in systematic inquiry that generates both empirical and contextual knowledge to create social change (Box 7.1).

Stage 3: Refreezing

During the final, and perhaps most important, stage of a change process, equilibrium is reestablished with the goal of promoting sustainability and permanency of the new behavior. Change will be short-lived if environmental forces are

BOX 7.1   Lewin's Principles of Action Research
1. **Employs systematic study (including experimental and nonexperimental) of a problem or opportunity as well as efforts to solve it**
2. **Includes data collection to identify goals, action to implement goals, and evaluation of the results of the intervention**
3. **Requires dissemination of intervention results with all stakeholders**
4. **Relies on continuous cooperation between researchers and practitioners**
5. **Emphasizes the critical role of group dynamics for decision making; anchored in the three change phases**
6. **Considers values, objectives, and power needs of all stakeholders**
7. **Generates scientific knowledge (quantitative) and actionable (contextual) knowledge**
8. **Emphasizes the recruitment, training, and support of change agents**

Source: Adapted from Bargal (2008).

insufficiently stabilized. Efforts to reinforce driving (helping) forces to maintain the change behavior and mitigate restraining (hindering) forces that undermine adoption are essential and ongoing. In the refreezing phase, change behavior is standardized and integrated into organizational culture, group norms, policy, and practice (Lewin, 1951).

Lippitt's Phases of Change Theory

Lippitt, Watson, and Westley (1958) expand Lewin's TPC and propose a seven-phase process to implement planned change. This process emphasizes the critical role of an objective (outside) change agent to facilitate change processes. Lippitt offers a dynamic systems approach to change that can occur on four levels: (a) individual, (b) face-to-face group, (c) organization, and (d) community, generally referred to as a *client system*. The Phases of Change Theory stresses communication, relationship building, and collaborative problem solving (Lippitt et al., 1958). Similar to Lewin, Lippitt describes the dynamic interplay of environmental forces and client system that influence change processes. *Change forces* encourage the client system to accept change, and *resistance forces* discourage the client system from accepting change. Recognizing that dynamic systems are constantly adapting, adjusting, and reorganizing, the change agent can facilitate the rate and direction of change by strengthening change forces that alter system structure and processes in a positive way and weakening resistance forces that oppose change (Lippitt et al., 1958). Enhancement of change stability occurs as change diffuses to other segments of the client system (Kritsonis, 2005; Lippitt et al., 1958).

Phase 1—Develop the Need for Change; Phase 2—Establish the Change Relationship

These early phases correspond to Lewin's "unfreezing" phase. The change agent focuses on problem awareness and assessment of the client system's motivation, capacity, and readiness for change. An evaluation of change and resistance forces is also completed. The quality of a client system/change agent relationship established during these phases is critical to the ultimate success of the change initiative (Lippitt et al., 1958).

Phases 3, 4, and 5—Work Toward Change

These three phases correspond to Lewin's "moving" stage. During Phase 3, the change agent helps explicate the problem. Once problem identification occurs, potential solutions are deliberated, and change goals become established in Phase 4. Phase 5 initiates the proposed change implementation with or without direct oversight of the change agent. The active work of changing is the underpinning of the change process (Lippitt et al., 1958).

Phase 6—Establish Generalization and Stabilization of Change; Phase 7—Achieve a Terminal Relationship

Phase 6 is perhaps the most critical phase, because success will be measured by improved performance and sustainability of the practice change. The change agent helps the client system to evaluate change outcomes, stabilize the change, and mitigate change resistance (Lippitt et al., 1958). Adoption and internalization of the new practice lead to Phase 7. Depending on the nature of the change agent/ client system relationship, Lippitt et al. (1958) contend that Phase 7 may begin as early as Phase 3. During Phase 7, the change agent helps the client system identify areas of additional support for change sustainability.

Rogers's Diffusion of Innovations Theory

In addition, building on Lewin's work, Rogers published the Diffusion of Innovations (DOI) Model in 1962 for furthering an understanding of the process of how a group adopts a new idea, practice, or innovation (Rogers, 2003; Roussel, 2013). Diffusion is a process by which an *innovation is communicated* over *time* and among members of a *social system* (Rogers, 2003). The four elements of diffusion theory are as follows:

1. Innovation: An idea, practice, or object that is perceived as new
2. Communication: The transfer of information among units (e.g., people and organizations)
3. Time: The passage of time necessary for an innovation to be adopted
4. Social system: A combination of internal (e.g., social relationships) and external (organizational mandates) influences that impact a potential adopter

Each of the four elements exists in every diffusion initiative and is integral to the decision-making process to adopt an innovation (Rogers, 2003).

According to Rogers, diffusion occurs through a five-stage decision-making process. The first stage is the *knowledge stage* in which the individual or "decision-making unit" learns about the proposed innovation, including what it is, how it works, and why it is important to practice (Rogers, 2003). Group characteristics, such as individual personalities and communication patterns, influence a group's openness to the proposition of new ideas or practices (Rogers, 2003).

The *persuasion stage* follows Stage 1 and is affect oriented with the processing of subjective influences, such as opinions from supervisors and colleagues. Perceived characteristics of the innovation occur during the persuasion stage, including relative advantage, compatibility, complexity, trialability, and observability (Table 7.2). According to Rogers (2003), the five perceived characteristics are the most important determinants of the rate of innovation adoption with relative advantage and compatibility being key.

During the *decision* stage, the individual/group determines whether to accept an innovation. Rogers (2003) classifies individuals into five classic adopter categories based on the rate of adoption over time (Figure 7.2). The earliest adopters are *innovators* who introduce the new practice to the group. Innovators are comfortable with uncertainty and willing to try new endeavors. Rogers (2003) describes innovators as the gatekeepers of new ideas flowing into a system. The next subgroup, *early adopters*, includes opinion leaders whom others turn to for information about the innovation. Early adopters receive respect within a social system and serve as change role models. Early adopter behavior positively influences others' attitudes, which helps reduce uncertainty and facilitate innovation adoption among

TABLE 7.2   Perceived Attributes of Innovations

Relative Advantage	Is the proposed innovation perceived by the organization's participants to be better than the current standard of organizational practice?
Compatibility	To what degree will the proposed innovation be perceived as consistent with the values and lived experiences of the organization's participants?
Complexity	How easy or difficult will the proposed innovation be for the organization's participants to implement?
Trialability	How easy will it be for the organization's participants to pilot and make needed modifications to the proposed innovation?
Observability	How easy will it be for the organization's participants to appreciate the potential outcomes of the proposed innovation?

Source: Adapted from Rogers (2003).

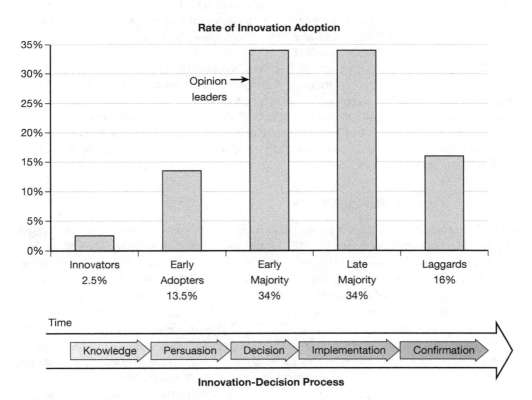

FIGURE 7.2   Rate of innovation adoption during innovation-decision process

Source: Adapted from Rogers (2003).

organizational participants (Rogers, 2003). The *early majority* and *late majority* subgroups represent roughly two-thirds of potential adopters. Early majority adopters are more deliberate in their decision making and require evidence and time to accept the innovation. Because of their proximity to later adopters, they have an important role in promoting diffusion to the remaining groups who have not adopted the innovation (Rogers, 2003). The late majority are skeptical. Members in the late majority will often decide to adopt the innovation because of organizational policy or peer pressure. Finally, *laggards* are the traditionalists who adhere to the status quo. Laggards remain reluctant to adopt innovation until they are convinced of the positive results and benefits for themselves (Rogers, 2003).

In the *implementation phase*, introduction of an innovation into practice occurs. Change agents energize support for the innovation effort and quell concern and uncertainty (Batras et al., 2014). During the implementation phase, Rogers (2003) describes the concept of *reinvention*, which refers to the degree to which an innovation changes during the adoption process. Reinvention is critical for the implementation of evidence-based initiatives, where successful adoption of new practices centers on contextual compatibility. Rogers (2003) asserts that innovation reinvention or modification by the users helps to assure the innovation will become accepted and standardized. Reinvention is an important aspect of nursing practice because evidence-based solutions to identified practice problems or improvement opportunities for specific practice enrich clinical implementations. The implementation stage ends once the innovation becomes standard practice within an organization (Rogers, 2003).

The final stage of the innovation–decision-making process is the confirmation stage, in which there is ongoing reinforcement of innovation adoption and minimization of what Rogers (2003) refers to as dissonance or disequilibrium that may lead to rejection of the innovation. A decision to reject an innovation can happen at any stage in the innovation–decision-making process (reversibility), underscoring the importance of ongoing efforts to support adaptation, adoption, and standardization of the new practice.

Havelock's Stages of Planned Change

In 1973, Havelock introduced a planned change approach as a resource for nurses engaged in education reform. In 1995, Havelock revised the theory for applicability to any planned change initiative (Havelock & Zlotolow, 1995). According to Havelock, the process of innovation involves the utilization of seven key concepts in a problem-solving cycle. Summarized by the acronym C-R-E-A-T-E-R, the concepts are (a) care, (b) relate, (c) examine, (d) acquire, (e) try, (f) extend, and (g) renew (Havelock & Zlotolow, 1995). The C-R-E-A-T-E-R concepts incorporate a six-stage framework facilitated by a change agent who engages and encourages participation of group members in all stages of the change process. The change agent is central to the innovation process and functions in four possible roles: (a) catalyst, (b) solution giver, (c) process helper, and (d) problem solver (Table 7.3) (Havelock & Zlotolow, 1995).

During the first stage of the planned stage cycle, *Stage 0—Care*, there is recognition of a problem or opportunity for positive change, such as the introduction of a new evidence-based clinical practice guideline. In *Stage 1 (Relate)*, the change agent establishes relationships with and among stakeholders, thereby creating a foundation for collaborative problem solving from which to *examine the situation* in detail (*Stage 2*). Once the problem is well defined, the change agent gathers needed resources (e.g., human, financial, technology, knowledge, and

TABLE 7.3   Change Agent Roles in Havelock's Planned Change Framework

Catalyst	Disrupts system status quo; energizes the initial problem-solving process and following change implementation to foster system self-renewal Stages: 0, 1, and 6
Solution Giver	Facilitates development of change plan based on system needs and concerns Stages: 3, 4, and 6
Process Helper	Assists each stage of the problem-solving process: identifying the need, building relationships, defining the problem, planning and implementing solutions Stages: 0, 1, 2, 3, 4, 5, and 6
Problem Solver	Gathers needed resources (financial, knowledge/skill, personnel) within and outside of the system; facilitates identification of resources to support independent problem solving Stages: 2, 3, and 6

Source: From Havelock and Zlotolow (1995).

infrastructure) to address the problem in *Stage 3 (Acquire)*. During *Stage 4 (Try)*, a solution is identified and designed for the specific setting. In *Stage 5 (Extend)*, the initiative is implemented, and the change agent facilitates adoption of the innovation with emphasis on effective communication and committed leadership. Finally, in *Stage 6 (Renew)*, the change agent reinforces the new practice and works to build capacity to sustain the change. Havelock and Zlotolow (1995) describe the *re*-C-R-E-A-T-E and *re*linquish aspects of this phase in which the change agent supports the continuation of effective problem solving while gradually diminishing his or her involvement in the change process. A comparison of change processes of Lewin, Lippitt, Rogers, and Havelock and their key theoretical concepts are outlined in Tables 7.4 and 7.5.

THEORY-INFORMED EVALUATION OF EBP CHANGE INITIATIVES

Evaluation is an indispensable component of the change process. Identification and measurement of process and outcome measures are essential to determine feasibility and identify potential program modifications prior to the formal adoption of change. Theory-informed evaluation provides a framework for determining the success or failure of change initiatives. Manchester et al. (2014) state that a quality gap in knowledge translation processes has been worsened by the lack of a unified and comprehensive framework for the planning and evaluation of EBP projects. An evaluation phase sets the foundation for ongoing monitoring of future change behavior compliance as well as measurement of long-term impact such as improved patient outcomes.

Evaluation efforts need to include an assessment of how well the theoretical framework guided the change process. Evaluation efforts must answer if main theoretical concepts were helpful in guiding each phase of the change process. Evaluation efforts need to indicate if application of a theory facilitated individual and/or group change. Questions to consider for the evaluation of a theoretical framework for change initiatives are described in Box 7.2.

TABLE 7.4 Comparison Chart of Planned Changes According to Key Theorists

	Lewin (1947)	Lippett (1958)	Rogers (1962)	Havelock (1973)
Systematic Approach to Change Process	Step 1: Unfreezing (destabilize)	Phase 1: Develop need for change Phase 2: Establish change relationship	Stage 1: Knowledge	Stage 0: Care (establish need for action) Stage 1: Relate (build relationships) Stage 2: Examine (define the problem) Stage 3: Acquire (find resources)
	Step 2: Moving (implement change)	Work Toward Change Phase 3: Clarify/diagnose the problem Phase 4: Examine alternatives; establish change goals Phase 5: Attempt change efforts	Stage 2: Persuasion Stage 3: Decision Stage 4: Implementation	Stage 4: Try (choose solution) Stage 5: Extend (expand acceptance and solidify adoption)
	Step 3: Refreezing (restabilize)	Phase 6: Generalize and stabilize the change Phase 7: Terminate the change relationship	Stage 5: Confirmation	Stage 6: Renew, re-CREATE, terminate (support self-renewal capacity and disengage from system)
Key Perspectives	The status quo (quasi-stationary equilibrium) exists as a balance of opposing environmental forces. Change results from a shift in the balance of forces. Change efforts should be aimed at group level to affect nurse behavior.	The environment is a dynamic system maintained by a balance of opposing forces. Change occurs as a deliberate effort to improve the client system with the help of an outside agent. The change agent creates a favorable balance of forces through communication, relationship building, and collaborative problem solving.	The spread of an innovation (new idea) occurs as a decision-making process (nurse/group) is influenced by innovation characteristics, communication channels, time, and social context.	Innovation (change) is an intentional process of cycles of rational problem solving within a specific social context guided by change agents who serve in one of four specialized roles: catalyst, solution giver, process helper, and problem solver.

Sources: From Batras et al. (2014), Havelock and Zlotolow (1995), Lippitt et al. (1958), and Roussel (2013).

TABLE 7.5 Common Elements of Planned Change Theoretical Frameworks

Element	Lewin	Lippitt	Rogers	Havelock
Systematic Approach	Three-step change process; eight-step action research model	Seven-phase systems approach	Five-stage decision-making process	Seven-stage problem-solving process
Change initiative is inseparable from the change context	Appropriate conditions are needed to sustain change. The environment is composed of opposing forces (driving/ resisting). Nurse behavior is a function of group behavior (group dynamics).	The environment is a balance of resistance and change forces. There is interdependence of the client system in determining solutions. There is system openness to new information, and the ability to create new responses leads to success.	Social system: interrelated units engaged in decision making; determines innovation adoption Characteristics of the decision-making unit (e.g., communication and personalities) Perceived characteristics of the innovation Antecedents: prior conditions that impact change Innovation (i.e., norms) Reinvention results from the interaction between context and innovation	Change does not exist in a social vacuum; context is an integral part of the problem-solving process. The interrelatedness of social elements is stressed
Change process takes time (Elasticity)	Environment (field) is time-dependent Completion of FFA before and after change takes time Change not an event but a process	Change process should not occur too rapidly, leads to partial solutions Collecting information during middle phases time consuming and labor intensive	Innovation–decision-making process determined by length of time spent in each stage. Rate of adoption is a function of time (early→late adopters) Time is most often ignored consideration in change efforts	Ample time is needed to complete rational problem-solving process, diffuse the change through system, and stabilize change

(continued)

TABLE 7.5 Common Elements of Planned Change Theoretical Frameworks *(continued)*

Element	Lewin	Lippitt	Rogers	Havelock
Change leadership is critical to success	*Change agent/leader actions:* • Disrupts status quo—introduces new practice • Prepares group (motivation, readiness) • Communicates change message (creates shared vision) • Provides feedback and encourages change behavior • Fosters integration of new behavior into group values	*Change agent/leader actions:* • Professional change agent who facilitates change process • Influences rate of change and direction/strength of forces • Maintains objectivity; respects system autonomy • Builds needed knowledge and skills for each phase • Promotes stabilization and permanence of change behavior	*Change agent/opinion leader actions:* • Facilitates every phase of the innovation-decision process • Focuses on time/resources needed to equip adopters with knowledge and skills • Change agent works through opinion leaders to achieve innovation adoption • Positively influences attitudes and reduces uncertainty; maintains client orientation • Communicates relative advantage of innovation	*Change agent/leader actions:* • Approaches change from total system view • Primary change agent roles: catalyst, solution giver, process helper, and problem solver • Builds capacity to sustain change and identify future change initiatives
Requires ongoing action (evaluation, monitoring, and reinforcement)	Iterative process that requires evaluation of the outcome and need for potential modification (action research) Reinforcement of change behavior	Evaluation of change outcomes essential for integration Generalization and stabilization activities determined by change agent and client system	Supportive messages given to reinforce adoption decision and prevent dissonance (conflict between behavior and attitudes) Reinvention activities support sustainability and minimize discontinuation	*Reinforcement* of change to ensure security and integration of behavior Promotion of *self-renewal* through ongoing problem-solving efforts

Sources: From Havelock and Zlotolow (1995), Lewin (1951), Lippitt et al. (1958), Rogers (2003), and Stichler (2011).

BOX 7.2   Guiding Questions to Evaluate Change Theory Efficacy in EBP Initiatives

---

Lewin

1. Is the simplicity of the three-step process easily understood by the group? How can the action research model be integrated into the three-step planned change process?

2. How is Lewin's emphasis on the influence of the group on nurse behavior important for your EBP change initiative?

3. How can FFA be utilized to assess the change environment both pre- and postimplementation?

4. Are the role and responsibilities of the change leader clearly articulated?

5. How does the theory inform ongoing activities to sustain the practice change?

Lippitt

1. How is the description of an interdependent "client system" operationalized in the proposed change project?

2. What role will the change agent play in assisting the change initiative?

3. Does identification of change and resistance forces facilitate group deliberation around change process planning?

4. Does the framework's expansion of Lewin's "moving" phase provide more specific guidance for project design?

5. Does Lippitt's theory address stabilization of the change behavior following termination of the change agent relationship in an actionable way?

Rogers

1. How well does Rogers's emphasis on antecedent conditions foster assessment of the change environment preintervention?

2. How does the identification of innovation characteristics facilitate implementation of an EBP?

3. Is Rogers's depiction of the rate of adoption helpful in promoting the spread and uptake of the change behavior?

4. Does Rogers's five-step decision-making process clearly guide activities for each stage of the change process?

5. How does Rogers's concept of "reinvention" inform the integration of best evidence into specific practice settings?

Havelock

1. Are change activities clearly defined in each stage to guide the change process?

2. How does the framework promote participation and consensus building around the change initiative?

3. Does the description of specific change agent roles foster development of change leadership? Has someone been identified to fulfill the role(s)?

4. In what ways does the framework foster collective problem solving related to current and future change initiatives?

5. How does the framework facilitate reinforcement and adoption of the change behavior?

EBP, evidence-based practice; FFA, force field analysis.

APPLICATION OF CHANGE THEORY EXEMPLAR USING SCENARIO 2

This chapter began with the presentation of two change scenarios. In Scenario 1, implementation of a practice change related to interprofessional simulation was ultimately unsuccessful. Loss of the change champion, a lack of demonstrated commitment by unit leaders, and the inability to eliminate emerging obstacles eroded motivation and enthusiasm for the change effort. In the end, capitulation triumphed over commitment.

In contrast, Scenario 2 illustrates a successful practice change initiative in which the approach to the proposed initiative was deliberate and systematic to ensure adoption in a dynamic and demanding practice environment. Lewin's three-step change model and FFA (Figure 7.1) along with Kotter's (1995) change management principles frame the discussion about this EBP organizational initiative.

Unfreezing

In Scenario 2, an opportunity to disrupt the status quo was largely due to the introduction of the new idea (innovation) by the DNP nurse (i.e., change agent). The DNP nurse had a clear understanding of department and organizational culture and received respect from all stakeholder groups. The DNP nurse was able to secure management support, in part, because she presented a change opportunity to enhance the organization's ability to meet strategic goals of clinical and nursing practice excellence through implementation of EBP. The change initiative also reinforced the nursing department's commitment to Magnet principles. The change agent built a broad base of support for the project by including all staff in the development and implementation of the change effort. The staff had a choice to identify their own EBP projects or work on an existing department priority, thereby fostering ownership.

Kotter (1995) emphasizes the importance of creating a compelling appeal for change achieved in this example. Aligning the project's aims with organizational and strategic imperatives to improve care and provide staff development was effective. The alignment enabled the DNP nurse to build a broad coalition for change that included administrative, education, and practice leaders.

Moving

Once the committee formed, the DNP nurse used monthly meetings and frequent touch points to role model EBP behaviors for nurses throughout the process. Role modeling involved providing education about critical appraisal of clinical literature and gathering important data to inform the design of each EBP initiative. The DNP nurse used group meetings to gather support and input for project development and promoted the opportunity for more-experienced nurses to work with less-experienced nurses. This form of role modeling exemplifies Kotter's (1995) "walking the talk" in which active engagement of staff as role models helps to diffuse the change vision beyond the original leadership team. Positive reports about the EBP initiative provided additional encouragement for nurses involved in EBP projects. Challenges encountered during the first few months included loss of a PIC member and interference with a few scheduled meetings. The initiative had early wins such as the successful completion of one EBP project that integrated easily into the standard of care and successful advancement of two nurses to the next level in the clinical ladder who were involved in the PIC initiative. Mindful that sustainable change takes time, these early successes can fuel commitment to the change project while reinforcing participation. The moving period, characterized by trial and error, provides real-time and real-world feedback that integrates into the change initiative. The DNP nurse made an effort to provide direct care nurses with the necessary knowledge and skill to engage in EBP, which also bolstered project support while reducing nurse change resistance.

Refreezing

During this phase, equilibrium reestablishes as the new initiative is adapted, adopted, and hard-wired into department culture. The process of change stabilization can take years. Change initiatives are most vulnerable to fail once the novelty has worn off (waning driving forces). Following early wins, committee enthusiasm began to fade when nurses who had successfully advanced in the clinical ladder started to lose interest in their projects. At the department level, multiple demands on staff time and the high patient volume and high-acuity clinical environment made it increasingly difficult to manage and support multiple EBP initiatives for both direct care nurses and practice leaders. After a number of staff discussions at the monthly PIC meetings and several conversations between the DNP nurse and department leadership, several program modifications came into effect. The group, including direct care nurses, nurse managers, medical director, clinical nurse specialist, and DNP mentor, agreed to identify and prioritize future EBP projects based on the department and medical center's quality and safety agenda and practice needs. The group decided subsequent EBP projects need to meet implemented requirements according to priority ranking and that the number of concurrent projects would be limited to two. In addition, the unit formed EBP teams to work on projects rather than relying on single nurse efforts. The modification promoted shared responsibility, increased change capacity, and created a mechanism by which direct care nurses could remain involved in their projects after achieving clinical promotion by serving as EBP team mentors.

LEADING CHANGE

Effective leadership is crucial to achieve sustained practice change (Mitchell, 2013). A lack of strong leadership is a major reason for organizational change failure. Lack of strong leadership positively correlates with increased change resistance (Oreg, 2003). Two distinct bodies of nursing literature have contributed to the current understanding of change leadership. The first of these describes nurses whose innate *leadership style* inspires support and active participation in the change process (i.e., transformational leader). The second describes situation-sensitive *leadership behaviors* (i.e., build a coalition) that are used in specific change situations (Alavi & Gill, 2017).

Leadership Styles and Change Leadership Strategies

Goleman, Boyatzis, and McKee (2013) identify six change leadership styles (Table 7.6) that are based on four dimensions of emotional intelligence. Emotional intelligence (EQ) is the ability to manage ourselves and our relationships effectively

TABLE 7.6   Leadership Styles for Planned Change Initiatives

Leadership Style	Focus	Emotional Intelligence Competency	Application to Change Process
Affiliative	People and relationships	Empathy Communication	• Builds emotional bonds and staff harmony • Supports motivation and innovation • *Highly positive* impact on setting
Authoritative	Achieving a vision	Self-confidence Empathy	• Change catalyst; integrates and creates shared vision • Provides clear change goals • *Most positive* impact on setting
Coaching	Employee development	Empathy Self-awareness	• Supports adoption of change behavior; models change behavior • Identifies area(s) of staff development to accomplish change behavior • *Positive* impact on setting
Coercive	Immediate compliance	Self-control Achievement	• Limits flexibility; dulls motivation • Useful during crisis • *Strongly negative* impact on setting
Democratic	Participation and communication	Collaboration Teamwork	• Builds broad base of support for change • Promotes staff feedback/input related to change initiative • *Positive* impact on setting
Pacesetting	Peak performance	Conscientious Initiative	• Urges quick results from highly motivated and self-directed staff • Demands excellence; lowers morale and weakens commitment • *Negative* impact on setting

Source: Adapted from Goleman, Boyatzis, & McKee (2013).

(Goleman, 2000). The foundational dimension of EQ is *self-awareness* and involves being aware of one's emotions, strengths, weaknesses, and level of self-confidence. The second dimension is *self-management* and includes exercising self-control, being conscientious, being adaptable, and being achievement oriented. *Social awareness* is the third EQ dimension and pertains to having organizational awareness and being empathetic and approachable. The fourth dimension is *relationship management* and is concerned with creating bonds, developing others, and collaborating and managing change and conflict (Goleman et al., 2013). Given the complex and dynamic work environment, effective change leaders rely on multiple leadership styles depending on the situation and the needs of the group.

Over the past decade, there has been considerable scholarly interest in the development of authentic leadership (AL). AL is not a leadership style per se, but it is a component of several leadership styles that focuses on values-based behavior (Alavi & Gill, 2016). Authentic leaders communicate openly and honestly and create a positive organizational environment by demonstrating a commitment to high ethical standards and developing others (Woolley, Caza, & Levy, 2011). Alavi and Gill (2016) propose that AL can enhance change leadership by positively influencing followers' attitudes and behaviors related to change commitment, change readiness, and change efficacy.

Chin and Benne developed the seminal work on change leadership strategies in 1961 and identified three leadership approaches: (a) *empirical-rational*, (b) *normative-reductive*, and (c) *power-coercive* (Szabla, 2007). Empirical-rational strategies are based on the assumption that nurses are rational, and if presented with the benefits of the proposed change will adopt new behaviors. Normative-reductive strategies are founded on the notion that nurse participation in the design and implementation of change will lead to adoption of the new behavior. Such strategies involve changes in attitudes, values, norms, and relationships. Finally, power-coercive strategies leverage organizational, social, economic, or political power to impose change without input from those affected (Burke, 2014; Szabla, 2007). Table 7.7 provides examples of strategies for each approach. Burke (2014) identifies key leadership activities for every phase of the organizational change process (Table 7.8).

TABLE 7.7 Change Leadership Strategies (Chin & Benne, 1961)

Rational-Empirical	1. Disseminate scientific evidence to others.
	2. Position nurses/experts in the system who will take action.
	3. Collect and disseminate context-specific data to drive change.
Normative-Reeducative	1. Improve the problem-solving capacity within the system.
	2. Involve nurses in all phases of the change process.
	3. Invest in nurse staff development.
Power-Coercive	1. Leverage influence (political, economic, social, and hierarchical) to impose change.
	2. Nurses are not involved in change process.

Source: From Burke (2014).

TABLE 7.8 Key Leadership Behaviors During the Change Process

Prelaunch Phase	Conduct self-assessment (self-awareness, motives, and values), collect relevant data from the practice setting, establish the need for change, create the change vision
Launch Phase	Communicate the need for change, initiate activities that excite group about change, mitigate resistant behavior
Postlaunch Phase	Seek honest feedback, demonstrate/verbalize commitment to the change behavior, persevere (remember change takes time), reinforce change behavior
Sustaining Phase	Manage unanticipated consequences, monitor practice setting for potential adaptations, mentor new change leaders (EBP champions), plan additional EBP initiatives

Source: From Burke (2014).

SUMMARY

This chapter provided an overview of planned change management to facilitate implementation of EBP in the clinical setting. Introduction of new evidence-based approaches in clinical practice can be challenging given that more than two-thirds of all organizational change efforts fail. Change resistance is a major reason for change failure; therefore, assessment of organizational readiness is a critical first step in any planned change project to minimize resistance. Participation of staff in the change effort from the onset as well as maintaining open and ongoing communication throughout the change process are essential to minimize resistance and promote sustainable, permanent change.

Implementation of EBP requires a systematic approach. Several change theorists' frameworks, whose efforts were largely influenced by the seminal work of Kurt Lewin, were presented to guide practice change projects. Key elements of change theories are summarized in Tables 7.5 and Box 7.2. Chief among them is the *inextricable relationship between the change initiative and the environment,* frequently conceptualized as forces within the change setting. Contextualization of evidence-based interventions is the cornerstone of successful adoption. Accordingly, the change process takes *time,* because developing a well-designed plan and evaluating project implementation require sustained commitment. *Ongoing monitoring* of longer-term results, which reinforces the change behavior and identifies potential modifications to the change behavior, is essential for long-term sustainability.

Finally, change leadership is critical to the success of any change project. The change leader can be an internal/external change agent, clinical expert, or formal/informal group leader. Goleman and others identify six leadership styles based on EI to guide the planned change process. Kotter (1995), Chin and Benne (1961), and Burke (2014) offer key strategies that lead EBP change initiatives.

REFERENCES

Alavi, S. B., & Gill, C. (2017). Leading change authentically: How authentic leaders influence follower responses to complex change. *Journal of Leadership & Organizational Studies, 24*(2), 157—171. doi:10.1177/1548051816664681

Bargal, D. (2008). Action research: A paradigm for achieving social change. *Small Group Research, 39*(1), 17–27.

Batras, D., Duff, C., & Smith, B. J. (2014). Organizational change theory: Implications for health promotion practice. *Health Promotion International, 31*(1), 1–11. doi:10.1093/heapro/dau098

Black, A. T., Balneaves, L. G., Garossino, C., Puyat, J. H., & Qian, H. (2015). Promoting evidence-based practice through a research training program for point-of-care clinicians. *Journal of Nursing Administration, 45*(1), 14–20.

Burke, W. W. (2014). *Organizational change: Theory and practice.* Thousand Oaks, CA: Sage.

Burnes, B. (2004). Kurt Lewin and the planned approach to change: A re-appraisal. *Journal of Management Studies, 41*, 977–1002.

Burnes, B. (2005). Complexity theories and organizational change. *International Journal of Management Reviews, 7*(2), 73–90.

Burnes, B. (2011). Why does change fail, and what can we do about it? *Journal of Change Management, 11*(4), 445–450.

Burnes, B. (2014). *Managing change* (6th ed.). Harlow, UK: Pearson.

Canning, J., & Found, P. A. (2015). The effect of resistance in organizational change programs: A study of lean transformation. *International Journal of Quality and Service Sciences, 7*(2/3), 274–296.

Chin, R., & Benne, K. D. (1961). General strategies for effecting changes in human systems. In W. G. Bennis, K. D. Benne, & R. Chin (Eds.), *The planning of change* (pp. 22–45). Austin, TX: Holt, Rinehart, and Winston.

Eccles, M. A., Grimshaw, J., Walker, A., Johnston, M., & Pitts, N. (2005). Changing the behavior of healthcare professionals: The use of theory in promoting the uptake of research findings. *Journal of Clinical Epidemiology, 58*, 107–112.

Erwin, D. G., & Garman, A. N. (2010). Resistance to organizational change: Linking research and practice. *Leadership & Organization Development Journal, 31*(1), 39–56.

Fineout-Overholt, E, Williamson, K. M., Kent, B., & Hutchinson, A. M. (2010). Teaching EBP: Strategies for achieving sustainable organizational change toward evidence-based practice. *Worldviews in Evidence Based Nursing, 7*(1), 51–53. doi:10.1111/j.1741-6787.2010.00185

Goleman, D. (2000, March-April). Leadership that gets results. *Harvard Business Review,* 78–90.

Goleman, D., Boyatzis, R., & McKee, A. (2013). *Primal leadership: Unleashing the power of emotional intelligence.* Boston, MA: Harvard Business Review Press.

Grol, R., Bosch, M. C., Hulscher, M. E., Eccles, M. P., & Wensing, M. (2007). Planning and studying improvement in patient care: The use of theoretical perspectives. *Milbank Quarterly, 85*(1), 93–138.

Havelock, R. G., & Zlotolow, S. (1995). *The change agent's guide* (2nd ed.). Englewood Cliffs, NJ: Educational Technology Publications.

Kanter, R. M. (2012, September). Ten reasons people resist change. *Harvard Business Review.* Retrieved from https://hbr.org/2012/09/ten-reasons-people-resist-chang%20oct%2028

Karp, T., & Helgø, T. (2008). From change management to change leadership: Embracing chaotic change in public service organizations. *Journal of Change Management, 8*(1), 85–96.

Kotter, J. P. (1995). Leading change: Why transformation efforts fail. *Harvard Business Review,* 59–67. Retrieved from http://www.gsbcolorado.org/uploads/general/Pre SessionReadingLeadingChange-John_Kotter.pdf

Kritsonis, A. (2005). Comparison of change theories. *International Journal of Scholarly Academic Intellectual Diversity, 8*(1), 1–7.

Krugman, M. (2010). Evidence-based practice and the Magnet journey. *Journal for Nurses in Staff Development, 26*(5), 239–241.

Levasseur, R. E. (2010). People skills: Ensuring project success—a change management perspective. *Interfaces, 40*(2), 159–162.

Lewin, K. (1951). Field theory and learning. In D. Cartwright (Ed.), *Field theory in social science* (pp. 60–86). New York, NY: Harper & Row

Lewis, L. (2006). Employee perspectives on implementation communication as predictors of perceptions of success and resistance. *Western Journal of Communication, 70*(1), 23–46.

Lippitt, R., Watson, J., & Westley, B. (1958). *The dynamics of planned change.* New York, NY: Harcourt, Brace & World.

Manchester, J., Gray-Miceli, D. L., Metcalf, J. A., Paolini, C. A., Napier, A. H., Coogle, C. L., & Owens, M. G. (2014). Facilitating Lewin's change model with collaborative evaluations in promoting evidence based practices of health professionals. *Evaluation and Program Planning, 47,* 82–90.

McClellan, J. G. (2014). Announcing change: Discourse, uncertainty, and organizational control. *Journal of Change Management, 14*(2), 192–209. doi:10.1080/14697017.2013.844195

McMillan, K., & Perron, A. (2013). Nurses admidst change: The concept of change fatigue offers an alternative perspective on organizational change. *Politics & Nursing Practice, 14*(1), 26–32.

Melnyk, B., & Fineout-Overholt, E. (2012). The state of evidence-based practice in US nurses. *Journal of Nursing Administration, 42*(9), 410–417.

Mitchell, G. (2013). Selecting the best theory to implement planned change. *Nursing Management, 20*(1), 32–37.

Oreg, S. (2003). Resistance to change: Developing a nurse differences measure. *Journal of Applied Psychology, (88)*4, 680–693.

Rogers, E. M. (2003). *Diffusion of innovations* (5th ed.). New York, NY: Free Press.

Rossi, P. H., Freeman, H. E., & Lipsey, M. W. (1999). *Evaluation: A systematic approach* (6th ed.) . Thousand Oaks, CA: SAGE.

Roussel, L. (2013). *Management and leadership for nurse administrators* (6th ed.). Burlington, MA: Jones & Bartlett.

Shirey, M. R. (2013). Lewin's theory of planned change as a strategic resource. *Journal of Nursing Administration, 43*(2), 69–72.

Smith, J. R., & Donze, A. (2010). Assessing environmental readiness: First steps in developing an evidence-based practice implementation culture. *Journal of Perinatal & Neonatal Nursing, 24*(1), 61–71.

Stichler, A. F. (2011). Leading change. *Nursing for Women's Health, 15*(2), 166–170.

Szabla, D. B. (2007). A multidimensional view of resistance to organizational change: Exploring cognitive, emotional, and intentional responses to planned change across perceived change leadership strategies. *Human Resource Quarterly, 18*(4), 525–558.

Van der Voet, J., Groeneveld, S., & Kuipers, B. S. (2014). Talking the talk or walking the walk? The leadership of planned and emergent change in a public organization. *Journal of Change Management, 14*(2), 171–191.

Vanhook, P. M. (2009). Overcoming the barriers to EBP. *Nursing Management,* 9–11.

Weiner, B. J. (2009). A theory of organizational readiness for change. *Implementation Science,* (4)67. doi:10.1186/1748-5908-4-67

Woolley, L., Caza, A., & Levy, L. (2011). Authentic leadership and follower development: Psychological capital, positive work climate, and gender. *Journal of Leadership & Organizational Studies, 18*(4), 438–448.

CHAPTER 8

How to Read and Assess for Quality of Research

Rene Love and Donna Behler McArthur

Objectives

After reading this chapter, learners should be able to:

1. Name the key elements of quantitative and qualitative research reports
2. Organize a critique of quantitative and qualitative research reports
3. Determine the quality of research reports

EVIDENCE-BASED PRACTICE (EBP) SCENARIOS

Scenario 1

A nurse practitioner group plans to evaluate outcomes of a brief group intervention related to physical activity for patients with newly diagnosed type 2 diabetes mellitus (DM). The sample would include patients at a large rural clinic in whom type 2 DM had been diagnosed within the last 3 months. The nurse practitioners in the clinic developed a 4-week group exercise intervention and a supportive phone app as a supplement for patient education. The clinic manager, unilaterally, decided which patients would participate in the study based on the patients' perceived interest when being interviewed by the manager. The physical activity level of the patients would be evaluated at the end of the intervention through the use of a Fitbit. Blood glucose levels would also be monitored daily during the 4 weeks. There was no comparison group identified despite the desire to use an experimental design because the manager believed that all patients with newly diagnosed type 2 DM should have access to the 4-week intervention.

Scenario 2

A practitioner group plans to evaluate outcomes of a brief group exercise intervention for patients with newly diagnosed type 2 DM. The practitioners have developed a 4-week group exercise intervention and a supportive phone app as a supplement to the intervention. The researcher invited all patients at the clinic with newly diagnosed type 2 DM to participate in the study. There were two randomized groups for the patients: (a) care as usual and (b) a 4-week intervention. Patient physical activity level would be evaluated at the end of the intervention through the use of a Fitbit. Blood glucose would be monitored daily during the 4 weeks. The comparison group (care as usual) would be offered the intervention after the study was completed. The outcomes would be analyzed within and between treatment and control groups.

Discussion

In Scenario 1, the clinic manager introduced bias into the study. It is important to obtain nonbiased data in studies to produce credible research evidence. By not having a comparison group, it is difficult to determine if the intervention was effective or if the patients would have shown similar improvement over the 4-week period without the intervention. To confirm efficacy of the intervention, patients needed to be randomized, rather than selected by the manager, and compared with a similar group not receiving the intervention.

Nursing research provides the scientific bases for practice, and nurses are interested in finding the most effective approaches to achieving and sustaining optimal patient-centered care (American Association of Colleges of Nursing [AACN], 2006). To help determine the credibility and usefulness of research to practice, this chapter provides basic guidelines for reviewing and critiquing quantitative and qualitative research reports.

Research and EBP

Research is an important component of the EBP triumvirate: *research, patient values,* and *practitioner expertise.* Because of nursing's proximity to patients and patient care decisions, nurses understand that research must be of high quality before applying research findings to patient care. Without sound research, patient care may be influenced by dogma, ideology, unconfirmed theory, and prejudice. Research reports in peer-reviewed journals frequently undergo a systematic and rigorous review process to help assure scientific quality. As with all discipline-specific journals (e.g., medicine, psychology, epidemiology), review standards among peer reviewers and journals vary, which means that not all research reports are thoroughly reviewed and scientifically sound (Kaplan, 2012). Because research provides evidence that guides clinical practice, it is important that nurses appraise research findings for soundness and credibility before applying those findings to patient care.

Nursing is a blend of art and science; thus, nurses learn about research to provide the best possible care for patients (Nightingale, 1860). The ability to identify sound research enables nurses to provide a higher standard of patient care. Chapter 3 provides a detailed description of how to determine a study's level of evidence. This chapter focuses on assessment of research quality. In research, quality is defined as the extent to which a study has minimized bias in the selection of participants, measurements, and external factors that may have an impact on the study's results (Glasofer, 2014).

The AACN has set educational research standards for all nursing practice programs that offer baccalaureate or higher degrees. The AACN requires that nursing practice programs be committed to teaching and integrating nursing research and relevant research from other disciplines (e.g., biomedical, business, or public health). To strengthen nursing's contribution to optimizing the health and healthcare services to patients and populations, the AACN has established research expectations and competencies for all nursing practice degree levels:

- *Baccalaureate programs* prepare nurses with a basic understanding of the processes of research. Graduates can understand and apply research findings from nursing and other disciplines in their clinical practice. They understand the basic elements of EBP, can work with others to identify potential research problems, and can collaborate on research teams (AACN, 2008).
- *Master's programs* prepare nurses to evaluate research findings and to develop and implement EBP guidelines. Their leadership skills enable them to form and lead teams within their agencies and professional groups. They identify practice and systems problems that require study, and they collaborate with scientists to initiate research (AACN, 2011).
- Practice-focused doctoral programs prepare graduates for the highest level of nursing practice beyond initial preparation in the discipline. Graduates obtain the highest level of practice expertise integrated with the ability to translate scientific knowledge into complex clinical interventions tailored to meet individual, family, and community health and illness needs. In addition, these professionals use advanced leadership knowledge and skills to evaluate the translation of research into practice and collaborate with scientists on new health policy research opportunities that evolve from the translation and evaluation processes. They are prepared to focus on the evaluation and use of research rather than the conduct of research (AACN, 2004).

Nurses have access to growing quantities of research, and access to research is becoming increasingly convenient (Squires et al., 2011). Boxes 8.1 and 8.2 provide a basic framework for nurses to use when appraising research quality. The quantitative and qualitative frameworks, Boxes 8.1 and 8.2, respectively, are each composed of three essential sections: (a) introduction, (b) methodology, and (c) results. Subsumed under each section are definitions, questions, discussion, and explanations to aid in the evaluation of research quality. A hierarchy of evidence reflective of quantitative and qualitative studies is presented in Figures 8.1 and 8.2, respectively. There are four primary types of quantitative designs (Box 8.3) and six primary types of qualitative designs (Box 8.4).

BOX 8.1 Guideline for Reviewing/Critiquing a Quantitative Research Report

I. Introduction Section

The introduction section should establish the context and significance of the research report. The introduction includes relevant background information to summarize current knowledge about the research topic. Though not always labeled, the introduction section usually includes the following subsections: problem/purpose statement, literature review, research question/hypothesis, and conceptual/theoretical framework.

Problem Statement

Defined: A problem statement is a *brief* description of a gap in current knowledge that a research project proposes to bridge. A nursing problem statement illustrates a gap between what is desired and what is observed in relation to patient care.

Key Questions for Analysis:

- Does the problem statement identify an area of concern for a specific patient group or population?
- Does the problem statement create an awareness of the problem's significance to nurses and patients?
- Is a context for the problem detectable, and does the context provide realistic parameters for the problem?

Discussion: A problem statement should address a problem that is topical and of interest to nursing and healthcare. It is important to consider if the identified problem is likely to continue, unless there is an intervention. Consider if studying the identified problem will extend nursing's body of knowledge and if outcomes will lead to useful changes in patient or population care.

Example: The most important and compelling nursing motivations for decreasing hospital central line-associated bloodstream infection (CLABSI) rates are to optimize quality of care and to promote patient wellness. With an unacceptable rate of 3.4 infections per 1,000 central line days in the cardiac unit, efforts were needed to reduce this rate. This study was conducted to investigate an intervention designed to reach this necessary goal (Hanson, 2017).

Purpose Statement

Defined: A purpose statement is a declarative *sentence* that summarizes a research topic and its goal(s).

Key Questions for Analysis:

- Does the purpose statement provide a concrete understanding of what the research project will cover?
- Is the purpose statement a nonambiguous goal-oriented statement?
- Does the purpose statement indicate a sample and/or setting?
- Does the purpose statement suggest how the study will improve nursing practice and/or add to nursing's body of knowledge?

Discussion: The purpose statement needs to be stated in the first few paragraphs of a research report so that readers can efficiently connect the purpose to both the research material they are seeking and the remainder of the research report. Purpose statements require contextualizing, which often occurs in a section identified as "introduction" or "background." The scope and breadth of background information differ, depending on the project topic and what is known about the topic. Regardless of the scope, the background information should be clear and succinct; elaboration of critical points or in-depth analysis of salient issues is usually found in the literature review section.

(continued)

BOX 8.1   Guideline for Reviewing/Critiquing a Quantitative Research Report *(continued)*

Example: We wanted to better understand the deployment process experience of individual family members in relationship to one another within the family system and to include the perspectives of children within military families. When available, we also were interested in the observations and reflections of teachers and other school personnel on how children responded to the experience of having a deployed parent (Yablonsky, Barbero, & Richardson, 2016).

Literature Review

Defined: A literature review is a systematic appraisal of a body of research and/or scholarly work that identifies and analyzes what is known about a PICOT question, research question, and/or a hypothesis (Bolderston, 2008).

Key Questions for Analysis:

- Does the literature review trace the intellectual progression of the research topic?

- Does the literature review identify contributions that each article under review makes to understanding the research topic?

- Does the literature review provide new interpretations of prior research (i.e., synthesis)?

- Does the literature review build a convincing case for conducting the research project?

- Are gaps and limitations in the body of existing knowledge about the research topic discussed?

Discussion: Articles reviewed in a literature review generally fall into one of three categories: (a) primary studies, (b) systematic reviews, and (c) opinions. Primary studies describe the findings of original research conducted by investigators. Systematic reviews are reviews of primary studies that systematically summarize and offer new insights and interpretations built from the primary studies. Opinions are an author's perceptions and interpretations of a topic and, therefore, are not considered scientific knowledge. A literature review for a research project in nursing should be composed of primary studies and systematic reviews.

Example: Although some recent information is available about how nursing faculty view their positions and resources, there is little literature describing the organizationally sanctioned ways in which junior nursing research track faculty in institutions offering research-focused doctorates are supported (Candela, Gutierrez, & Keating, 2013; Cash, Daines, Doyle, von Tettenborn, & Reid, 2009; Derby-Davis, 2014; Yedidia, Chou, Brownlee, Flynn, & Tanner, 2014). In addition, no recent public data describe how well new faculty meet nursing administrators' expectations regarding their ability to use the research supports offered and simultaneously fulfill other faculty roles. These gaps in the literature make it difficult to determine if maintenance or improvements are necessary to meet the scientific and training needs of the discipline (Minnick, Norman, & Donaghey, 2017).

Research Question or Hypothesis

Quantitative reports may have a research question and/or a hypothesis. Qualitative reports will not have a hypothesis.

Defined:

Research Question: An interrogative statement, designed to answer a research problem, which guides a study's literature review and methodology (Haynes, 2006)

Hypothesis: A conjectural statement about the relationship of two or more variables (Kerlinger, 1973)

Key Questions for Analysis:

Research Question:

- Does the research question inspire inquiry that will generate discipline-specific knowledge?

- Is the research question feasible to answer?

(continued)

BOX 8.1 Guideline for Reviewing/Critiquing a Quantitative Research Report (*continued*)

- Will the research question contribute to improvement in patient care?
- Is the research question ethical?

Hypothesis:

- Is the hypothesis testable? If using a hypothesis, the study design will need to be experimental or quasi-experimental.
- Does the hypothesis have an identifiable independent variable (i.e., intervention that is manipulated by the researcher) and a dependent variable (i.e., the variable caused by the independent variable)?
- Is the hypothesis safe for human experimentation and ethical?

Discussion: Research questions and hypotheses should contain the population, topic, and variables to be studied. Research questions analyze and investigate a topic. Hypotheses are predictive and are generally used when a significant amount of knowledge already exists about the topic. The existing knowledge aids in predicting the hypothetical relationship proposed for investigation.

Example:

Research Questions

1. What is the level of emotional intelligence (EI) among nurse managers (NMs) in a large academic medical center in the northeast?
2. What is the relationship between the level of EI among the NMs and demographic variables (Prufeta, 2017)?

Hypothesis: It is hypothesized that the utilization of the primary care–posttraumatic stress disorder (PC-PTSD) screening tool by bedside nurses will help identify more patients who are at risk for maladaptive traumatic stress. In addition, use of the screening tool by bedside nurses will trigger more readily available inpatient resources for these patients before they are discharged (Frank, Schroeter, & Shaw, 2017).

Conceptual/Theoretical Framework

Defined: Frameworks interconnect abstractions (i.e., concepts) that abridge and organize knowledge for the purpose of describing, explaining, or predicting phenomena (Davidson, 1971).

Key Questions for Analysis:

- Are key concepts in the purpose statement present in the framework?
- Are there logical linkages between concepts in the framework and concepts in the study?
- **Important:** Does the author(s) relate the study findings to the framework in the *discussion section*?

Discussion: *Conceptual framework* and *theoretical framework* are sometimes used interchangeably. Technically, a theoretical framework is based on theories that have been tested. A conceptual framework represents the researcher's idea of how a research problem will be explained and shows the relationship among concepts used in a study.

Example: The theoretical framework underlying the Fall Prevention Collaborative is based on problem-based and cooperative learning approaches, espoused by Knowles's self-directed learning. This approach encourages peer collaboration and the teacher's role as a group facilitator. Groups work together where participants engage to problem solve and share ideas, ultimately developing one agreed-upon fall prevention solution (Gray-Miceli, Mazzia, & Crane, 2017).

(*continued*)

BOX 8.1   Guideline for Reviewing/Critiquing a Quantitative Research Report *(continued)*

II. Methods Section

The methods section should provide a clear and precise description of how the study was conducted. The methods section describes both the study's procedures and procedural rationale. The methods section focuses on how data were generated and/or collected and analyzed.

Project Design

Defined: A project design is an inclusive strategy used to coordinate and integrate the different elements of a study. A design provides logical and coherent guidelines for the way a study will be conducted. A design outlines the processes for collection, measurement, and analysis of data. A strong design enhances the credibility of a study's finding and/or outcomes (de Vaus, 2001).

Key Questions for Analysis:

- Is the design nonexperimental (i.e., descriptive)? If the design is descriptive, how were observations of phenomena conducted? How many observation points are there?

- Is there a treatment or intervention (i.e., experiment)? If so, was the treatment described so that it could be replicated? Were treatments conducted with consistency and fidelity?

- If there was a treatment, were participants randomized to control or experimental groups? Were participants, researchers, and associated staff blinded to those who were assigned to either a control or treatment group?

Discussion: Nurses use evidence from various disciplines to provide the best patient-centered care. Design terminology varies among disciplines such as medicine, epidemiology, psychology, and social psychology. For example, medicine typically uses *case-control study*, while the corresponding social science term is *retrospective study*. Awareness and understanding of discipline-specific design terminology enable nurses to select the highest-quality designs to guide patient care decisions. For further discussion of design methodology, see Chapter 3.

Example: The current study used a descriptive correlational design to examine the relationships between the variables of familial socialization and ethnic identity, and the physical activity and eating behaviors of a sample of African American adolescents in Detroit (N. H. Tate, Davis, & Yarandi, 2015).

Study Population and Sampling

Definition: A sample is a subset of participants from a larger population. Sampling is the process of taking a subset of participants, representative of the entire population, to enroll in the project.

Key Questions for Analysis:

- What justification did the authors provide for the sample size? *Note:* The sample must have sufficient size to merit statistical analysis.

- Were eligibility criteria appropriate for the project question?

- Did the sampling plan (e.g., convenience, random, or stratified) provide for the most representative sample?

Discussion: Samples are either probability (e.g., random or stratified) or nonprobability (e.g., purposive, convenience, or quota). Probability samples are representative of the population and provide the most valid or credible results, because they most closely reflect the characteristics of the population. Nonprobability samples are not necessarily representative of the population and may produce less generalizable findings or outcomes than probability samples.

(continued)

BOX 8.1   Guideline for Reviewing/Critiquing a Quantitative Research Report *(continued)*

Example: Stratified balanced sampling is a technique that uses an auxiliary variable to attain a probability sample. Auxiliary variables are observed events in a population used to predict the value for unobserved events. A stratified balanced design allows for even distribution of a study sample in both urban and rural areas, with higher and lower levels of population density. The goal of stratified balanced sampling in the current study is to create a nationally representative sample of nurses who have been identified with a substance use problem (Monroe, Kenaga, Dietrich, Carter, & Cowen, 2013).

Data Collection

Definition: Data collection describes the tools and methods used to collect information necessary to answer a project's question or hypothesis. Data collection helps develop new or deeper understandings of the project's phenomenon.

Key Questions for Analysis:

- Do the data help answer the research question or hypothesis?
- Is there congruency between the conceptual and operational definitions (i.e., description of how a concept or variable will be measured)?
- Are the instruments valid and reliable? Validity refers to how well an instrument reflects the phenomenon being measured. Reliability indicates the degree of dependability an instrument has in measuring a phenomenon.
- Could data collection procedures be replicated?

Discussion: Readers should be aware that the development of measurement questions by a study's researchers might lead to answers that reflect the views of the researchers instead of the participants. Researcher-developed instruments are prone to "structural bias" and can lead to false representation of the phenomena being studied.

Example: The Memorial Symptom Assessment Scale (MSAS) 7Y12 was selected for the study to minimize the burden of frequent symptom assessments in a sample of hospitalized children and adolescents and to support comparison across the entire study sample. The authors of the MSAS 10Y18 noted that some adolescents had difficulty completing the lengthier tool and that the availability of a simpler version might be useful. An additional item, "numbness/tingling or pins and needles feeling in hands or feet," commonly associated with vincristine administration, was added to address peripheral neuropathy. This symptom has been added to the MSAS in a previous study with a reported frequency of 39%. The recall period was also adapted for this study to reflect "the previous shift" rather than "the last 2 days" to support the identification of shift-by-shift changes (Linder, Al-Quaaydeh, & Donaldson, 2017).

III. Results

The project's findings or outcomes are described in the results section.

Data Analysis and Findings

Definition: Data analysis is a process of cleaning (i.e., removing incomplete or inaccurate data), condensing, organizing, and finding meaning in a study's results or outcomes.

Key Questions for Analysis:

- Are the data analysis procedures described?
- Are each of the project's questions or hypotheses addressed in the analysis?
- Are findings described coherently in the narrative and presented in graphics that are understandable?
- Do the findings reflect the intent of the question or hypothesis?

(continued)

BOX 8.1   Guideline for Reviewing/Critiquing a Quantitative Research Report (*continued*)

Discussion: Nurse scientists and researchers live in a relative world; therefore, a project's findings do not "prove" anything. Answers to a research question should provide a more complete understanding of the identified problem. A study's findings aid in confirming or rejecting the hypothesis.

Example: Results showed a significant decrease in mean systolic blood pressure, pulse rate, and respiration rate after intervention in the two groups, compared to before intervention ($P = 0.001$), but the mean difference was not significant before and after intervention between the two groups. Results showed a significant correlation between the plasma cortisol level and the anxiety score before intervention ($r = 0.566$, $P < 0.001$) as well as after intervention ($r = 0.536$, $P < 0.001$). In fact, the subjects with higher plasma cortisol obtained higher scores on the Spielberger anxiety questionnaire (which shows their higher anxiety). There was a significant correlation between mean difference of plasma cortisol and anxiety score ($r = 0.355$, $P < 0.001$).

Discussion

Definition: The discussion section interrupts the significance of the findings in light of what is already known about the research topic.

Key Questions for Analysis:

- Are key findings discussed within the context of prior research related to the topic?
- Are the study's limitations presented?
- Are recommendations or implications for nursing care discussed?
- *Based on the overall quality of the research, would you be comfortable using the findings to initiate or contribute to practice change?*

Discussion: The discussion section is not rote reporting of objective, numeric information. A well-done discussion section provides nurses a means to critically think about an evidence-based interpretation and application of findings.

Example: Our study provides valuable insight into the adherence behaviors and personal perceptions about diabetes medication taking among African Americans with type 2 diabetes living in economically distressed rural counties in southeastern North Carolina. The majority of participants in this study (62%) reported low levels of adherence to their diabetes medications, while 30% indicated moderate adherence. Only 5% reported high levels of adherence. This finding contrasts with previous research by Mann, Ponieman, Leventhal, & Halm. (2009), where the majority of predominantly African American and Latino patients receiving care through a primary care clinic in New York reported higher levels of adherence (72%) to their diabetic medications. This finding may reflect increased resources available in urban areas. In this study, diabetes control was significantly poorer in males than females. The finding is consistent with previously published research that found female gender was associated with increased glycemic control in a family medicine practice in North Carolina (Blackmon, Laham, Taylor, & Kemppainen, 2016).

BOX 8.2   Guidelines for Analyzing a Qualitative Research Report

I. The *Introduction Section* establishes the context and significance of the exploration into individual experiences, discovery of meaning, or theory development. It usually includes background information and the current nature of understanding the phenomenon of interest. It may include a statement of the phenomenon of interest or a problem statement, the purpose or significance of the study, and the conceptual framework, if used. Qualitative research may or may not have a research question.

(continued)

BOX 8.2   Guidelines for Analyzing a Qualitative Research Report *(continued)*

Phenomenon of Interest Statement

Defined: The statement of the phenomenon of interest identifies the abstract encounters or experiences to be observed or explored.

Key Questions for Analysis:

- Does the statement of the phenomenon of interest identify the specific area of exploration for a specific population or group of individuals?

- Does the statement of the phenomenon of interest clearly indicate significance to nursing?

- Is the context for the phenomenon of interest identified?

- If a research question is proposed, does it clearly link to the phenomenon of interest?

Discussion: Qualitative research is dependent on acknowledgment of a subjective reality; therefore, the phenomenon of interest may be sufficiently abstract. Although qualitative research is not intended to be generalizable to the population, the area of interest should be of concern to nursing and provide useful insight and knowledge to the body of evidence in the care of specific individuals or groups of patients.

Example: Dementia is characterized by nonreversible cognitive decline. Approximately 11% (5 million people) of older adults over 65 years old in the United States have dementia, and with the aging population, the number is expected to triple by 2050 (Alzheimer's Association, 2013). Caregivers of individuals with dementia must endure continuous cycles of physical, psychological, financial, and emotional challenges related to long-term dementia care. However, variations in reports of caregiver experiences exist from negative to positive. These variations can be somewhat explained by the ways in which caregivers derive meaning from their particular caregiving situations (Ayres, 2000; Kim, Shultz, & Carver, 2007). Finding meaning is considered a critical aspect of being able to grow as a result of stressful events (Davis & Morgan, 2008), and the meaning an individual attributes to a circumstance plays a significant role in his or her affective responses to the situation (Frankl, 1959; Shim, Barroso, Gilliss, & Davis, 2013)

Purpose Statement

Defined: The purpose statement can be considered the research question. It is the specific aim that reflects the phenomenon of interest and drives the research.

Key Questions for Analysis:

- Is the purpose of the research clearly identified?

- Does the purpose statement reflect the need for a qualitative approach?

Discussion: Because qualitative research is exploratory, there is usually no hypothesis; however, the purpose statement directs the methods to best explore the phenomenon of interest.

Example: Thus, the purpose of this study was to describe the experience of spousal caregivers of individuals with dementia who reported having found meaning in their care. Understanding how these caregivers found meaning in their caregiving experiences may reveal insights or strategies that can be helpful to other caregivers who may be struggling to find meaning of their own (Shim et al., 2013).

Literature Review

Defined: The literature review is a systematic appraisal of the body of research and other scholarly work that addresses the phenomenon of interest.

(continued)

BOX 8.2 Guidelines for Analyzing a Qualitative Research Report (*continued*)

Key Questions for Analysis:

- Is a literature review present?

- Does the body of literature represented in the review adequately and objectively establish current understanding or emerging themes for the phenomenon of interest?

- Does the literature review help illustrate the need for exploration into the phenomenon of interest?

Discussion: Because qualitative research is concerned with inductive reasoning and exploration, the literature review may not be present prior to data collection and analysis.

Example: The measures to prevent surgical site infection (SSI) are well established, and professionals should know and implement them while providing healthcare (Harrop et al., 2012). Specific protocols for orthopedic units include actions regarding internal procedures and strategies for epidemiological surveillance (Răuția & Nemet, 2015). However, a literature review on the characteristics of studies that addressed readmissions for SSI after orthopedic surgeries did not find studies that assessed the repercussions for affected individuals (Torres, Turrini, Merighi, & Cruz, 2015). Pujol et al. (2015) highlight the importance of investigating revision surgery and its consequences at the global level. From the individual's perspective, being in the hospital represents a major disruption in routine (Santos & Carlo, 2013), even with scientific and technological advances in health recovery (Sanches et al., 2013). In this context, the associated physical frailty and emotional vulnerability are potential problems that the individual must experience in the presence of strangers. For example, few studies have demonstrated experiences related to being in a hospital due to SSI, regardless of being the first hospitalization in people's lives or subsequent occurrences. However, admissions or readmissions are unique experiences that do not repeat in the same manner. The results of a qualitative study that analyzed 14 testimonials from individuals who developed SSIs detected significant pain, isolation, insecurity, and negative economic, social, physical, and emotional impacts, some of which were long-standing (Andersson, Bergh, Karlsson, & Nilsson, 2010). Seventeen patients who underwent surgery in three hospitals in the United Kingdom reported experiencing despair and a desire to die when describing how SSIs affected their lives and the lives of their family members (Tanner, Padley, Davey, Murphy, & Brown, 2013; Torres, Turrini, & Merighi, 2017).

Theoretical or Conceptual Framework

Defined: A theoretical or conceptual framework is used to frame the study, providing boundaries for understanding concepts and providing focus about the phenomenon of interest. The theoretical or conceptual framework may also provide parameters for the methods used.

Key Questions for Analysis:

- Is a theoretical or conceptual framework identified?

- Is there rationale for using the selected theoretical or conceptual framework?

- Is the theoretical or conceptual framework described in enough detail to determine appropriate links approaching the phenomenon of interest?

Discussion: The aim of some qualitative research is to generate theory; thus, an existing theoretical or conceptual framework would not be used. Additionally, in some instances, there is not enough knowledge of the phenomenon of interest for an appropriate theoretical or conceptual framework to exist.

Example: A theoretical framework for a qualitative study can refine researchers' ideas about the topic and guide but not constrain interpretation of the data (Wu & Volker, 2009). We chose a biopsychosocial approach as a lens through which to view the participant's experience of poststroke sexuality. According to Daniluk (1998), an individual constructs a "sexual self" throughout her life, consisting of "physical and biological capacities, cognitive and emotional development and is influenced by past experiences and current circumstances" (p. 15). The sexual self is continually shaped as a woman faces new life events

(*continued*)

BOX 8.2   Guidelines for Analyzing a Qualitative Research Report *(continued)*

and developmental changes and receives messages from society about the meaning of these events and changes for her sexuality (Beal & Millenbruch, 2015; Daniluk, 1998; Koert & Daniluk, 2010).

II. The *Methods Section* should give a clear and precise description of the data collection and analysis procedures used in the study.

Research Methodology

Defined: The research methodology is the overall approach or design used in the study.

Key Questions for Analysis:

- Does the report adequately describe the chosen method?
- Does the report include justification for the methodological approach?
- Is the methodological approach consistent with what is already known about the phenomenon of interest?
- Is the methodological approach congruent with the purpose statement?

Discussion: There are a variety of approaches in naturalistic inquiry, and each reveals a certain set of beliefs. The description of the methodology should include rationale and justification for the approach that are congruent with both the purpose and the phenomenon of interest. Research methodology in qualitative research usually reflects an inductive approach.

Example: We used existing data from an ethnographic study of 30 critically ill patients who were weaning from prolonged mechanical ventilation. The dataset for the parent study included observational, interview, and medical record data. The periods of observation ranged from 3 to 65 days per patient, with a total of 655 days in the dataset for the cohort (Happ et al., 2007). We chose qualitative secondary analysis for this study because (a) the phenomena of anxiety and agitation were frequently occurring in the existing dataset, (b) the dataset was extensive, and (c) use of the dataset maximized participation of this vulnerable population (Heaton, 2004). We expanded the analysis to include questions about anxiety and agitation as common and important phenomena that occurred both within and outside of weaning events. The principal investigator (Judith Tate) and two research team members (Mary Beth Happ and Leslie Hoffman) were part of the original study team; three members with prior qualitative experience were involved in analysis (Judith Tate, Mary Beth Happ, and Annette Devito Dabbs). We conducted fieldwork from November 2001 to July 2003 (J. Tate, Dabbs, Hoffman, Milbrandt, & Happ, 2012).

Philosophical Underpinnings

Defined: Qualitative research has a rich tradition in philosophy. The philosophical underpinnings described can indicate the researcher's beliefs, goals, understandings, assumptions, worldviews, and stance that influence the approach to methodology.

Key Questions for Analysis:

- Is a philosophical approach identified?
- If a philosophical approach is identified, is it described in adequate detail to facilitate understanding?
- Is the rationale for the philosophical approach identified?

Discussion: The philosophical underpinnings may be explicitly presented or assumed with the research methodology. The methods used should be true to the philosophical origins.

(continued)

BOX 8.2   **Guidelines for Analyzing a Qualitative Research Report** (*continued*)

Example: An example is qualitative research with a phenomenological focus based on Martin Heidegger's theoretical framework. This framework has been shown to be consistent with and adequate for nursing research because of its humanistic principles and study domains, which involve the theory and practice of care as an attempt to understand how phenomena impact the health of individuals, their families, and the community (de Paula, Padoin, Terra, Souza, & Cabral, 2014). A phenomenon, according to Heidegger (2008), must be understood as something that manifests in itself and that constitutes one's way of being; thus, it is understood as an encounter and not as an outward projection. First, this understanding is achieved through the factual dimension, which in our case relates to the testimonials. Next, it involves hermeneutics, which through interpreting and seeking meanings reveals the uncovered, which emerges as a phenomenon (de Paula et al., 2014). Heidegger's hermeneutics is a method of interpreting reality that leads to comprehension (Almeida, 2014). Using this process, understanding the human being who experiences a readmission for SSI after being subjected to an orthopedic surgical procedure becomes a practice of care. Because humans are not detachable from the world (Roehe & Dutra, 2014), experience affects the relationality between this individual and the surrounding readmission environment. The methodology of this study enabled an understanding of the study's subject: the readmission for SSI after an orthopedic surgical procedure, from a subjective point of view (Torres, Turrini, & Merighi, 2017).

Sample

Defined: The sample is the group of participants in the study.

Key Questions for Analysis:

- Is the sampling strategy clearly identified and appropriate?
- Are participant inclusion and exclusion criteria clearly identified?
- Is the sample size appropriate for qualitative research and method?
- Is there an indication of data saturation that explains sample size?
- Is the sample adequately described, including key characteristics that will allow for assessment of transferability?
- Do the sample and setting adequately represent those who will be able to provide insight into the phenomenon of interest?

Discussion: In qualitative research, the individuals participating in the study are known as participants, as opposed to subjects. They are purposefully recruited to provide insight because of their specific experience with the phenomenon of interest. Sample size in qualitative research is usually, practically, and intentionally small, and should not be considered a limitation, as the objective is not generalization of findings, but transferability. Data saturation is noted to occur when the researcher has reason to believe no new information is emerging from participants about the phenomenon of interest.

Example: Inclusion criteria were to be an adult (18 years or older) parent of a child (of any age ranging from infancy through adulthood) who had been diagnosed with Prader-Willi syndrome (PWS) and able to converse in English. A flyer announcing the study had the researcher's contact information. Interested individuals contacted the researcher to volunteer and were enrolled sequentially. There were 15 mothers and 5 fathers. They resided in rural, suburban, and urban areas throughout New York State. Occupations varied with 53% ($n = 8$) of mothers reporting that they were not working so as to care for their young child with PWS. All self-declared themselves as non-Hispanic/Caucasian. The ages of their children with PWS ranged from 2 to 17 years. They were diagnosed before entering school. All of the children with PWS lived at home except one who attended a residential school setting but still

(continued)

BOX 8.2   Guidelines for Analyzing a Qualitative Research Report (*continued*)

returned home for periods of time. All had other children living in the home except for one who had other grown children living outside of the home. Saturation of data was achieved at 20 participants (Vitale, 2016).

Ethical Considerations

Defined: For the purpose of critique, ethical considerations comprise the processes in place to assure adherence to ethical principles and protection of participants from harm.

Key Questions for Analysis:

- Were participants fully informed about the research purpose and methods?
- How was the autonomy and confidentiality of participants ensured?
- Was appropriate permission granted for undertaking the study?

Discussion: There are unique ethical considerations and dilemmas in qualitative research that require specific assurances. Data are usually generated from a small number of participants through interviews or observation, where there is no anonymity and there is expectation that the participants share personal, potentially uncomfortable experiences. Researchers must ensure informed consent, have a plan for managing potential participant distress, and assure that data generated will not be disseminated in such a manner as to reveal their identity. Institutional board review must be explicit in the report of research.

Example: A qualitative descriptive study was used to determine nurses' perceptions of family practice (FP) in an emergency department where a FP protocol has been well established. The study was approved by the appropriate institutional review boards. Subjects signed written consent forms prior to participating in the study (Lowry, 2012).

Data Collection

Defined: Data collection refers to the strategies used to collect or generate data about the phenomenon of interest.

Key Questions for Analysis:

- Are data collection strategies described?
- Are data collection strategies appropriate for capturing the phenomenon of interest?
- Is the role of the researcher in collection of data described?
- Were data collection strategies consistent with the method?
- What were the steps used to ensure accuracy of the data?
- Does the author describe the role of the researcher in the study?

Discussion: Data collection in qualitative research is usually accomplished through structured or semistructured interviews (individual and/or focus groups, face to face, or technologically mediated); nonnumerical questionnaires with open-ended, narrative responses; text documents; or observation. The data collection strategy should be consistent with the methodological approach and philosophical underpinnings, and the rationales for the decisions made should be clearly presented. In qualitative approaches, the researcher as interviewer is integrated into data collection. The report should address any steps the researcher undertook to reduce bias in data collection and analysis.

(*continued*)

BOX 8.2   Guidelines for Analyzing a Qualitative Research Report *(continued)*

Example: Data were collected over an 18-month period between 2013 and 2015. In-depth interviews (unstructured and semistructured) were used as the main tool for data collection. The first stage of data collection consisted of unstructured interviews, using open-ended questions: What is your experience with sexuality in the nursing home? After the performance of unstructured interviews, a first analysis was performed with the participant covering thematic development and the clarification of themes. After that, it was necessary to deepen our understanding of several relevant topics that arose and required further study. Thus, it was necessary to include a second stage of data collection. The second stage consisted of semistructured interviews based on a question guide, in order to gather information regarding specific topics of interest (Box 8.1).

During interviews, study participants vividly described their experiences and perspectives to the researchers. All residents participating in the study were asked to write personal letters or share extracts from their journals related to the study subject (their experience regarding sexuality within the nursing home), which were part of the analyzed data. During both stages, personal documents (letters and journal extracts) were collected, provided by participants, together with researcher field notes. Throughout data collection, these sources supported the previous ones and were often used for triangulation.

The interviews were audio-recorded and transcribed verbatim. Thirteen of the residents were interviewed twice. For eight of these cases, a repeat interview was necessary because of interruptions by visiting relatives; for another three, the first interview was stopped due to exhaustion; and in two cases a medical situation arose during the interview. Ultimately, a total of 33 interviews took place, producing a total of 45.58 hours of recordings. Ten personal letters and six journal entries were collected from the residents, together with the researcher's field notes (Palacios-Ceña et al., 2016).

Data Analysis

Defined: Data analysis is the process used to transform and organize raw data into themes or other formats for final presentation. Data analysis is also concurrent with data collection.

Key Questions for Analysis:

- Is the data analysis method adequately described in enough detail to be repeated?
- Is the data analysis method consistent with the method and approach?
- Is the data analysis method consistently and appropriately applied?

Discussion: There are a variety of structured and unstructured data analysis approaches in qualitative research, including computer software. Data analysis is usually described in terms of coding, or constant comparison. Data analysis is the key feature of qualitative research, and the processes that led to theme emergence should be sufficiently detailed for the reader to assess the outcomes in light of the generated data. Data analysis should also be consistent with the methodological approach and philosophical underpinnings.

Example: We conducted qualitative coding of text and matrices within and between cases. The units of analysis were phrases and sentences that described dimensions of anxiety or agitation. Once we completed descriptions and coding for several cases, we compared cross-case events of anxiety and agitation. Each event generated questions such as, "What is going on here?" "With whom?" and "What are the circumstances?" (Kools, McCarthy, Durham, & Robrecht, 1996). Patterns within and between cases were examined using constant comparative analysis (Strauss & Corbin, 1990). This led to the collapsing of codes into themes or categories. We saw no new themes or patterns. We examined graphic displays of data to confirm patterns (see Figure 8.1). For instance, sedation and analgesia administration were redisplayed in a graphic, with an overlay of anxiety descriptions. The analytic process also included diagramming relationships between concepts (J. Tate et al., 2012).

(continued)

BOX 8.2   Guidelines for Analyzing a Qualitative Research Report *(continued)*

III. The *Results Section* presents the findings and outcomes of the study.

Findings

Defined: Findings in qualitative research can be stories, themes, or descriptions that represent a description or interpretation of the final outcome.

Key Questions for Analysis:

- Are major themes described?
- If there are excerpts of data, do they represent the theme appropriately?
- Do the findings seem to reflect accurate interpretation and conceptualization?
- Do the findings adequately capture meaning and give a clear picture?

Discussion: Qualitative findings are usually presented as themes, with narrative quotes from the participants as examples of data related to each theme.

Example: The flipside of the problem was the parents' right to express their joy. They felt like they had to put a lid on their feelings in case these were seen to be inappropriate in an open-spaced environment with other ill infants and their families. One father to a 3.5 months premature girl expressed this concern as follows:

"You felt like you didn't have the right to smile. The baby was certainly very small but you still had to change [her] diaper, and you'd feel good about it all. But there were other parents who were sitting down and crying nearby over a faulty heart valve and you knew they were facing very serious problems."

Several of the parents aired their frustrations over the lack of privacy to express their joy and sorrow. Many of them experienced difficulties with witnessing expressions of joy and sorrow from others. One mother had the following experience when accessing the kitchen for parents:

"That was the only place you could go if you had company, so you could risk going out there and finding a party with about 15 people in full swing, presents being unwrapped and a lot of congratulations, and I just wanted to scream, just scream at them to disappear."

Another mother who had her infant in one of the smaller rooms described the value of being able to hide away. She was on her way to the milk kitchen and described the sound of another mother crying that forced her to turn around without getting the milk she required:

"When you've experienced several crises and lived through several incidents and are trying to regain your composure, it doesn't take a lot to tip you off balance again, like [hearing] deep sobbing from a mother. It goes straight to your heart and deeply affects you." (Beck, Weis, Greisen, Andersen, & Zoffman, 2009)

Discussion

Defined: The discussion offers a description of the findings that is placed back in the context of what is known about the phenomenon of interest.

Key Questions for Analysis:

- Is discussion of the findings placed in the context of the previous literature review?
- Does discussion of the findings reflect the original purpose/significance of the study?

Discussion: If a literature review was not provided as part of the background for the study, then it may be done for the first time as part of the discussion. The discussion should clearly link the findings to the statement of purpose.

(continued)

BOX 8.2 Guidelines for Analyzing a Qualitative Research Report *(continued)*

Example: Despite the limitations, these findings have implications for helping healthcare personnel who care for veterans with combat experience. They also offer insights that are useful to the American Academy of Nursing's "Have you ever served in the military?" campaign (Collins, Wilmoth, & Schwartz, 2013). An affirmative response to "Have you ever served in the military?" requires follow-up questions about whether individuals have deployed, and if yes, further inquiry to understand their deployment experience and the potential for hidden or invisible combat-related injuries. Although the visible wounds of war gain attention (e.g., amputations and disfigurement), they affect fewer than 1,700 service members (0.06% of those deployed to combat; Fischer, 2015). By contrast, hidden or invisible injuries (e.g., posttraumatic stress disorder, chronic pain, binge drinking, and sleep problems) have affected more than 100,000 service members (Crum-Cianflone, Powell, LeardMann, Russell, & Boyko, 2016; Fischer, 2015). The prevalence of invisible injury diagnoses after combat deployment is estimated to be 12% to 29% (Cesur, Sabia, & Tekin., 2013; Jennings, Melvin, & Belew, 2017)

Trustworthiness

Defined: Trustworthiness refers to the establishment of integrity, or rigor, of the study though various criteria.

Key Questions for Analysis:

- Does the study report efforts to assure quality in the documentation of the process steps, of the data, and of interpretation of the data?
- Does the study discuss elements of trustworthiness including credibility, dependability, confirmability, and transferability?
- Are limitations of the study addressed?

Discussion: There are multiple ways to demonstrate trustworthiness in qualitative approaches that may be integrated into different sections of the report, or may be presented in a separate section. There are also various criteria that may be used both in the report of and in appraisal of the study. The decisions and actions of the researcher should be explicit. Criteria commonly used include credibility (consistency of participant views and researcher representation of them), dependability (sufficient information and detail of decisions made about methods), transferability (sufficient detail of context to allow for application of findings), and confirmability (consistency of interpretation and conclusions with the data). These are demonstrated through reporting on specific practices of the researcher.

Example: We maintained methodologic rigor and trustworthiness in four ways (Lincoln & Guba, 1985; Morse & Field, 1995; Sandelowski, 1986). An audit trail of methodologic notes and analytic memos was recorded systematically to detail thoughts and establish dependability. Multiple data sources were cross-checked or triangulated to support confirmability. Credibility was established through member checks with five clinician participants and consultation with critical care colleagues to determine if the analysis accurately reflected critical care practice. Prolonged engagement within the intensive care unit enhanced the potential to achieve a thorough understanding of the phenomenon. Weekly analysis meetings established credibility and fittingness as findings were validated (Morse & Field, 1995); this included review and critique of analytic lines as the analysis progressed. The purposive sample as well as thick descriptive data and rich description of context established transferability (J. Tate et al., 2012).

Conclusions, Implications, and Recommendations

Defined: The conclusion provides key summary points and specifies how the new information about the phenomenon of interest is of value to nursing and healthcare.

(continued)

BOX 8.2   Guidelines for Analyzing a Qualitative Research Report (*continued*)

Key Questions for Analysis:

- Is the importance of the findings identified?

- Are the implications of the findings identified?

- Are recommendations for further exploration or for patient care provided?

- *Based on the overall quality of this research, would you be comfortable using the findings to initiate or contribute to practice change?*

Discussion: The last section of the report should offer the reader more than just a summary or highlights of the implications for practice. It should convey the significance of the study and how it contributes to nursing knowledge. Recommendations for innovative or expanded ways to approach the phenomenon of interest that reflect the objectives of study are usually included.

Example: This qualitative descriptive study adds to the body of knowledge about the postoperative distress of patients and caregivers after orthopedic ambulatory surgery and how they manage symptoms, which is a unique focus. Nurses and other healthcare providers do not fully assess home readiness (e.g., knowledge of or skill in using assistive devices). This is a new finding that has far-reaching implications to alleviate the distress of patients at home. A more holistic educational approach is needed for these patients, with multidisciplinary involvement (e.g., surgeons, anesthesia professionals, physical therapists, athletic trainers, nurses, and pharmacists). The authors plan to design an interventional study using the knowledge gained from this study to increase the self-management of symptoms and quality of life and decrease the intensity of symptoms such as pain (Odom-Forren, Reed, & Rush, 2017).

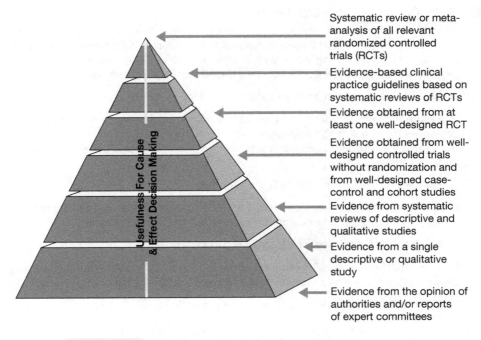

FIGURE 8.1   Hierarchy of evidence for quantitative research

Source: From Fineout-Overholt, Melnyk, and Schultz (2005).

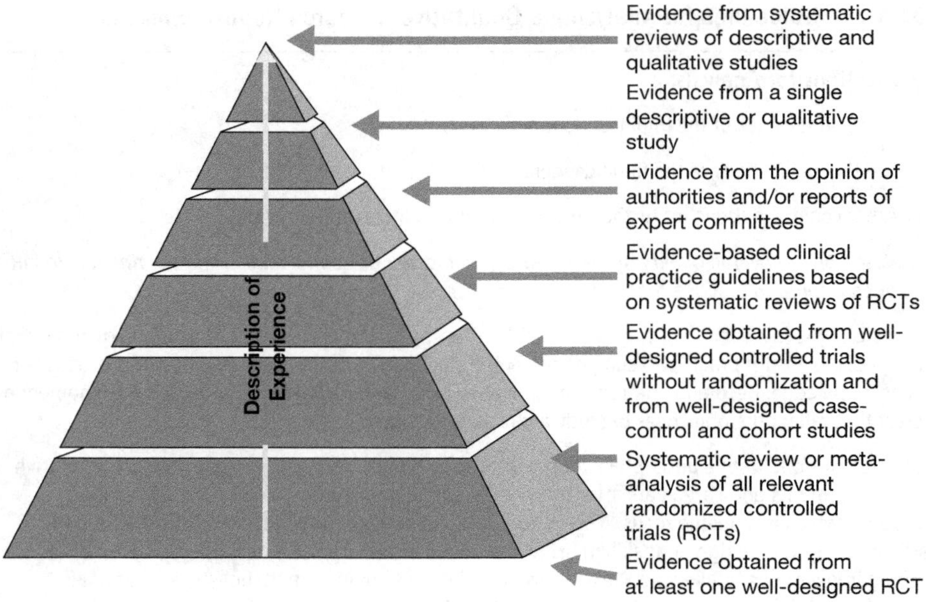

FIGURE 8.2   **Hierarchy of evidence for qualitative research**

Source: From Fineout-Overholt et al. (2005).

BOX 8.3   **Quantitative Research Designs**

- **Descriptive:** Seeks to portray the present status of a phenomenon and the frequency with which a phenomenon occurs. A hypothesis is not seen with a descriptive study; however, information gleaned from descriptive studies often generates hypotheses for future research.

  - Example: Description of tobacco use habits of middle-school students.

- **Correlational:** Seeks to determine the extent of a relationship between two or more variables. Determines the type of relationship (i.e., positive or negative) and the strength of the relationship. Helps to detect trends and patterns of phenomena but does not attempt to find cause and effect.

  - Example: The relationship between EI and self-esteem.

- **Quasi-experimental:** Seeks to identify cause-and-effect relationships for intervention studies but does not have the benefit of random assignment to control and treatment groups.

  - Example: The effect of gender on RN-NCLEX® pass rates.

- **Experimental:** Seeks to establish cause and effect. Considered the only form of true experimental study because participants are randomized to control and treatment groups.

  - Example: Differences in temperature perception comparing patients with fibromyalgia and healthy controls).

> **BOX 8.4 Qualitative Research Approaches**
>
> - **Ethnography:** Originated in the discipline of anthropology. Seeks to explore cultures and communities through the collection, description, and analysis of data and artifacts to develop deeper understandings of cultural behavior.
>
>   - Example: Medication communication among nurses, physicians, pharmacists, and patients.
>
> - **Phenomenology:** Originated in phenomenological philosophy. Seeks to describe the meaning, structure, and essence of experiences as they are lived by participants without recourse to a researcher's theories, assumptions, or deductions.
>
>   - Example: The experience of living with persistent hiccups.
>
> - **Grounded Theory:** Originated in the social sciences. Inductive research that seeks to explain what has been observed about problems that exist in society and strategies for coping with identified problems.
>
>   - Example: Men in nursing and their development of professional relationships.
>
> - **Case Study:** Seeks to provide an in-depth description or analysis for understanding a single aspect of a phenomenon. The case may be an individual, family, social unit, process, or activity.
>
>   - Example: Bridging the gap in discharge planning for homeless HIV patients and community psychosocial services.
>
> - **Narrative Inquiry:** Originated in the social sciences and literary criticism. Seeks to interpret human phenomenon through examination of personal stories and narratives.
>
>   - Example: Parent stories of the decision to vaccinate their children.
>
> - **Historical:** Seeks to systematically explore causes, effects, and trends of past events through examination of narrative artifacts to help understand present phenomena and anticipate future phenomena.
>
>   - Example: Historical study of treatments for intractable cancer pain.

HELPFUL SUGGESTIONS FOR REVIEWING RESEARCH ARTICLES

1. Assess the title of the article to determine if the article is aligned with your phenomenon of interest. Do a quick check to see if concepts in the title are present in the research question or hypothesis. This will help you assess the author's fidelity with conceptual usage.
2. Consider the authors, their institutional affiliations, and the funding sources. This will assist you in determining if biases may occur in the study. For example, if a hospital bed comfort study was funded by a mattress company, then the rigor of the study should be a priority concern to determine if biases occurred in the study's design.
3. Read the article's abstract to determine if the study is truly aligned with your phenomenon of interest. The article should not be discounted if the outcomes do not align with your question or hypothesis. Finding conflicting results is an important aspect of a literature review in EBP. It is important to remember that authors generally do not convey a study's flaws and limitations in an abstract, which means it is imperative to read beyond the abstract.
4. Determine what question the researcher is attempting to answer.

5. Read the introduction and background to the research study. This section should provide foundational information depicting why the research was conducted. Is the study needed (what is the significance of the problem)? What is the theory/framework that the study is based on? Are the concepts in the framework the same as those in the problem statement? Does the synthesis of the literature identify the strengths/weaknesses and gaps of previous studies? The literature review is generally composed of articles published within the last 3 to 5 years. However, it may take 2 years or longer to get an article published, which may make some of the literature in the review seem outdated for the topic.

6. Methodology: What is the design of the study? Based on the information provided in the article, could the study be replicated? What are the study participants' demographics? Does the study's statistical analysis align with the study design?

7. Results sections: Are the findings statistically significant or statistically nonsignificant? What is the sample size? (A quantitative study may have a larger sample size than a qualitative study.) Do the results suggest an answer to the proposed research question?

8. Conclusions/discussions: How do the authors interpret the study findings? Are there other ways to interpret the findings? What do the authors propose as the next steps, and are there other future steps that are not discussed? Are the limitations of the study discussed?

SUMMARY

This chapter emphasizes the role of nurses' use of research as a component of EBP to answer practice questions, solve problems, enhance the quality of patient care, and shape important healthcare decisions. *To deliver high-quality patient care, nurses need high-quality research as a foundation for EBP*. It is important for nurses to appraise quantitative and qualitative research studies to provide the highest-quality patient-centered care. This chapter reviews basic terms and provides checklists and suggestions that support nurses in the appraisal of research prior to translating the research into practice.

REFERENCES

Almeida, F. S. (2014). Meaning and novelty of the notions of phenomenology and hermeneutics in the thought of Heidegger. *Think-Electronic Journal of FAJE, 5*, 197–207.

Alzheimer's Association. (2013). 2012 Alzheimer's disease facts and figures. Retrieved from http://www.alz.org/downloads/facts_figures_2013.pdf

American Association of Colleges of Nursing. (2004). *AACN position statement on the practice doctorate in nursing*. Washington, DC: Author.

American Association of Colleges of Nursing. (2006). *AACN position statement on nursing research*. Washington, DC: Author.

American Association of Colleges of Nursing. (2008). *The essentials of baccalaureate education for professional nursing practice*. Washington, DC: Author.

American Association of Colleges of Nursing. (2011). *The essentials of master's education in nursing.* Washington, DC: Author.

Andersson, A. E., Bergh, I., Karlsson, J., & Nilsson, K. (2010). Patients' experiences of acquiring a deep surgical site infection: An interview study. *American Journal of Infection Control, 38,* 711–717.

Ayres, L. (2000). Narratives of family caregiving: The process of making meaning. *Research in Nursing & Health, 23,* 424–434.

Beal, C., & Millenbruch, J. (2015). A qualitative case study of poststroke sexuality in a woman of childbearing age. *Journal of Obstetrical, Gynecological, and Neonatal Nursing, 44,* 228–235.

Beck, S., Weis, J., Greisen, G., Andersen, M., & Zoffman, V. (2009). Room for family-centered care: A qualitative evaluation of a neonatal intensive care unit remodeling project. *Journal of Neonatal Nursing, 15,* 88–99.

Blackmon, S., Laham, K., Taylor, J., & Kemppainen, J. (2016). Dimensions of medication adherence in African Americans with type 2 diabetes in rural North Carolina. *Journal of the American Association of Nurse Practitioners, 28*(9), 479–486.

Bolderston, A. (2008). Writing an effective literature review. *Journal of Medical Imaging and Radiation Sciences, 39*(2), 86–92. doi:10.1016/j.mir.2008.04.009

Candela, L., Gutierrez, A., & Keating, S. (2013). A national survey examining the professional work life of today's nursing faculty. *Nurse Education Today, 33,* 853–859.

Cash, P. A., Daines, D., Doyle, R. M., von Tettenborn, L., & Reid, R. C. (2009). Recruitment and retention of nurse educators: A pilot study of what nurse educators consider important in their workplaces. *Nursing Economic$ 27,* 384–389.

Cesur, R., Sabia, J. J., & Tekin, E. (2013). The psychological costs of war: Military combat and mental health. *Journal of Health Economics, 32,* 51–65.

Collins, E., Wilmoth, M., & Schwartz, L. (2013). "Have you ever served in the military?" campaign in partnership with the Joining Forces Initiative. *Nursing Outlook, 61*(5), 375–376.

Crum-Cianflone, N. F., Powell, T. M., LeardMann, C. A., Russell, D. W., & Boyko, E. J. (2016). Mental health and comorbidities in U.S. military members. *Military Medicine, 181*(6), 537–545. doi:10.7205/MILMED-D-15-00187

Daniluk, J. C. (1998). *Women's sexuality across the life span: Challenging myths, creating meanings.* New York, NY: Guilford Press.

Davidson, R. P. (1971). *A primer in theory construction.* Boston, MA: Allyn & Bacon.

Davis, C. C., & Morgan, M. S. (2008). Finding meaning, perceiving growth, and acceptance of tinnitus. *Rehabilitation Psychology, 53*(2), 128–138.

de Paula, C. C., Padoin, S. M. M., Terra, M. G., Souza, I. E. O., & Cabral, I. E. (2014). Driving modes of the interview in phenomenological research experience report. *Brazilian Journal of Nursing Research, 67,* 468–472.

de Vaus, D. A. (2001). *Research design in social research.* London, UK: Sage.

Derby-Davis, M. J. (2014). Predictors of nursing faculty's job satisfaction and intent to stay in academe. *Journal of Professional Nursing, 30,* 19–25.

Fineout-Overholt, E., Melnyk, B. M., & Schultz, A. (2005). Transforming health care from the inside out: Advancing evidence-based practice in the 21st century. *Journal of Professional Nursing, 21*(6), 335–344.

Fischer, H. (2015). *A guide to U.S. military casualty statistics: Operation Freedom's Sentinel, Operation Inherent Resolve, Operation New Dawn, Operation Iraqi Freedom, and Operation Enduring Freedom.* Retrieved from http://news.usni.org/2015/08/14/document-guide-to-u-s-military-casualty-statistics

Frank, C. A., Schroeter, K., & Shaw, C. (2017). Addressing traumatic stress in the acute traumatically injured patient. *Journal of Trauma Nursing, 24*(2), 78–84

Frankl, V. (1959). *Man's search for meaning.* Boston, MA: Beacon Press.

Glasofer, A. (2014). Searching with critical appraisal tools. *Nursing Critical Care, 9*(2), 18–22. doi:10.1097/01.CCN.0000444001.11581.a2

Gray-Miceli, D., Mazzia, L., & Crane, G. (2017.) Advanced practice nurse-led statewide collaborative to reduce falls in hospitals. *Journal of Nursing Care Quality, 32*(2), 120–125.

Hanson, D. (2017). Reducing central line-associated bloodstream infection rates in the context of a caring healing environment: A patient safety program evaluation. *Journal of Infusion Nursing, 40*(2), 101–110. doi:10.1097/NAN.0000000000000212

Happ, M. B., Swigart, V. A., Tate, J. A., Arnold, R. M., Sereika, S. M., & Hoffman, L. A. (2007). Family presence and surveillance during weaning from prolonged mechanical ventilation. *Heart & Lung, 36*(1), 47–57.

Harrop, J. S., Styliaras, J. C., Ooi, Y. C., Radcliff, K. E., Vaccaro, A. R., & Wu, C. (2012). Contributing factors to surgical site infections. *Journal of the American Academy of Orthopedic Surgeons, 20*, 94–101.

Haynes, B. (2006). Forming research questions. *Journal of Clinical Epidemiology, 59*(9), 881–886.

Heaton, J. (2004). *Reworking qualitative data.* London, UK: Sage.

Heidegger, M. (2008). *Being and time.* New York, NY: HarperPerennial.

Jennings, B. M., Melvin, K. C., & Belew, D. L. (2017). Underpadding deployment from the perspective of those who have served. *Nursing Outlook, 65*(4), 455–463. doi:10.1016/j.outlook.2016.12.005

Kaplan, L. (2012). Reading and critiquing a research report. *Americana Nurse Today, 7*(10). Retrieved from https://www.americannursetoday.com/reading-and-critiquing-a-research-article

Kerlinger, F. N. (1973). *Foundations of behavioral research* (2nd ed.). New York, NY: Holt, Rinehart and Winston.

Kim, Y., Shultz, R., & Carver, C. S. (2007). Benefit finding in the cancer caregiving experience. *Psychosomatic Medicine, 69*, 283–291.

Koert, E., & Daniluk, J. C. (2010). Sexual transitions in the lives of adult women. In T. W. Miller (Ed.), *The handbook of stressful transitions across the lifespan* (pp. 235–252). New York, NY: Springer.

Kools, S., McCarthy, M., Durham, R., & Robrecht, L. (1996). Dimensional analysis: Broadening the conception of grounded theory. *Qualitative Health Research, 3*, 312–330.

Lincoln, Y., & Guba, E. (1985). *Naturalistic inquiry* (pp. 289–331). Newbury Park, CA: Sage.

Linder, L. A., Al-Quaaydeh, S., & Donaldson, G. (2017). Symptom characteristics among hospitalized children and adolescents with cancer. *Cancer Nursing.* Advance online publication. doi:10.1097/NCC.0000000000000469

Lowry, E. (2012). "It's just what we do": A qualitative study of emergency nurses working with well-established family presence protocol. *Journal of Emergency Nursing, 38*(4), 329–334.

Mann, D., Ponieman, D., Leventhal, H., & Halm, E. (2009). Predictors of adherence to diabetes medications: The role of disease and medication beliefs. *Journal of Behavioral Medicine, 32*, 278–284.

Minnick, A. F., Norman, L. D., & Donaghey, B. (2017). Junior research track faculty in the U.S. schools of nursing: Resources and expectations. *Nursing Outlook, 65*(1), 18–26.

Monroe, T. B., Kenaga, H., Dietrich, M. S., Carter, M. A., & Cowen, S. L. (2013). The prevalence of employed nurses identified or enrolled in substance use mentoring programs. *Nursing Research, 62*(1), 10–15.

Morse, J. M., & Field, P A. (1995). *Qualitative research methods for health professionals.* Cheltenham, UK: Chapman & Hall.

Nightingale, F. (1860). *Notes on nursing: What it is and what it is not.* New York, NY: D. Appleton.

Odom-Forren, J., Reed, D. B., & Rush, C. (2017). Postoperative distress of orthopedic ambulatory surgery patients. *AORN Journal, 105*(5), 463–477.

Palacios-Ceña, D., Martínez-Piedrola, R. M., Pérez-de-Heredia, M., Huertas-Hoyas, E., Carrasco-Garrido, P., & Fernández-de-las-Peñas, C. (2016). Expressing sexuality in nursing homes. The experience of older women: A qualitative study. *Geriatric Nursing, 37*(6), 470–477.

Prufeta, P. (2017). Emotional intelligence of nurse managers: An exploratory study. *Journal of Nursing Administration, 47*(3), 134–139.

Pujol, N., Merrer, J., Lemaire, B., Boisrenoult, P., Desmoineaux, P., Oger, P., . . . Beaufils, P. (2015). Unplanned return to theater: A quality of care and risk management index? *Orthopaedics & Traumatology: Surgery & Research, 101,* 399–403.

Răuţia, C., & Nemet, C. (2015). The impact of nosocomial infections on orthopedic patients' quality of life. *Acta Medica Transilvanica, 20,* 10–12.

Roehe, M. V., & Dutra, E. (2014). Dasein, Heidegger's conception of human being. *Advances in Latin American Psychology, 32,* 105–113.

Sanches, I. C. P., Couto, I. R. R., Abrahao, A. L., & Andrade, M. (2013). Hospital treatment: Right or concession to the hospitalized user? *Science & Collective Health, 18,* 67–76.

Santos, C. A. V., & Carlo, M. M. R. P. (2013). Occupational therapy in the hospital context: An integrative literature review. *Occupational Therapy Notebooks, 21,* 99–107.

Shim, B., Barroso, J., Gilliss, C., & Davis, L. (2013). Finding meaning in caring for a spouse with dementia. *Applied Nursing Research, 26,* 121–126.

Squires, J. E., Hutchinson, A. M., Bostrom, A. M., O'Rourke, H. M., Cobban, S. J., & Estabrooks, C. A. (2011). To what extent do nurses use research in clinical practice: A systematic review. *Implementation Science, 6*(21). Retrieved from http://implementationscience.biomedcentral .com/articles/10.1186/1748-5908-6-21

Strauss, A. L., & Corbin, J. (1990). *Basics of qualitative research: Grounded theory procedures and techniques.* Newberry Park, CA: Sage.

Tanner, J., Padley, W., Davey, S., Murphy, K., & Brown, B. (2013). Patient narratives of surgical site infection: Implications for practice. *Journal of Hospital Infection, 83,* 41–45.

Tate, J., Dabbs, A., Hoffman, L., Milbrandt, E., & Happ, M. (2012). Anxiety and agitation in mechanically ventilated patients. *Qualitative Health Research, 22*(2), 157–173.

Tate, N. H., Davis, J. E., & Yarandi, H. N. (2015). Sociocultural influences on weight-related behaviors in African American adolescents. *Western Journal of Nursing Research, 37*(12), 1531–1547.

Torres, L. M., Turrini, R. N. T., & Merighi, M. A. B. (2017). Patient readmission for orthopaedic surgical site infection: An hermeneutic phenomenological approach. *Journal of Clinical Nursing, 26,* 1011–1020.

Torres, L. M., Turrini, R. N. T., Merighi, M. A. B., & Cruz, A. G. (2015). Readmission from orthopedic surgical site infections: An integrative review. *Journal of School of Nursing - University of Sao Paulo, 49,* 1008–1015.

Vitale, S. A. (2016). Parent recommendations for family functioning with Prader-Willi syndrome: A rare genetic cause of childhood obesity. *Journal of Pediatric Nursing, 31,* 47–54.

Wu, H.-L., & Volker, D. L. (2009). The use of theory in qualitative approaches to research: Application in end-of-life studies. *Advances in Nursing Science, 65*(12), 2719–2732. doi:10.1111/ j.1365-2648.2009.05157.x

Yablonsky, A. M., Barbero, E. D., & Richardson, J. W. (2016). Hard is normal: Military families' transitions within the process of deployment. *Research in Nursing and Health, 39,* 42–56. doi:10.1002/nur.21701

Yedidia, M. J., Chou, J., Brownlee, S., Flynn, L., & Tanner, C. A. (2014). Association of faculty perceptions of work-life with emotional exhaustion and intent to leave academic nursing: Report on a national survey of nurse faculty. *Journal of Nursing Education, 53,* 569–579.

CHAPTER 9

Clinical Practice Guidelines

Molly Bradshaw

Objectives

After reading this chapter, learners should be able to:

1. Explain the significance of clinical practice guidelines (CPGs)
2. Describe the relationship between CPGs and evidence-based practice (EBP)
3. Describe the Institute of Medicine (IOM) standards for CPG development
4. Discuss CPG appraisal and implementation
5. Identify factors that promote or inhibit CPG adoption

EVIDENCE-BASED PRACTICE (EBP) SCENARIOS

Scenario 1

Substance abuse is a growing clinical problem, and nurses do not assess and manage substance abuse consistently across clinical settings. To address inconsistencies of assessment and management about substance issue, nurses at a healthcare setting wrote a clinical practice guideline (CPG). The CPG provided nurses instruction on systematically screening patients for substance abuse. In addition, patients who were assessed as positive for substance abuse were provided a brief counseling session and then referral for further intervention (Tran, Stone, Fernandez, Griffiths, & Johnson, 2009). The CPG was distributed to organizational departments, and direct care nurses throughout the organization completed a substance abuse assessment and management in-service. The in-service was a half-day experience of lecture, handouts, and role play to discuss substance abuse in the community, improve knowledge on the process for screening and referral, and demonstrate brief counseling points. To assess for in-service effectiveness, nurses conducted a quality improvement (QI) chart audit before and after the in-service. The nurses assumed audit data would indicate an increase in substance abuse CPG use following the in-service. However, the post in-service chart audit demonstrated no significant changes. Screening for illicit drug abuse improved slightly; however, direct care nurses were not documenting that they offered counseling or provided referrals to patients with substance abuse concerns. What happened? There was a clinical problem, and a CPG was developed to ensure direct care nurses were providing consistency and continuity of care surrounding substance abuse. Yet, these initiatives did not seem to change nurses' clinical practice in caring for patients with substance abuse issues (Tran et al., 2009).

Scenario 2

The Centers for Medicare and Medicaid Services (CMS) identified a need to prevent recurrent hospital admissions for patients with chronic obstructive pulmonary disease (COPD), stating that COPD should be managed in outpatient settings (CMS, 2011). In 2016, the American Lung Association developed a COPD Action Plan to promote guideline adherence, improve patient self-management of symptoms, and ultimately reduce unnecessary hospital admission. Action plans are demonstrated to be an effective strategy for reinforcing patient and provider adherence to the CPG for COPD management (Choi, Chung, & Han, 2014).

A team of DNP students identified a gap in practice for a COPD patient: The outpatient pulmonology clinic was not using the new COPD action plans. With the help of nursing faculty and support of healthcare organization leadership, the DNP students developed a quality improvement project. Unlike Scenario 1, the DNP students' strategy was comprehensive. First, the DNP students completed a practice analysis to determine current practice standards of care for patients with COPD. Second, the nurses conducted a series of in-services to demonstrate proper use of COPD action plans and to follow up on barriers to using the plans in clinical practice. The nurses developed a chart flag system for reminding providers to adhere to salient points of the CPG, such as promoting smoking cessation, pneumococcal vaccination, referral to pulmonary rehabilitation, and incorporation of COPD action plans into each clinic visit.

To assess for compliance to CPG recommendations, chart audits were conducted before and after the project started. As a team, the DNP students discussed the findings and made adjustments to improve CPG compliance. The DNP students helped the unit to accomplish a successful Joint Commission on Accreditation of Healthcare Organizations review when the clinic was asked to produce documentation of utilization of COPD action plans.

Discussion

Differences in the approach to implementation of CPGs in Scenario 1 compared to Scenario 2 are salient, and the clinical outcomes and matrices are markedly different. Reasons for the success and failure between the two scenarios warrant further discussion in this chapter.

OVERVIEW OF CLINICAL PRACTICE GUIDELINES

Nurses are demonstrating commitment to EBP and the most effective methods for translating appropriate evidence into a clinical context (Kitson & Harvey, 2016). CPGs are an effective method to facilitate appropriate patient-centered care based on best evidence and broad expert consensus. CPGs are systematically and rigorously developed clinical recommendations intended to optimize patient care (IOM, 2011). The content of credible CPGs arises from systematic reviews of clinical evidence and is designed to support healthcare providers in making specific patient care decisions (Taylor, 2014). Use of CPGs helps limit unscientific variation in practice and enable healthcare team members to use sound clinical decision-making criteria (IOM, 2011). In addition, credible CPGs promote the practice of high-quality evidence-based healthcare and provide a means to underscore nurses' responsibilities and accountabilities for clinical decision making (Thomas, 1999).

Healthcare providers have used guidelines as a means for making clinical decisions for centuries to guide the diagnosis, management, and care of patients (IOM, 2011). Guidelines, prior to systematic reviews (circa 1980), were based on specialist opinions and traditions. The first formalized CPGs in nursing emerged in the early 1980s with the 10 nursing care interventions outlined by the Conduct and Utilization of Research in Nursing (CURN) project (Haller, Reynolds, & Horsley, 1979). In the 21st century, clinical practice guidelines have become widely used in nursing to promote EBP and improve patient care outcomes. In fact, many nurses in healthcare organizations have developed CPGs as a means for direct care nurses to efficiently use EBP in clinical decision making (Mackey & Bassndowski, 2016).

The growing demand for high-quality interventions in healthcare helped bring about an escalation of clinical guideline development (Figure 9.1). In 2011, the Guidelines International Network (GIN) and the National Guideline Clearinghouse (NGC) accommodated 3,700 and 2,700 guidelines, respectively, in their databases (IOM, 2011). Currently, those numbers have more than doubled. With rapid development of CPGs, it is challenging to determine which guidelines are of high quality (IOM, 2011). If CPGs are unsystematically developed, based on weak evidence, and improperly disseminated, they are unhelpful in

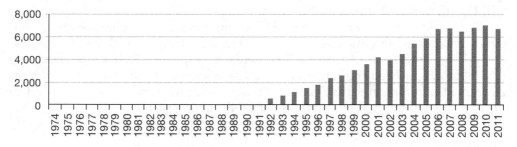

Derived from: U.S. National Library of Medicine National Institutes of Health
PubMed.gov, available at: http://www.ncbi.nlm.nih.gov/pubmed.

FIGURE 9.1 Number of clinical practice guidelines from 1974 to 2011

Source: Reprinted with permission from Taylor (2014).

clinical practice and create untoward outcomes for patients (IOM, 2011; Woolf, Grol, Hutchinson, Eccles, & Grimshaw, 1999).

A provision of the Medicare Improvements for Patients and Providers Act of 2008 recommended the Institute of Medicine (IOM) develop standards for both systematic review of evidence and CPG development. As an outcome of this recommendation, in March 2011 the IOM released a report titled *Clinical Practice Guidelines We Can Trust*, which can be accessed in full and without cost at www.nationalacademies. org/hmd/Reports/2011/Clinical-Practice-Guidelines-We-Can-Trust.aspx. In the next section, the IOM standards for CPG development are reviewed.

CLINICAL PRACTICE GUIDELINE DEVELOPMENT

CPGs are developed locally (e.g., internal guidelines) or regionally/nationally (e.g., external guidelines). CPGs are generally developed by national groups such as the Oncology Nursing Society or the American Thoracic Society (National Institutes of Health, 2015). Local CPGs often require fewer resources and are adopted into practice more rapidly related, in part, to local ownership. Local CPGs are sometimes developed by groups who do not have a requisite skillset to develop sound, credible guidelines. A reasonable alternative to local CPG development is use of regional and national guidelines with subsequent adoption and modification at the local level to suit organization-specific circumstances.

The purpose of developing a CPG must be clearly articulated and include the population and audience for the CPG's intended use. Absolute transparency in CPG development is critical. Transparency includes public awareness that the CPG development team is clinically diverse, free of conflicts of interest, and has a credible and well-established process for systematic review of relevant evidence. Presentation of the final CPG must be concise, visually appealing, and user friendly (IOM, 2011). As CPG standards are introduced throughout this section, clinical examples illustrate salient concepts.

IOM Standard 1: Establishing Transparency

The IOM defines *Standard 1: Establishing Transparency* as making sure that when a CPG is developed, the process used to develop it is open to the public and explained in detail (IOM, 2011). Understanding the CPG process provides context to help ascertain quality. Transparency provides healthcare providers an opportunity to fully assess for CPG trustworthiness, thus enabling providers to make informed decisions about whether or not to use/adopt a CPG recommendation. *Transparency is required in all steps of the CPG development process* (Talwalkar, 2014).

In commitment to EBP, consider this situation. A registered nurse (RN) has a new job in the emergency department (ED). The RN quickly observes that it is more difficult to get intravenous (IV) access in the ED patient population than on general medical unit patient populations, especially during codes. Nurse and physician colleagues are giving tips and advice, and saying to the RN, "This is the way we've always done it." But, the RN is determined to know what *best evidence* recommends for best practice IV insertion in the ED.

The RN notices the hospital's policy on starting IVs has no reference list, which raised concern because it is unknown who wrote the policy, how recommendations were determined, or if the policy is current. In other words, the information is untrustworthy. The RN decides to turn to a professional organization, the Emergency Nurses Association (ENA). On the ENA website, the RN finds a CPG titled *Difficult Intravenous Access* (ENA, 2015). The CPG is referenced, has full disclosure of how it was developed, and has a short version for use at the patient's bedside. This concise CPG boosts the confidence of the RN. The information is trustworthy. Examine the guideline *Difficult Intravenous Access* at www.ena.org/practice-research/research/CPG/Pages/Default.aspx. Do you agree?

IOM Standard 2: Management of Conflict of Interest (COI)

A COI is defined as a relationship or reason that may contribute to biasing a person's judgment (Cosgrove et al., 2017). COI is an ongoing concern in both clinical research and development of CPGs (Ross, Gross, & Krumholz, 2012). COI engenders mistrust in the healthcare system for both healthcare providers and patients (Perry, Cox, & Cox, 2014). Consider the example, in Standard I, about IV access. If you were asked to select a team to revise or develop a new CPG about IV insertion, which person(s) is least likely to have a potential conflict: (a) a nurse-manager with 25 years of ED experience, (b) a direct care nurse who is married to the salesman for the IV company, or (c) a physician who is paid to promote a topical anesthetic cream for IV insertion?

The IOM (2011) *Standard 2* addresses the *Management of Conflicts of Interest* by making four specific recommendations:

1. Before selecting a team to develop a CPG, each potential team member must disclose current financial, intellectual, organizational, and patient/public activities pertinent to the CPG (IOM, 2011).
2. When the COIs are disclosed, each team member must explain how the relationship might affect the work.
3. Team members must divest themselves of conflicts of interest.
4. Team members with a COI should be excluded or at least not represent the majority of the group.

Several federal mandates, such as the *Sunshine Act* (2010) and the *Patient Protection and Affordable Care Act* (2010), require improved disclosure procedures, specifically of financial relationships between industry and healthcare providers (Perry et al., 2014). Conflicts of interest may exist in terms of academic, political, social, or personal relationships. Transparency, full disclosure, and careful selection of team members promote development of trustworthy CPGs.

IOM Standard 3: Guideline Development Group Composition

Referring to the question in *Standard 2* about selecting a new team to develop a new/revised CPG for IV access, the team member least likely to have a COI is the experienced nurse manager. The direct care nurse and physician have noticeable

COIs, family influence, and financial gain, respectively. There are other important COI considerations. The IOM (2011) *Standard 3* for developing CPG, *Guideline Development Group Composition*, states that a clinically diverse group is needed. Preferably, a CPG group should be multidisciplinary and have expertise in the identified population. An ideal CPG group includes a former patient or patient representative (IOM, 2011). The organization developing the CPG must select the most appropriate and diverse team, and the authors of the CPG are acknowledged with full credentials in the publication.

Review the list of authors from the ENA guideline on *Difficult Intravenous Access* listed in Table 9.1. In this example, all levels of nursing are well represented, including ADN (associates degree in nursing), BSN (bachelor of science in nursing), MSN (master of science in nursing), DNP (doctor of nursing practice), and PhD. Because obtaining IV access has become primarily a nursing responsibility, it is logical the ENA CPG development team consisted of nurses. However, when creating CPG(s) with broad context, such as tobacco cessation or COPD, one should find greater professional diversity among the guideline developers.

The U.S. Preventive Services Task Force (USPSTF) is an example of a federal entity that appoints interdisciplinary teams to develop clinical guidelines. The USPSTF organizational mission has a strong emphasis on health promotion and disease prevention. The mission requires multidisciplinary input from

TABLE 9.1   Comparison of Guideline Development Group Composition

Title	Select Members and Their Credentials*
Difficulty With IV Access (ENA, 2015)	Anna Maria Valdez, PhD, MSN, RN, CEN, CFRN Alysa Reynolds, RN Mary Alice Vanhoy, MSN, RN, CEN, CPEN Marsha Cooper, MSN, RN, CEN Karen Gates, DNP, RN, NE-BC Mary Kamienski, PhD, APRN, CEN, FAEN, FAAN David McDonald, MSN, RN, APRN, CEN, CCNS Janis Provinse, MS, RN, CNS, CEN *This list is not comprehensive.
Title	**Select Members, Their Credentials, and Organizational Affiliation***
Behavioral and Pharmacotherapy Interventions for Tobacco Smoking Cessation in Adults (Siu, 2015)	Albert Siu, MD, MSPH: Mount Sinai School of Medicine, New York, NY James Peters, MD: Veterans Affairs Medical Center, Bronx, NY David Grossman, MD, MPH: Group Health, Seattle, WA Linda Ciofu Baumann, PhD, RN, APRN: University of Wisconsin, Madison, WI Francisco A. R. Garcia, MD, MPH: Pima County Department of Health, Tucson, AZ Michael P. Pignone, MD, MPH: University of North Carolina, Chapel Hill, NC Jessica Herzstein, MD, MPH: Independent Consultant, Washington, DC *This list is not comprehensive.

Source: Adapted from the previously referenced guidelines.

medicine, nursing, public health, and private and public entities from across the country. Compare the list of authors from the CPG, *Behavioral and Pharmacologic Interventions for Tobacco Abuse for Adults*, to the ENA group (Table 9.2). This is a salient illustration of diversity of professions, geography, and organizations in CPG development. It is understandable that a CPG developed to address tobacco cessation would have a more clinically diverse development team than a CPG developed to advise best practice for IV access.

TABLE 9.2 Comparison Grading System Definitions

ENA Grading System Definitions (Adapted from ENA, 2015)		
A	Level A (High)	Based on credible and consistently sound evidence. Evidence is appropriate for given emergency department nursing care.
B	Level B (Moderate)	Limited number of inconsistencies found in creditable research evidence. Remains appropriate for use in select emergency nursing situations.
C	Level C (Weak)	Evidence is scant and and/or primarily of low-quality. Effectiveness of evidence is yet to be soundly determined.
NR	Not recommended	Evidence is based on poor quality studies. Not recommended for practice.
I/E	Insufficient evidence	Sound evidence is lacking, therefore not recommended for practice until further quality studies are conducted.
N/E	No evidence	No existing evidence can be determined.
USPSTF Grading System Definitions (USPSTF, 2012)		
Grade A	The USPSTF recommends the service.	There is high certainty that the net benefit is substantial. Suggestion for Practice: Offer the service.
Grade B	The USPSTF recommends the service.	There is high certainty that the net benefit is moderate or substantial. Suggestion for Practice: Offer the service.
Grade C	The USPSTF recommends selectively offering this service based on professional judgment and patient preference.	There is moderate certainty the net benefit is small. Suggestion for Practice: Offer this service for selected patients depending on the individual circumstances.
Grade D	The USPSTF recommends against this service.	There is modest or high certainty that there is no net benefit or that the harms outweigh the benefits. Suggestion for Practice: Discourage use of this service.
Grade I	The USPSTF concludes the evidence is insufficient to make a recommendation.	Evidence is lacking or is of poor quality, or is conflicting, and the balance of benefits and harms cannot be determined. Suggestions for Practice: Read the clinical considerations section. If the service is offered, the patient should understand the uncertainty about the balance of benefits and harms.

ENA, Emergency Nurses Association; USPSTF, U.S. Preventive Services Task Force.

IOM Standard 4: CPG Systematic Review Intersection

Developing quality guidelines follows a process that is led by a clinical guideline development team, such as the appointed ENA team or the USPSTF group. As part of the CPG process, teams are required to have a systematic method for reviewing and appraising the quality of reviewed research. The search strategy, key terms, databases used, and inclusion/exclusion criteria must be clearly stated to promote CPG transparency and quality. Nurses should not confuse summarizing literature (i.e., literature review) with completing an actual systematic review. Literature review and systematic review are distinct concepts and should not be used interchangeably. A literature review is a much weaker source of evidence than a systematic review (see Chapter 3). The IOM (2011) *Standard 4: Clinical Practice Guideline–Systematic Review Intersection* helps distinguish the difference.

Clinical guideline development groups may systematically review evidence as a single entity or interact with a systematic review team. A systematic review team generally seeks to answer a more singular clinical question using a defined methodology, such as the *Cochrane Database of Systematic Reviews* or *Joanna Briggs Institute Database of Systematic Reviews and Implementation Reports* (refer to Chapter 3). For example, Stolz, Stolz, Howe, Farrell and Adhikari (2015) completed a systematic review and meta-analysis to determine if using ultrasound to guide IV insertion reduced the number of unsuccessful IV attempts. The question(s) analyzed in this systematic review process did not encompass the full scope of the clinical problem being examined by the ENA team who were developing a guideline on difficult IV access. The ENA guideline development group wanted to examine other strategies for IV access as well, such as skin warming, intraosseous, and subcutaneous alternatives (ENA, 2015). Therefore, the guideline development group reviewed evidence and used evidence developed by a systematic review team. On the topic of ultrasound utilization, there was an intersection between the goals of the guideline team and the systematic review team.

Evidence used to inform a guideline must meet the requirements described in the IOM (2011) *Standards for Systematic Reviews of Comparative Effectiveness Research*. The term *intersection* refers to the point at which a systematic review question meets, intersects, or aligns with the goal and scope for a clinical practice guideline. In our example, it is clear that both the ENA and the Stolz team had a common interest in improving IV access.

IOM Standard 5: Foundations for Rating Strength of Recommendations

The IOM recommendations must include a full description, expression of confidence, rating of strength, and explanation of any differences of opinion (IOM, 2011). Organizations often write more than one CPG and have developed a grading system that is used standardly for rating the strength of recommendations. Clinicians must read the definitions of the grading systems and recognize variation. As an exercise, compare and contrast the differences in the systems used by the ENA and the USPSTF (Table 9.2).

IOM Standard 6: Articulation of Recommendations

Communication impacts organizational missions, participants, and work; therefore, it is important for leaders to be clear when communicating. Clinical practice guidelines are developed, in part, by leaders in organizations or external agencies. The IOM (2011) *Standard 6: Articulation of Recommendations* states that communication should be clear, standardized, and precisely articulated to ensure compliance. The ease of use, formatting, and visual appeal are among some of the most important factors in promoting the adoption of CPGs by clinicians. Consumption of information is correlated to the clinical role, age generation, and learning preference (Bellato, 2013). Therefore, it is helpful to have multiple media to best suit the consumer.

IOM Standard 7: External Review

The purpose of external review is to allow others not associated with the CPG an opportunity to cross-check the work. In *Standard 7*, the IOM suggests that a process of external review needs to include public, individual, organizational, and governmental reviews. A record of the external feedback should be securely archived. The CPG development group should keep notes regarding any amendments or decisions about their work based on external reviewer feedback.

IOM Standard 8: Updating

According to *Standard 8: Updating* (IOM, 2011), when a CPG is published, it must include the date of publication, date of evidence review, and a proposed date for future revision. The CPG for *Difficulty With IV Access* was originally developed in 2011 and revised in 2015 (ENA, 2015). The current CPG from the USPSTF about interventions for tobacco cessation, released in 2015, was updated from 2009 recommendations (Siu, 2015). Customarily, 3 to 5 years is the time frame for CPG updates and revisions as observed by many organizations. The development of new therapies, technologies, or scientific discoveries may prompt early CPG revision. Natural disasters, epidemics, or unforeseen events may draw early attention for a need to update or revise CPGs. Recent examples of CPG revision and update include that made for Ebola and Zika virus outbreaks.

There are alarming examples of failure to update CPG in a timely manner, and guidelines are sometimes only partially updated. A classic example of CPG update misuse is the National Heart, Lung, and Blood Institute's (NHLBI) Joint National Committee (JNC) guidelines on the diagnosis and treatment of hypertension. The hypertension guidelines underwent a series of periodic revisions until 2003, which was the seventh version. The *2014 Evidence-Based Guideline for Management of Hypertension for Adults* was published by members of the JNC 8 team (James et al., 2014). An astute nurse would notice the 2014 update examined only medical management of hypertension. The hypertension CPG does not revisit every recommendation in the JNC 7 guideline, such as the hypertension diagnosis, lifestyle modification, or classification of hypertension, which are elements extremely important to nursing care. Critics commonly and acerbically refer to the full JNC 8 update as "JNC Late" (Jancin, 2013).

To summarize, IOM Standards for CPG development describe various components required to create high-quality CPGs. Other models and methodologies for CPG development exist. For example, the World Health Organization (WHO) endorses the GRADE methodology, which stands for "Grading of Recommendations, Assessment, Development and Evaluations" (Austin, Richter, & Sebelski, 2014; Davoli et al., 2014). In comparison, among CPG development guidelines there are similarities in the emphasis on transparency, process for evidence review, and recommendations for implementation. The next sections explore how topics are identified, appraised, and implemented.

Identification of Topics for Clinical Practice Guideline Development

Organizations that develop CPGs have varying systems for selecting guideline topics. For example, the American Academy of Family Physicians develop CPGs based on relevance to practice, absence of a current guideline, availability of a formal systematic review of evidence, and importance of the topic to overarching organizational strategic objectives (American Academy of Family Physicians [AAFP], 2017). The USPSTF solicits new guideline topics. USPSTF topics receive priority if topics are significant to public health and have the potential to impact clinical practice (USPSTF, 2008).

Patients and consumer advocates may also be involved in topic selection, CPG development, review, and dissemination. Consumer involvement is sometimes challenging, because consumers may not understand the technical language, science of healthcare, and/or evidence appraisal processes. However, nurses need to include consumers, as stakeholders, in CPG development whenever possible. Tong et al. (2011) recommend incorporating consumer roles in parallel to the review process and in the development of consumer information surrounding the guideline. The stakeholder-centered approach has the potential to improve guideline adherence (van Dulmen et al., 2013).

Differentiation of Clinical Practice Guidelines

Other words may seem synonymous with the term *Clinical Practice Guideline*. The key to differentiation is to understand the differences in the process for development of these recommendations, the audience they are intended for, the means in which they will be used, and the person/team developing them. A summary of clarifying definitions is offered in Table 9.3.

SOURCES OF CLINICAL PRACTICE GUIDELINES

This section explores some of the better-known sources of CPGs, which will include both national and international groups. Awareness of these organizations provides a foundational point for practitioners who seek to incorporate CPG(s) into their clinical practice.

TABLE 9.3 Clinical Practice Guideline Terms

Term	Definition
CPG	A standard developed by an organization to eliminate practice variation and improve quality of care (IOM, 2011). Guidelines are official recommendations to address a specific practice situation (Levin & Lewis-Holman, 2011). **Examples:** 1. ENA (2015) *Difficulty With Intravenous Access* 2. USPSTF (2015) *Behavioral and Pharmacotherapy Interventions for Tobacco Cessation in Adults*
Protocol	A set of specific practices to be followed that are often viewed as stricter than a guideline. The term can also refer to a description of a method to be used during a research study (Levin & Lewis-Holman, 2011). **Example:** Following surgery, the nurses follow the protocol for nine steps of prevention of deep-vein thrombosis (Van Wicklin, 2011).
Clinical pathway	A method for the patient-care management of a well-defined group of patients during a well-defined period of time (De Bleser et al., 2006, p. 553). Popular in the late 1990s, the idea was to improve quality and contain use of resources. **Example:** After coronary artery bypass surgery (well-defined group of patients), the nursing staff will follow the clinical pathway until discharge (well-defined period of time; Zevola, Raffa, & Brown, 2002).
Care plan	An individualized plan of care developed by a nurse to reflect basic nursing activity (Englebright, Aldrich, & Taylor, 2014; Radwin & Alster, 2002). **Example:** A patient wants to quit smoking, so the nurse added elements of education to the patient's care plan on smoking cessation strategies.

CPG, clinical practice guidelines.

National Guideline Clearinghouse

The U.S. Department of Health and Human Services requires the Agency for Healthcare Research and Quality (AHRQ) to lead the nation in achieving excellence in healthcare (AHRQ, 2017). The National Guideline Clearinghouse (NGC) is a subsidiary of the AHRQ. The NCG is a public resource for evidence-based CPGs and is available, free, online at www.guideline.gov.

To be published by the NGC, CPGs must meet certain inclusion criteria. In 1998, the first criteria were published and later revised when the IOM published the 2011 *Clinical Practice Guidelines We Can Trust* recommendations. The most recent revision of the guideline inclusion criteria was adopted in 2014 (NGC, 2017). According to the current standards, CPGs published by the NGC must meet six requirements:

1. Statements must be synthesized to optimize patient care and help healthcare providers make clinical decisions
2. Standard must be developed by an organization or entity, not an individual

3. Evidence must be based on systematic reviews, which include descriptions of explicit methodology
4. Harms and benefits must be assessed and a discussion of alternative care options provided
5. Full text must be provided in English
6. Guideline must be developed, revised, and/or reviewed within the last 5 years

The NGC website offers healthcare providers tools and matrices to compare and contrast guidelines. There are also commentaries from clinical experts, Rich Site Summary (RSS) feeds (i.e., a format for delivering regularly changing web content), and other relevant resources. The guidelines include issues relevant to direct care nurses, advanced practice nurses, physicians, and ancillary healthcare providers. It is imperative that nurses at all levels of practice be familiar with NCGs. Please explore this resource further at www.guideline.gov.

Professional Organizations

This chapter has examined CPGs developed by professional organizations, such as the Emergency Nurses Association and the U.S. Preventive Service Task Force. The mission, funding sources, affiliations, population(s) of interest, and members of these organizations are influential factors in setting priorities for CPGs to be developed, revised, and sustained. As CPG appraisal is introduced, notice the questions asked about the sponsoring professional organization in the AGREE II appraisal tool.

It is typical to see multiple professional organizations either work collaboratively to develop CPGs or endorse CPGs developed by others. For instance, the 2013 *Guideline for the Management of Overweight and Obesity in Adults* (Jensen et al., 2013) CPG was developed by a CPG taskforce representing the American Heart Association, American College of Cardiology, and the Obesity Society. The resultant CPG is endorsed by a number of other organizations such as the American Pharmacists Association, National Lipid Association, and The National Coalition for Women with Heart Disease (Jensen et al., 2013). To further examine this CPG, visit http://circ.ahajournals.org/content/early/2013/11/11/01.cir.0000437739.71477.ee.

Professional organizations that develop guidelines may also have a scope beyond healthcare. Consider the Veterans Administration (VA). The mission of the VA is to support veterans in a number of capacities, such as with burial benefits, mortgage insurance, and student loans (Veterans Administration, 2017). The primary healthcare goal of the VA is to support a veteran for life, starting at the time of separation from active service. To ensure quality and high standards of care, the VA has been developing CPGs since the early 1990s. The VA is an organization with a fundamental interest in a holistic view of veterans that extends beyond healthcare. Explore VA guidelines further at www.healthquality.va.gov.

G-I-N

The Guidelines International Network (G-I-N) is a global organization, founded in 2002 and dedicated to using sound evidence to improve lives (G-I-N, 2016).

The G-I-N website provides a platform for the international community to share expertise, connect with healthcare leaders, facilitate workgroups, access training opportunities, and share clinical guidelines. As of January 2017, the G-I-N guideline database housed 6,187 documents (G-I-N, 2017). G-I-N promotes implementation of science and strategies to promote use of guidelines in practice. Promoting use of guidelines is discussed further in a later section. The resources offered by G-I-N can be further investigated by accessing their website at www.g-i-n.net.

CPGs are developed to reduce inconsistent clinical practice and improve the quality of healthcare. When a clinical problem or practice gap is identified, a nurse can use CPGs to foster optimal decision making for patient care. Identifying CPG sources and understanding the processes for CPG development provide context for nurses to critically appraise guideline content. Informed decisions must be made to determine if CPG information will be used, if it should be adapted to a local context, and the best strategies for implementation in the clinical setting (Peterson et al., 2014).

GUIDELINE APPRAISAL

In 2003, the Appraisal of Guidelines for Research and Evaluation (AGREE) collaboration published an instrument to help appraise and evaluate guidelines. The AGREE II Instrument, Appraisal of Guidelines for Research and Evaluation, was revised in 2013 and currently includes 23 items divided into six domains (Brouwers et al., 2010). The domains are as follows: (a) scope and purpose, (b) stakeholder involvement, (c) rigor of development, (d) clarity of presentation, (e) applicability, and (f) editorial independence (Brouwers et al., 2010). At the AGREE organization website, free training is offered to ensure the instrument is understood and used properly. The full instrument and instructions can be accessed at www.agreetrust .org/agree-ii. Using the instrument provides a standardized method to examine the quality and scope of critical healthcare recommendations.

From a clinical perspective, the AGREE II instrument helps to clarify conflicting information. For example, there are two major CPGs about treatment of type 2 diabetes in the United States. One guideline was developed by the American Diabetes Association (ADA), and the other guideline was developed by the American Association of Clinical Endocrinology (AACE). If the AGREE II criteria were applied, one would find differences in the scope, purpose, and options for management of type 2 diabetes. The ADA sets the cost of medication as a high priority (ADA, 2017). The AACE sets obesity and weight gain as a high priority, stating those factors are more important than treatment cost (AACE, 2017). What should a healthcare provider do? Which guideline should be followed?

Imagine you are a primary care advanced nurse practitioner treating a patient with metformin who has a current A1c of 8.1 mg/dL. In this case, both diabetes guidelines recommend adding a second medication. Yet, the guidelines do not recommend the same order of add-on therapy. The ADA guideline recommends adding an inexpensive, oral sulfonylurea (ADA, 2017). But, the AACE guideline favors medications that may have a more positive effect on weight loss, such as a

GLP-1 (AACE, 2017). Understanding the values and perspectives of each organization, teased out in using the AGREE II tool, helps explain the clinical discrepancy between organizational CPG priorities. However, it is incumbent upon the nurse practitioner to take both recommendations under advisement and make the best decision for the select clinical situation. Having CPGs available does not replace the imperative need for *critical thinking*. Likewise, a CPG does not negate the importance of involving patients in their medical decision making. In this case, a collaborative decision must be made involving the provider and patient with diabetes.

In summary, the AGREE II Instrument provides a vetted series of questions to ask when evaluating CPGs. The answers to these questions may help practitioners, or an organization, determine if implementing a recommendation is appropriate within a given clinical context. The next section elaborates the challenges of guideline implementation.

GUIDELINE IMPLEMENTATION

It takes, on average, 17 years for new information to be implemented into clinical practice, even when the information is found to be of highest quality (Westfall, Mold, & Fagnan, 2007). Implementation science is a type of research consigned to the examination of best methods for efficient and effective research utilization in healthcare to promote optimal practice changes (Glasgow et al., 2012). Implementation science seeks to understand system barriers, characteristics of stakeholders, and cause/effect relationships of interventions on healthcare outcomes. Nurses educated with the DNP degree are emerging as leaders in this area of implementation science (Riner, 2015). Implementation frameworks are discussed in Chapter 13. The Promoting Action on Research Implementation in Health Services (PARIHS) and Knowledge to Action (KTA) are examples that illuminate the concept of implementation science (Kitson & Harvey, 2016).

Implementation strategies for CPGs are gaining acceptance. High-quality information helps no one if the information is not utilized. Wang, Norris, and Bero (2016) conducted a review of guidelines endorsed by the World Health Organization. The authors observed that *passive* implementation strategies, such as providing information on the Web or written handouts, were described in 21% of the published implementation strategies. Passive implementation strategies are regarded as being less effective than *active* strategies, such as audit and feedback, reminder systems, and use of champions/opinion leaders (IOM, 2011; Wang et al., 2016). Therefore, as CPGs are implemented, a multifaceted approach, including both passive and active strategies, should be used (IOM, 2011). Strategies should be expanded beyond education to include policy, financial, and even patient-mediated solutions (Wang et al., 2016).

Factors That Influence or Inhibit CPG Adoption

The IOM (2011) *Clinical Practice Guidelines We Can Trust* discussed factors that influence and inhibit adoption of guidelines in Chapter 6 of the document. The basic recommendation for implementation of a CPG requires a multidimensional approach, which targets individuals and the healthcare delivery system.

Providers are more likely to use CPGs if CPGs are trustworthy, easy to use, have clinical relevance, and are supported by a clinical leader or practice champion (IOM, 2011; Wang et al., 2016). Table 9.4 presents a summary of factors that promote and inhibit CPG adoption.

On an individual level, nurses may have a personal bias about guideline(s). If a CPG is recommending the use of medication to help a patient quit smoking cigarettes, a nurse might take issue with the recommendation based on whether or not the nurse smokes cigarettes (Ritchie, Evans, & Matthews, 2010). The literature indicates that nurses educated at the BSN level and employed by academic medical centers tend to adopt guidelines more easily (Bourgault et al., 2014). When nurses view a CPG as high priority, translation to practice more readily occurs (Ganz et al., 2013).

At an organizational level, a culture of leadership and organizational adaptability are key. Leaders must be visible, supportive, and role model the change process (see Chapter 7). Leaders, as CPG champions, must influence organizational structure by reporting to administration, ensuring follow-up, and participating in policy development. In fact, effective leadership seems to be the most reliable predictor of long-term use of a CPG (Gifford, Davies, Tourangeau, & Lefebre, 2011). The organization must ensure that training for CPG adoption is adequate and provide performance feedback that is nonpunitive (IOM, 2011).

CPGs may be translated to fit a local context. CPGs must have straightforward language and visual appeal (Saunders, 2015). Pause for a moment to consider the following statistics. In the acute care setting, patients receive the care recommended by a CPG only 54.9% of the time. In the primary care setting, providers have demonstrated an ability to deliver 61% of CPG recommendations to patients. Among mental health providers, guideline adherence occurs only 27% of the time (IOM, 2011). Clearly, it is not enough to develop a CPG; a plan for successful implementation in the local context is imperative.

The GuideLine Implementability Appraisal (GLIA)

The *GuideLine Implementability Appraisal* tool is an example of an instrument developed and validated to provide feedback to CPG developers about potential barriers of the implementation process (Shiffman et al., 2005). In GLIA, there are

TABLE 9.4 Factors That Promote/Inhibit Adoption of CPG

Promote	Inhibit
Ease of use and visual appeal	Passive distribution
Ease of access	Difficult use during direct patient care
Electronic support: EHR, CDS, CPOE	Workload and time limitations
Pilot testing	Staff readiness for change
Trustworthy development	Requirements for new skills
Support from clinical leader/champion	Lack of clinical leader/champion
Support from organization	Lack of support by organization

CDS, clinical decision support; CPG, clinical practice guidelines; CPOE, computerized provider order entry; EHR, electronic health records.
Source: Adapted from Bahtsevani et al. (2010), Bourgault et al. (2014), Gifford et al. (2011), IOM (2011), and Ploeg et al. (2010).

two domains of criteria. The CPG must meet standards for both "decidability" and "executability" to be fully ready for implementation. The GLIA has 27 questions, with the first seven questions focusing on the CPG. The remaining 20 items address readiness for implementation (Hill & Lalor, 2009; Shiffman et al., 2005). In real-world application, Hill and Lalor (2009) utilized the GLIA for the implementation of stroke guidelines. The feedback from study participants noted ease of use and practical application in planning educational sessions and other roll-out activities. Environmental surveillance and taking inventory of the resources required to implement a CPG promote adoption.

Electronic Decision Support Systems

Use of electronic medical records provides a platform for incorporation of CPGs into daily clinical practice. Healthcare providers are prompted to document key quality indicators, reminded of contraindications to practice, and assisted to make clinical decisions. Use of electronic decision support systems has a positive effect on utilization of CPG (IOM, 2011). In a systematic review, Jamal, McKenzie, and Clark (2009) examined the impact of electronic health records (EHRs), decision support systems (DSSs), and computerized provider order entry (CPOE) and noted that compliance to CPGs was increased with these systems in the majority of studies.

CPG challenges remain. For example, clinicians may lack sufficient computer skills (Toth-Pal, Wardh, Strender, & Nilsson, 2008). Computer systems may not be standardized, and in some cases they are not in use. *In the outpatient setting, only 80% of providers are using electronic documentation despite financial incentives to use them* (Monegain, 2015). Computers have not eliminated human error (Cipriano, 2011; Classen & Bates, 2011).

Still, evidence suggests that computer support systems have the potential for a positive impact on clinical tasks, such as antibiotic prescribing (Linder et al., 2009), management of patients taking nonsteroidal anti-inflammatory medication (Gill et al., 2011), and lipid management (Gill, Chen, Glutting, Diamond, & Lieberman, 2009). Certainly, organizational factors (Bourgault et al., 2014), team leadership by clinical champions (Gifford et al., 2011; Ploeg et al., 2010), and attitudes toward CPG all inform the extent of CPG adoption and utilization (Bahtsevani, Willman, Stoltz, & Ostman, 2010; Ritchie, Evans, & Matthews, 2010).

To review, recall the opening clinical scenarios in this chapter. In Scenario 1, the implementation of the CPG for tobacco cessation was not successful. In Scenario 2, the implementation and compliance to the COPD guideline were enhanced by a diverse, multifactor implementation strategy. It is important to consider what factors may influence adoption and use of a CPG as it is rolled out to healthcare providers. As translational and implementation sciences evolve, this drives the need for more doctorly educated nurses and direct care nurses who are committed to the use of evidence in practice.

LIMITATIONS OF CLINICAL PRACTICE GUIDELINES

CPGs have limitations. A CPG should never replace good judgment on behalf of the nurse or other healthcare providers. A CPG is only as "good" as the evidence and development process. This reinforces the critical need to appraise the information and determine if information is adoptable for particular clinical situations. Guidelines may set fair/unfair measures of behavior. Nurses could be legally accountable for both compliance and noncompliance to a CPG depending on the situation. In other words, nurses are not legally "safe" simply for doing everything a guideline indicates (Taylor, 2014).

It cannot be expected that every patient situation will translate perfectly into a CPG context. This is not realistic. CPGs often overlap. CPGs primarily focus on only one disease state (Woolf et al., 1999) and do not always consider comorbidities. CPGs carry a burden of cost and resources for development (Garrison, 2016) with no guarantee that they will provide a cost benefit to the healthcare organization (Drummond, 2016). CPGs can be taken out of context by nonmedical entities and demonstrate negative effects on healthcare policy, reimbursement, and other aspects of professional practice (Woolf et al., 1999).

SUMMARY

In summary, CPGs are primarily developed to improve quality by reducing variation in practice. The nurse and healthcare organization deciding to use a guideline must ensure the CPG was developed appropriately using a standardized and acceptable methodology. By understanding the factors that influence adoption and utilization of a CPG, better planning for implementation in the clinical setting can occur. Ideally, a CPG assists nurses with clinical decision making and makes the implementation of evidence-based practice easier and realistic.

REFERENCES

Agency for Healthcare Research and Quality. (2017). National guideline clearinghouse. Retrieved from https://www.guideline.gov

American Academy of Family Physicians. (2017). *Clinical practice guideline manual*. Retrieved from http://www.aafp.org/patient-care/clinical-recommendations/cpg-manual.html

American Association of Clinical Endocrinologists. (2017). AACE/ACE comprehensive type 2 diabetes management algorithm 2017. Retrieved from https://www.AACE.com/publications/algorithm

American Diabetes Association. (2017). Standards of care in diabetes care. Retrieved from http://professional.diabetes.org/content/clinical-practice-recommendations

Austin, T. M., Richter, R. R., & Sebelski, C. A. (2014). Introduction to the GRADE approach for guideline development: Considerations for physical therapist practice. *Physical Therapy, 94*(11), 1652–1659. doi:10.2522/ptj.20130627

Bahtsevani, C., Willman, A., Stoltz, P., & Ostman, M. (2010). Experiences of the implementation of clinical practice guidelines: Interviews with nurse managers and nurses in hospital care. *Scandinavian Journal of Caring Sciences, 24*, 514–522.

Bellato, N. (2013). Infographics: A visual link to learning. *ELearn, 2013*(12), 1.

Bourgault, A., Heath, J., Hooper, V., Sole, M., Waller, J., & NeSmith, E. (2014). Factors influencing critical care nurses' adoption of the AACN practice alert of verification of feeding tube placement. *American Journal of Critical Care, 23*(2), 134–143.

Brouwers, M., Kho, M., Browman, G., Burgers, J., Cluzeau, F., Feder, G., … Zitzelsberger, L. (2010). AGREE II: Advancing guideline development, reporting and evaluation in healthcare. *Canadian Medical Association Journal, 182*, e839–e842. doi:10.1503/cmaj.090449

Centers for Medicare and Medicaid Services. (2011). COPD readmission methodology report. Retrieved from https://www.cms.gov/Medicare/Quality-Initiatives-Patient-Assessment -Instruments/HospitalQualityInits/Measure-Methodology.html

Choi, J. Y., Chung, H.-I. C., & Han, G. (2014). Patient outcomes according to COPD action plan adherence. *Journal of Clinical Nursing, 23*(5/6), 883–891. doi:10.1111/jocn.12293

Cipriano, P. F. (2011). The future of nursing and health IT: The quality elixir. *Nursing Economic$, 29*(5), 282, 286–289.

Classen, D. C., & Bates, D. W. (2011). Finding the meaning in meaningful use. *New England Journal of Medicine, 365*(9), 855–858. doi:10.1056/NEJMsb1103659

Cosgrove, L., Krimsky, S., Wheeler, E., Peters, S., Brodt, M., & Shaughnessy, A. (2017). Conflict of interest policies and industry relationships of guideline development group members: A cross-sectional study of clinical practice guidelines for depression. *Policies and Quality Assurance, 24*(2), 99–115.

Davoli, M., Amato, L., Clark, N., Farrell, M., Hickman, M., Hill, S., ... Schunemann, H. (2014). The role of Cochrane reviews in informing international guidelines: A case study of using the Grading of Recommendations, Assessment, Development and Evaluation system to develop World Health Organization guidelines for the psychosocially assisted pharmacological treatment of opioid dependence. *Addiction, 110*, 891–898.

De Bleser, L., Depreitere, R., Waele, K., Vanhaecht, K., Vlayen, J., & Sermeus, W. (2006). Defining pathways. *Journal of Nursing Management, 14*, 553–563.

Drummond, M. (2016). Clinical Guidelines: A NICE way to introduce cost-effectiveness considerations? *Value in Health, 19*, 525–530.

Emergency Nurses Association (2015). Difficulty with intravenous access. Retrieved from https://www.ena.org/docs/default-source/resource-library/practice-resources/cpg/ difficultivaccesscpg.pdf?sfvrsn=9944da58_8

Englebright, J., Aldrich, K., & Taylor, C. (2014). Defining and incorporating basic nursing care actions into the electronic health record. *Journal of Nursing Scholarship, 46*(1), 50–57.

Ganz, F., Ofra, R., Khalaila, R., Levy, H., Arad, D., Kolpak, O., ... Benbenishty, J. (2013). Translation of oral care practice guidelines into clinical practice by intensive care nurses. *Journal of Nursing Scholarship, 45*(4), 355–362.

Garrison, L. (2016). Cost-effectiveness and clinical practice guidelines: Have we reached a tipping point?—An overview. *Value in Health, 19*, 512–515. doi:10.1016/j.jval.2016.04.018

Gifford, W., Davies, B., Tourangeau, A., & Lefebre, N. (2011). Developing team leadership to facilitate guideline utilization: Planning and evaluating a 3-month intervention strategy. *Journal of Nurse Management, 19*, 121–132.

Gill, J., Chen, Y., Glutting, J., Diamond, J., & Lieberman, M. (2009). Impact of decision support in electronic medical records on lipid management in primary care. *Population Health Management, 12*(5), 221–226. doi:10.1089/pop.2009.0003

Gill, J., Mainous, A., Koopman, R., Player, M., Everett, C., Chen, Y., ... Lieberman, M. (2011). Impact of EHR-based clinical decision support on adherence to guidelines for patients on NSAIDs: A randomized controlled trial. *Annals of Family Medicine Web, 9*(1), 22–30. doi:10.1370/afm.1172

Glasgow, R., Vinson, C., Chambers, D., Khoury, M., Kaplan, R., & Hunter, C. (2012). National Institutes of Health approaches to dissemination and implementation science: Current and future directions. *Framing Health Matters, 102*(7), 1274–1281.

Guidelines International Network. (2016). Home page. Retrieved from http://www.g-i-n.net/home

Haller, K. B., Reynolds, M. A., & Horsley, J. A. (1979). Developing research-based innovation protocols: Process criteria and issues. *Research in Nursing and Health, 2*, 45–51.

Hill, K., & Lalor, E. (2009). How useful is an online tool to facilitate guideline implementation? Feasibility study of using eGLIA by stroke clinicians in Austraila. *Quality and Safety Health Care, 18*, 157–159.

Institute of Medicine. (2011, March). *Clinical practice guidelines we can trust.* Retrieved from http://www.nationalacademies.org/hmd/Reports/2011/Clinical-Practice-Guidelines-We -Can-Trust.aspx

Jamal, A., McKenzie, K., & Clark, M. (2009). The impact of health information technology on the quality of medical and health care: A systematic review. *Health Information Management Journal, 38*(3), 26–37.

James, P., Oparil, S., Carter, B., Cushman, W., Dennison-Himmelfarb, C., Handler, J., ... Ortiz, E. (2014). 2014 evidence-based guideline for the management of high blood pressure in adults: Report from the panel members appointed to the Eighth Joint National Committee (JNC 8). *Journal of the American Medical Association, 311*(5), 507–520. doi:10.1001.jama.2013.284427

Jancin, B. (2013). Critics dub JNC-8 as 'JNC-late'. *Cardiology News*. Retrieved from http://www .mededge.com/ecardiologynews/article/57721

Jensen, M., Ryan, D., Apovian, C., Ard, J., Comuzzie, A., Donato, K., ... Yanovkski, S. (2013). 2013 AHA/ACC/TOS guideline for the management of overweight and obesity in adults. *Circulation*. doi:10.1161.cir0000437739.71477.ee

Kitson, A., & Harvey, G. (2016). Methods to succeed in effective knowledge translation in clinical practice. *Journal of Nursing Scholarship, 48*(3), 294–302.

Levin, R., & Lewis-Holman, S. (2011). Developing guidelines for clinical protocol development. *Research and Theory for Nursing Practice, 25*(4), 233–237.

Linder, J., Schnipper, J., Tsurikova, R., Yu, T., Volk, L., Melnikas, A., ... Middleton, B. (2009). Documentation-based clinical decision support to improve antibiotic prescribing for acute respiratory infections in primary care: A cluster randomized controlled trial. *Informatics in Primary Care, 17*, 231–240.

Mackey, A., & Bassndowski, S. (2016). The history of evidence-based practice in nursing education and practice. *Journal of Professional Nursing, 33*(1), 51–55. Published ahead of print. doi:10.1016/j.profnurs.2016.05.009

Monegain, B. (2015). More than 80 percent of docs use EHR. *Healthcare IT News*. Retrieved from http://www.healthcareitnews.com/news/more-80-percent-docs-use-ehrs

National Institute of Health. (2015). Clinical practice guidelines. Retrieved from https://nccih .nih.gov/health/providers/clinicalpractice.htm

Perry, J. E., Cox, D., & Cox, A. D. (2014). Trust and transparency: Patient perceptions of physicians' financial relationships with pharmaceutical companies. *Journal of Law, Medicine, & Ethics, 42*(4), 475–491.

Peterson, M., Barnason, S., Donnelly, B., Hill, K., Miley, H., Rigges, L., & Whiteman, K. (2014). Choosing the best evidence to guide clinical practice: Application of AACN levels of evidence. *Critical Care Nurse, 34*(2), 58–68.

Ploeg, J., Skelly, J., Rowan, M., Edwards, N., Davies, B., Grinspun, D., ... Downey, A. (2010). The role of nursing best practice champions in diffusing practice guidelines: A mixed methods study. *World Views on Evidence-Based Nursing, 7*(4), 238–252. doi: 10.1111/j.1741-6787.2010.00202.x

Radwin, L., & Alster, K. (2002). Individualizing nursing care: An empirically generated definition. *International Nursing Review, 49*, 54–63.

Riner, M. (2015). Using implementation science as the core of the doctor of nursing practice inquiry project. *Journal of Professional Nursing, 31*(3), 200–207.

Ritchie, L., Evans, M., & Matthews, J. (2010). Nursing students' and clinical instructors' perceptions of the implementation of a best practice guideline. *Journal of Nursing Education, 49*(4), 223–227.

Ross, J., Gross, C., & Krumholz, H. (2012). Promoting transparency in pharmaceutical industry-sponsored research. *American Journal of Public Health, 102*(1), 72–80.

Saunders, H. (2015). Translating knowledge into best practice care bundles: A pragmatic strategy for EBP implementation via moving postprocedural pain management nursing guidelines into clinical practice. *Journal of Clinical Nursing, 24*, 2035–2051.

Shiffman, R. N., Dixon, J., Brandt, C., Essaihi, A., Hsiao, A., Michel, G., & O'Connell, R. (2005). The GuideLine Implementability Appraisal (GLIA): Development of an instrument to identify obstacles to guideline implementation. *BMC Medical Informatics and Decision Making, 5*, 23. doi:10.1186/1472-6947-5-23

Siu, A. L. (2015). Behavioral and pharmacotherapy interventions for tobacco smoking cessation in adults including pregnant women: U.S. Preventive Services Task Force recommendation statement. *Annales of Internal Medicine, 163*(8), 40. doi:10.7326/P15-9032

Stolz, L. A., Stolz, U., Howe, C., Farrell, I. J., & Adhikari, S. (2015). Ultrasound-guided peripheral venous access: A meta-analysis and systematic review. *Journal of Vascular Access, 16*(4), 321–326. doi:10.5301/jva.5000346

Talwalkar, J. A. (2014). Improving the transparency and trustworthiness of subspecialty-based clinical practice guidelines. *Mayo Clinic Proceedings, 89*(1), 5–7.

Taylor, C. (2014). The use of clinical practice guidelines in determining standard of care. *Journal of Legal Medicine, 35*, 273–290.

Thomas, L. (1999). Clinical practice guidelines. *Evidence Based Nursing, 2*, 38–39.

Tong, A., Lopez-Vargas, P., Howell, M., Phoon, R., Johnson, D., Campbell, D., ... Craig, J. (2011). Consumer involvement in topic and outcome selection in the development of clinical practice guidelines. *Health Expectations, 15*, 410–423.

Toth-Pal, E., Wardh, I., Strender, L., & Nilsson, G. (2008). Implementing a clinical decision-support system in practice: A qualitative analysis of influencing attitudes and characteristics among general practitioners. *Informatics for Health & Social Care, 33*(1), 39–54.

Tran, D., Stone, A., Fernandez, R., Griffiths, R., & Johnson, M. (2009). Does implementation of clinical practice guidelines change nurses' screening for alcohol and other substance use? *Contemporary Nurse, 33*(1), 13–19.

U.S. Preventive Services Task Force. (2008). *U.S. Preventive Services Task Force procedure manual* (AHRQ Publication No. 08-05118-EF). Retrieved from https://www.uspreventiveservicestaskforce.org/Page/Name/procedure-manual

U.S. Preventive Services Task Force. (2012). Grade definitions. Retrieved from https://www.uspreventiveservicestaskforce.org/Page/Name/grade-definitions#grade-definitions-after-july-2012

van Dulmen, S., Lukersmith, S., Muxlow, J., Mina, E., Nijhuis-van der Sanden, M., & van der Wees, P. (2013). Supporting a person-centered approach in clinical guidelines. A position paper of the Allied Health Community Guidelines International Network. *Health Expectations, 18*, 1543–1558.

Van Wicklin, S. (2011). Implementing AORN recommended practices for prevention of deep vein thrombosis. *AORN Journal, 94*(5), 443–454. doi:10.1016/j.aorn.2011.07.018

Veterans Administration. (2017). Mission, vision, core values, & goals. Retrieved from http://www.va.gov/about_va/mission.asp

Wang, Z., Norris, S., & Bero, L. (2016). Implementation plans included in World Health Organization guidelines. *Implementation Science, 11*(76), 1–9. doi:10.1186/s13012-016-0440-4

Westfall, J., Mold, J., & Fagnan, L. (2007). Practiced-based research: "Blue highways" on the NIH roadmap. *Journal of the American Medical Association, 297*, 403–406.

Woolf, S., Grol, R., Hutchinson, A., Eccles, M., & Grimshaw, J. (1999). Potential benefits, limitations, and harms of clinical guidelines. *British Medical Journal, 318*, 527–530.

Zevola, D. R., Raffa, M., & Brown, K. (2002). Using clinical pathways in patients undergoing cardiac valve surgery. *Critical Care Nurse, 22*, 31–50.

CHAPTER 10

Identifying Significant Evidence-Based Practice Problems Within Complex Health Environments

Nancy Wells and Elizabeth Borg Card

Objectives

After reading this chapter, learners should be able to:

1. Describe aligning practice problems with organizational priorities and strategic goals
2. Determine key stakeholders and organizational resources needed to change practice
3. Describe the benefits of interdisciplinary teams in practice change
4. Explain how continuous improvement strategies lead to standardization of processes

EVIDENCE-BASED PRACTICE (EBP) SCENARIOS

Scenario 1

Two nurses who worked on a general care surgical unit noted that some of their patients became nauseated after receiving analgesics to control their pain. One nurse, who had worked in the postanesthesia care unit (PACU) before transferring to the general care surgical unit, commented that they used smelling alcohol wipes to control nausea in the PACU. It was his impression that this intervention worked. Patients seemed less nauseated and more comfortable after smelling the alcohol for a minute or two. Armed with this anecdotal evidence, these nurses began using alcohol wipes for patients who became nauseated after pain medication. The nurses talked to their coworkers; their enthusiasm for the intervention was mixed. When they approached the manager about changing practice on the unit, she asked a number of questions: (a) How many patients experience this side effect and do not have or respond to antiemetic orders? (b) What is the evidence of the effectiveness of this intervention? (c) And, was there any evidence that nausea affected overall patient satisfaction? From the manager's perspective, this was a low-occurrence problem with other evidence-based effective interventions (antiemetics) available. Most importantly, the intervention did not address any of the organizational priorities. The two nurses did not have good answers to any of these questions, but they continued to use the alcohol wipe inhalation when patients became nauseated. The practice ended when a surgeon on rounds found patients "sniffing alcohol."

Scenario 2

A pair of nurse case managers working in a 918-bed urban academic medical center wanted to optimize safe outcomes for patients. The case managers sought to increase early ambulation and nurses' documentation inclusive of distance ambulated for the colorectal and urology surgical patients by promoting an evidence-based nursing intervention. The Early Ambulation project was launched to improve their patients' outcomes. A literature search revealed early ambulation can decrease complications (e.g., development of paralytic ileus, pneumonia), as well as hospital length of stay and costs. The two case managers examined if their practice question aligned with the institution's strategic goals—available through the nursing department's home webpage. Finding agreement, they identified the key stakeholders (i.e., those impacted by an initiative to improve early ambulation and increase nursing documentation): surgeons and advance practice providers, unit nurse managers and unit direct care nurses, the electronic health record (e.g., system support nurse specialist and database analyst), the office of evidence-based practice (EBP), and nursing research. They met, agreed this project was a priority, and assembled a team. The interventions implemented to increase early ambulation included: (a) revising the evidence-based order set, (b) measuring and posting the exact distances on the four general care units, (c) creating fields within the electronic health record to display the ambulation distances, (d) educating the nurses on the importance of early ambulation with clear documentation, and (e) adding a visual cue on whiteboards (e.g., screen savers at every clinical workstation) indicating completed ambulation. Findings from the 12 months of data revealed an increase in the number of patients who ambulated early as well as increased distances individuals ambulated, and an overall decrease in occurrence of paralytic ileus on the units with the intervention compared to the control units (i.e., those who did not implement the early ambulation project). Through ensuring that all of those affected by the project were included early and that the focus of the project was in alignment with the organization's priorities, the nurses gained support and access to the resources needed: physicians changing order sets, changes in the electronic health record, access to the data, and statistical analysis (Kibler et al., 2012).

Discussion

Nurses engaged in EBP understand that their role requires them to identify "trade-offs." Choosing what *not* to do is as important as what *to* do. Appraising the importance of various patient care initiatives in complex healthcare environments with finite resources is a primary goal of nurses engaged in EBP (Lidow, 2017).

ORGANIZATIONAL GOALS AND PRIORITIES

Changing nursing practice requires time, collaborative efforts among staff within the organization, and resources. In today's climate of fiscal restraint, practice change projects need to address at least one, and ideally all, of these criteria: (a) quality of care, (b) patient safety, (c) patient experience, and (d) cost of care. "High-impact" projects improve the quality/safety of care delivered to a large number of patients with the potential to reduce the cost of care. Alternatively, projects that affect a small number of patients but have the potential to substantially reduce cost also are considered to have a "high impact." Practice changes that are based on evidence are more likely to be implemented than those based on opinion or beliefs.

The Centers for Medicare and Medicaid Services (CMS) have implemented reimbursement programs that provide incentives for high-quality care delivery. In 2008, CMS stopped paying for costs from hospital-acquired conditions, such as catheter-associated bloodstream infections and pressure ulcers. These "never events" fall under the umbrella of value-based care, which rewards hospitals that provide high-quality safe patient care and penalizes hospitals that do not (Blesch, Rice, & McKinney, 2014). In 2010, 30-day readmission rates were added to the events that would affect reimbursement to hospitals for care delivered. At present, this system of reimbursement adversely affects the larger, more complex hospital systems (Blesch et al., 2014). Thus, prevention of these poor quality events is a high priority for many healthcare organizations, particularly the large health systems. One strategy adopted by healthcare organizations to improve quality and patient safety is to implement best practices used by high-reliability organizations.

National patient safety goals provide another source of healthcare priorities. The 2017 patient safety goals are consistent with the CMS reimbursement program, and one of the five safety goals for nursing is preventing hospital-acquired infections. Additional goals include patient identification, safe medication use, preventing falls, and preventing pressure ulcers (Joint Commission Nursing Care Centers, 2017). These national goals contribute to priorities set by healthcare organizations.

EVIDENCE-BASED PRACTICE

EBP involves the use of the best evidence, in conjunction with clinician expertise and patient preference, to make healthcare decisions (Sackett, Rosenberg, Gray, Haynes, & Richardson, 1996). Originally, EBP was promoted as a means of improving quality and reducing the cost of care through standardization of care delivery processes. As concern about patient safety grew, it became evident that process standardization, through EBP, also reduced the risk of healthcare errors.

EBP Models and Frameworks

A wide range of models and frameworks have been developed to explain how research is translated into clinical practice (Gawlinski & Rutledge, 2008; Poe & White, 2010). Models and frameworks can be extremely useful in finding solutions to practice problems. Models/frameworks (a) direct attention to the important aspect of the problem, (b) explain the possible mechanism(s) involved in achieving a successful solution, and (c) provide a link between the solution and the desired outcome(s) (Brown, 2014; Gawlinski & Rutledge, 2008) (see Appendix).

The Johns Hopkins Nursing Evidence-Based Practice (JHNEBP) Model outlines the steps to change practice as linear and process oriented (Dearholt & Dang, 2012). The model highlights internal and external forces that uncover practice problems (Figure 10.1). This model is scalable—that is, the scope of the problem or project is defined and can be local (e.g., a clinic or unit), departmental, or institution wide. The Practice question–Evidence–Translation (PET) phases identify the need to assemble an interdisciplinary team (Step 1) and identify the stakeholders (i.e., those who would be affected by the change in practice) (Step 4). Once the team has been assembled, evidence is appraised and synthesized, and recommendations are developed. Then, the team determines the fit and feasibility of making recommended practice changes in the organization (Step 11) (Figure 10.2). This means the project team reviews the organization's goals to ensure their project is in alignment with the strategic goals.

A second framework that explicitly directs attention to the organizational fit is the Iowa Model of Evidence-Based Practice to Produce Quality Care (Titler, 2014).

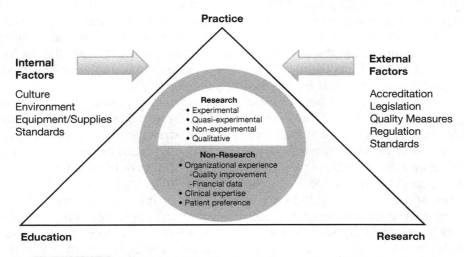

FIGURE 10.1   Johns Hopkins Nursing Evidence-Based Practice Model

The Johns Hopkins Nursing Evidence-Based Practice (EBP) Process
PET (Practice Question-Evidence-Translation)

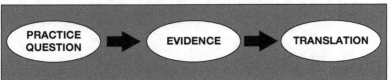

PRACTICE QUESTION

STEP 1:   Identify an EBP question
STEP 2:   Define scope of practice question
STEP 3:   Assign responsibility for leadership
STEP 4:   Recruit multidisciplinary team
STEP 5:   Schedule team conference

EVIDENCE

STEP 6:   Conduct internal and external search for evidence
STEP 7:   Critique all types of evidence
STEP 8:   Summarize evidence
STEP 9:   Rate strength of evidence
STEP 10:   Develop recommendations for change in processes or
             systems of care based on the strength of evidence

TRANSLATION

STEP 11:   Determine appropriateness and feasibility of translating
             recommendations into the specific practice setting
STEP 12:   Create action plan
STEP 13:   Implement change
STEP 14:   Evaluate outcomes
STEP 15:   Report results of preliminary evaluation to decision makers
STEP 16:   Secure support from decision makers to implement
             recommended change internally
STEP 17:   Identify next steps
STEP 18:   Communicate findings

FIGURE 10.2   Johns Hopkins Nursing Evidence-Based Practice process

This model is an algorithm with multiple decision points (Figure 10.3). Similar to the JHNEBP model, the scope of the practice change is scalable. In the Iowa Model, however, the decision point for organizational importance and support occurs early in the process—right after the problem has been defined (Brown, 2014). This model also emphasizes the importance of an interdisciplinary team that includes the critical stakeholders (Brown, 2014). Thus, these two examples of EBP models incorporate organizational fit into the implementation process.

The scenarios at the beginning of this chapter depict how the success of a project can be impacted by external and internal organizational pressures. Understanding an organization's priorities and strategic goals is paramount in the success of projects, whether large or small. Alignment between the practice problem and the priorities of the institution is critical to obtaining resources and support necessary to complete a project (Brown, 2014).

The scenarios also address the importance of interdisciplinary teams—in current healthcare environments, few practice problems involve only one of the healthcare team disciplines. Including stakeholders on the project team ensures that all who are affected have a voice in the solution. The involvement of all of those affected provides the opportunity to develop an understanding of the problem

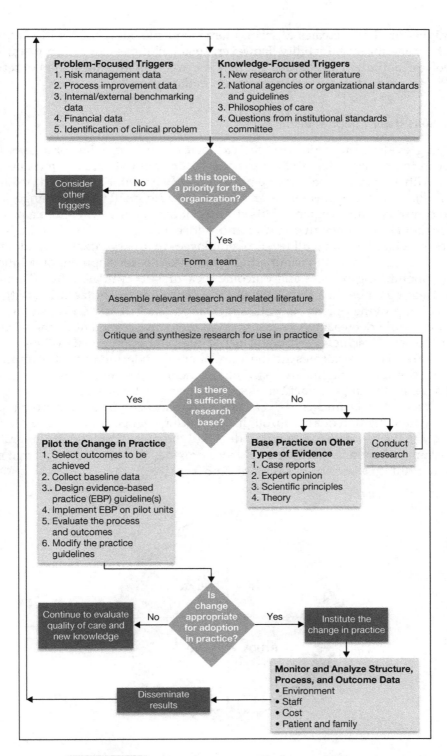

FIGURE 10.3 Iowa Model of Evidence-Based Practice

at a higher level and creates a richer, more eloquent solution. This involvement sets the stage for sustainability. However, sustainability is an action word, and it involves continually evaluating the new process with an anticipation of refinement through small changes to the process in the future.

Continuous Quality Improvement

Applying evidence to a practice change focuses on improving processes that will lead to desired outcomes. For example, a desired outcome for nursing that aligns with a strategic goal may be prevention of ventilator-associated pneumonia (VAP). Process improvements are completed with small tests of change, leading to continual improvements. This strategy of continually evaluating a process stems from Dr. Deming, an engineer and statistician in the 1950s. Deming's tactics included (a) involving all levels of employees in an organization in identifying process problems, (b) encouraging input into the development of solutions, and (c) monitoring process and outcome measures to evaluate effect (Deming, 1986). Deming embedded statistical process control into manufacturing with the vision of improving quality, as well as increasing productivity and customer satisfaction, while decreasing expenses. Continuous improvement of the systems and processes is achieved through use of the plan-do-study-act (PDSA) cycle (Figure 10.4). These strategies are the foundation of modern-day quality improvement. LEAN and Six Sigma are based on his theories (Deming, 1986).

These quality improvement strategies are primary tools used to change practice in healthcare. Deming's 14-point philosophy focused on standardizing processes, achieving high quality through anticipating change, and being vigilant in monitoring the processes and end product (i.e., the desired outcome). Integrating quality improvement and EBP, the evidence provides the intervention(s) that predictably result in a specific desired outcome (see Chapter 14).

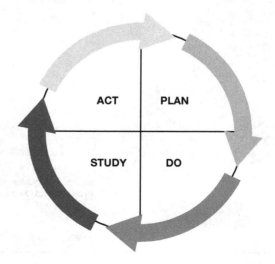

FIGURE 10.4   Plan-do-study-act model

Care Bundles

Care bundles are a series of care delivery tasks that, when used in combination, reduce the risk of an adverse event and improve the quality of care through the standardization of practice. The bundles exemplify the use of best evidence to develop interventions that have demonstrated a positive relationship with the desired outcome. For example, there is consistent evidence that when we provide oral care to ventilated patients, there is a reduction in the incidence of VAP (Li, Xie, Li, & Yue, 2013). The VAP bundle, developed by the Institute for Healthcare Improvement (IHI), consisted of four discrete interventions: (a) elevate head of bed 45°, (b) provide daily sedation vacation and assessment of readiness to wean, (c) prevent peptic ulcer, and (d) prevent deep vein thrombosis (IHI, 2017). The bundle, when implemented consistently, results in a reduction in VAP rates for ventilated adult patients (e.g., Caserta et al., 2012; Sulis, Walkey, Abadi, Campbell Reardon, & Joyce-Brady, 2014), although some negative trials have been reported (e.g., Croce et al., 2013). Although the bundle can be effective, research and monitoring has led to modifications to the bundle that improved its efficacy. In a critical systematic review of VAP research, Keyt, Faverio, and Restrepo (2014) concluded that there are four measures that consistently prevent VAP: (a) elevate head of bed 30° to 45°, (b) ensure daily sedation holiday, (c) provide oral care with chlorhexidine, and (d) perform subglottal suctioning. Successful bundle care implementation is dependent on clear key processes with team agreement on who is responsible for what process measures, compliance, and continuous monitoring. This bundle has been updated several times as newer evidence became available, demonstrating the continuous improvement nature of evidence-based bundles.

The VAP bundle is one example of standardization through monitoring and process improvement strategies. These strategies are integral to high-reliability organizations. Successful organizations have embedded these ideas with the concept of error-free processes, creating a platform for repeated high-quality results within complex, large healthcare organizations.

HIGH-RELIABILITY ORGANIZATIONS

The science of high reliability is the study of organizations that maintain low error rates despite operating in dangerous or hazardous conditions under tight time constraints. For example, the airline industry, aerospace (NASA), and nuclear power companies present substantial safety risks to the public (La Porte & Thomas, 1995; Rochlin, La Porte, & Roberts, 1998). The goal of high reliability organizations is to avoid serious errors in operations and processes.

Healthcare organizations are complex and highly regulated, and they do pose risks to patient safety. Similar to other industries, errors occurring in healthcare are primarily caused by a series of events that lead to system, rather than individual, failure (Leonard & Frankel, 2010; Riley, 2009). A number of factors contribute to developing a high-reliability healthcare organization. These factors include leadership commitment, effective communication, interdisciplinary teamwork, standardized processes, and a structure for process improvement (Melnyk, 2012).

Leadership Commitment

Leaders must communicate the importance of safety and support the activities needed to ensure high reliability within an organization. Clear and frequent communication from leadership to the front-line staff on strategic goals and frequent review of performance toward goal attainment communicates the organizational commitment to patient safety and quality care (Chassin & Loeb, 2013; Leonard & Frankel, 2010). In addition to commitment to safety and quality care, each individual and team is empowered and accountable to maintain the processes that produce desired outcomes (Leonard & Frankel, 2010).

Through a series of incremental steps, an organization can increase reliability. This requires leadership commitment to "zero patient harm." Establishing this belief and value may spark a culture of safety and the additional adoption of process improvement tools, such as LEAN, which provide structure and accountability for employees at all levels (Chassin & Loeb, 2013).

Effective Communication

Effective communication is essential at all levels of healthcare organizations. Regular communication from interdisciplinary leaders to the frontline staff is necessary to ensure all employees are aligned with the priorities and goals of the organization. In addition, clear and respectful communication between team members is needed for teams to function efficiently. Interdisciplinary team communication is a key component in the culture of safety.

Frequent, yet brief communication is critical if a team is to function optimally. Team huddles, or briefings, occur at the beginning of a shift or clinic to ensure all team members are "on the same page." They also provide the opportunity to discuss and plan for high-risk situations (i.e., those where errors are likely to occur). Debriefings take place after an error, or near miss, has occurred. Debriefings are a useful tool to identify steps in the process that require modification to improve safety and/or quality of care.

Debriefings should occur soon after the event, while it is fresh in the team members' minds. A more formal debriefing process is a root cause analysis, which is guided by a facilitator to determine the series of events or processes that led to system failure that resulted in a medical error (Makary & Daniel, 2016). Openness, honesty, and respect for all team members are important during debriefings and root cause analysis if the organization is to learn and grow. In the culture of safety paradigm, any member of the team, regardless of role, should feel free to voice concerns (Deming, 1986; Leonard & Frankel, 2010; Melnyk, 2012). The use of these communication tools will help ensure that the team, and the organization, learns from their mistakes (Leonard & Frankel, 2010).

Interdisciplinary Teamwork

The foundation of effective interdisciplinary teamwork is team training. Interdisciplinary teamwork ensures that each team member has a thorough understanding of the key processes necessary to achieve safety or quality outcomes (Deming, 1986; Melnyk, 2012; Riley, 2009). Team training also needs to address backup plans to be used when a system failure is identified (Melnyk, 2012). Involvement of discipline experts in the use of process improvement tools within the organization and collaboration with healthcare providers who are familiar with and embrace EBP provides additional rigor to the process. A well-functioning interdisciplinary team requires both effective communication and a commitment to a culture of safety.

Standardized Processes

Following standardized processes means that clinicians do the same thing every time for every patient. Examples of standardized processes are use of a template to hand off a patient from one level of care to another, use of the VAP bundle for ventilated patients in critical care, and time out to review patient identification and procedure before starting surgery (Al-Tawfiq & Abed, 2010; Haynes et al., 2009; Leonard, Graham, & Bonacum, 2004). Research evidence is the best way to standardize processes (Schriefer & Leonard, 2012), specifically research that demonstrates a clear relationship between the intervention and the outcome. For example, the measures recommended in the VAP bundle by Keyt et al. (2014) have demonstrated a positive impact on VAP rates (Caserta et al., 2012). The key processes used across an organization should be mapped out (Melnyk, 2012; Riley, 2009) in a flowchart, algorithm, or checklist; this will ensure that all clinicians understand the process and know their part in the process. Clearly, this is the point at which EBP and high-reliability organizations intersect.

Monitoring for Continuous Improvement

Monitoring the processes and outcomes completes the loop and provides feedback to clinicians on their performance. Compliance with the steps in the key processes is an important metric; research demonstrates that higher compliance with processes results in the desired outcome. For example, São Paulo [Brazil] hospital's medical ICU (Caserta et al., 2012) reported that when compliance with the VAP bundle was at 90%, they had no occurrences of VAP. Maintaining this high level of compliance, however, is time and effort intensive (Al-Tawfiq & Abed, 2010; Caserta et al., 2012). Monitoring and disseminating outcome metrics is important feedback of clinicians; if the outcome is trending up (indicating a worse outcome), then a review of compliance and the process(es) will help to identify corrections needed. For example, if the rate of VAP begins to rise in the medical ICU, are patients getting a sedation vacation daily? If this specific task in the bundle is falling short, interventions should be instituted to the next bundle recommendation, for example, increase handwashing. If clinicians are following all of the tasks in the bundle, a search for new evidence on strategies to prevent VAP should be undertaken. Continuous improvement requires monitoring, review of data, feedback, and adjustments to behaviors and processes. Monitoring occurs at all levels of the organization; executive leadership reviews the organizational rates, while managers review their unit/clinic rates. When planning change, the local level (e.g., unit, clinic) will be the most useful in adapting processes to improve quality (Leonard & Frankel, 2010).

High-reliability organizations recognize unsafe conditions and errors early through monitoring near misses as well as adverse events; near-miss reporting prevents systems from progressing into a dangerous incident through rapid remediation (La Porte & Consolini, 1991). The focus must be on the quality and standardization of the process itself, not the production targets—a focus on output increases output while decreasing quality. In the typical healthcare environment, medical errors are not valued as an avenue to improve patient safety and quality of care. In order to improve practice, near misses and errors must be reported, reviewed, and discussed among teams. Modifications in monitoring, process(es), or performance may be required to improve practice. This continuous improvement framework is a hallmark of a high-reliability organization.

Putting these principles of high-reliability organizations into place will bring the organization closer to being "error proof" (Melnyk, 2012; Riley, 2009). This translates into a safer healthcare experience for patients, and one that is high in quality and cost effectiveness.

SUMMARY

EBP supports standardized practice, which leads to decreased cost and improved patient outcomes (Umscheid et al., 2011). EBP projects should align with organizational goals and be inclusive of all stakeholders in defining the problem as well as creating the solution. Healthcare institutions adopt the philosophies of high-reliability organizations to support EBP through

- Standardizing practice (process) based on best available evidence
- Being vigilant about new research and adjusting practice as new evidence is available
- Training/educating all staff in readiness for change
- Creating a culture of ownership and shared success of process/outcomes
- Establishing a goal of "zero patient harm"

REFERENCES

Al-Tawfiq, J. A., & Abed, M. S. (2010). Decreasing ventilator-associated pneumonia in adult intensive care units using the Institute for Healthcare Improvement bundle. *American Journal of Infection Control*, 38(7), 552–556. doi:10.1016/j.ajic.2010.01.008

Blesch, G., Rice, S., & McKinney, M. (2014). CMS names hospital winners, losers on quality incentives. *Modern Healthcare*, 44(51), 10.

Brown, C. G. (2014). The Iowa Model of Evidence-Based Practice to Promote Quality Care: An illustrated example in oncology nursing. *Clinical Journal of Oncology Nursing*, 18(2), 157–159. doi:10.1188/14.cjon.157-159

Caserta, R. A., Marra, A. R., Durao, M. S., Silva, C. V., Pavao dos Santos, O. F., Neves, H. S., . . . Timenetsky, K. T. (2012). A program for sustained improvement in preventing ventilator associated pneumonia in an intensive care setting. *BMC Infectious Diseases*, 12, 234. doi:10.1186/1471-2334-12-234

Chassin, M. R., & Loeb, J. M. (2013). High-reliability health care: Getting there from here. *Milbank Quarterly*, 91(3), 459–490. doi:10.1111/1468-0009.12023

Croce, M. A., Brasel, K. J., Coimbra, R., Adams, C. A., Jr., Miller, P. R., Pasquale, M. D., . . . Tolley, E. A. (2013). National Trauma Institute prospective evaluation of the ventilator bundle in trauma patients: Does it really work? *Journal of Trauma and Acute Care Surgery, 74*(2), 354–360; discussion 360–362. doi:10.1097/TA.0b013e31827a0c65

Dearholt, S., & Dang, D. (2012). Johns Hopkins nursing evidence-based practice: Models and guidelines. Indianapolis, IN: Sigma Theta Tau.

Deming, W. E. (1986). *Out of the crisis* (p. 510). Cambridge, MA: Massachusetts Institute of Technology, Center for advanced engineering study.

Gawlinski, A., & Rutledge, D. (2008). Selecting a model for evidence-based practice changes: A practical approach. *AACN Advanced Critical Care, 19*(3), 291–300. doi:10.1097/01 .aacn.0000330380.41766.63

Haynes, A. B., Weiser, T. G., Berry, W. R., Lipsitz, S. R., Breizat, A. H., Dellinger, E. P., . . . Gawande, A. A. (2009). A surgical safety checklist to reduce morbidity and mortality in a global population. *New England Journal of Medicine, 360*(5), 491–499. doi:10.1056/NEJMsa0810119

Institute for Healthcare Improvement. (2017). Retrieved from http://www.ihi.org/resources/ Pages/Tools/HowtoGuidePreventVAP.aspx

The Joint Commission Nursing Care Center. (2017). 2017 National patient safety goals. Retrieved from https://www.jointcommission.org/ncc_2017_npsgs

Keyt, H., Faverio, P., & Restrepo, M. I. (2014). Prevention of ventilator-associated pneumonia in the intensive care unit: A review of the clinically relevant recent advancements. *Indian Journal of Medical Research, 139*(6), 814–821.

Kibler, V. A., Hayes, R. M., Johnson, D. E., Anderson, L. W., Just, S. L., & Wells, N. (2012). Cultivating quality: Early postoperative ambulation: Back to basics. *American Journal of Nursing, 112*(4), 63–69. doi:10.1097/01

La Porte, T. R., & Consolini, P. M. (1991). Working in practice but not in theory: Theoretical challenges of "high-reliability organizations." *Journal of Public Administration Research and Theory, 1*, 19–48.

La Porte, T. R., & Thomas, C. W. (1995). Regulatory compliance and the ethos of quality enhancement: Surprises in nuclear power plant operations. *Journal of Public Administration Research and Theory, 5*(1), 109–137.

Leonard, M. W., & Frankel, A. (2010). The path to safe and reliable healthcare. *Patient Education Counseling, 80*(3), 288–292. doi:10.1016/j.pec.2010.07.001

Leonard, M. W., Graham, S., & Bonacum, D. (2004). The human factor: The critical importance of effective teamwork and communication in providing safe care. *Quality and Safety in Health Care, 13*(Suppl. 1), i85–90. doi:10.1136/qhc.13.suppl_1.i85

Li, J., Xie, D., Li, A., & Yue, J. (2013). Oral topical decontamination for preventing ventilator-associated pneumonia: A systematic review and meta-analysis of randomized controlled trials. *Journal of Hospital Infection, 84*(4), 283–293. doi:10.1016/j.jhin.2013.04.012

Lidow, D. (2017). A better way to set strategic priorities. *Harvard Business Review*. Retrieved from https://hbr.org/2017/02/a-better-way-to-set-strategic-priorities

Makary, M. A., & Daniel, M. (2016). Medical error—the third leading cause of death in the US. *British Medical Journal, 353*, i2139. doi:10.1136/bmj.i2139

Melnyk, B. M. (2012). Achieving a high-reliability organization through implementation of the ARCC model for systemwide sustainability of evidence-based practice. *Nursing Administration Quarterly, 36*(2), 127–135. doi:10.1097/NAQ.0b013e318249fb6a

Poe, S., & White, K. M. (2010). *Johns Hopkins nursing evidence-based practice: Implementation and translation*. Indianapolis, IN: Sigma Theta Tau.

Riley, W. (2009). High reliability and implications for nursing leaders. *Journal of Nursing Management, 17*(2), 238–246. doi:10.1111/j.1365-2834.2009.00971.x

Rochlin, G. I., La Porte, T., R., & Roberts, K. H. (1998). The self-designing high-reliability organization: Aircraft carrier flight operations at sea. *Naval War College Review, 51*(3), 97–113.

Sackett, D. L., Rosenberg, W. M., Gray, J. A., Haynes, R. B., & Richardson, W. S. (2007). Evidence based medicine: What it is and what it isn't. 1996. *Clinical Orthopedics and Related Research*, *455*, 3–5.

Schriefer, J., & Leonard, M. S. (2012). Patient safety and quality improvement: An overview of QI. *Pediatrics in Review, 33*(8), 353–359; quiz 359–360. doi:10.1542/pir.33-8-353

Sulis, C. A., Walkey, A. J., Abadi, Y., Campbell Reardon, C., & Joyce-Brady, M. (2014). Outcomes of a ventilator-associated pneumonia bundle on rates of ventilator-associated pneumonia and other health care-associated infections in a long-term acute care hospital setting. *American Journal of Infection Control, 42*(5), 536–538. doi:10.1016/j.ajic.2014.01.020

Titler, M. G. (2014). Overview of evidence-based practice and translation science. *Nursing Clinics of North America, 49*(3), 269–274. doi:10.1016/j.cnur.2014.05.001

Umscheid, C. A., Mitchell, M. D., Doshi, J. A., Agarwal, R., Williams, K., & Brennan, P. J. (2011). Estimating the proportion of healthcare-associated infections that are reasonably preventable and the related mortality and costs. *Infection Control and Hospital Epidemiology, 32*(2), 101–114. doi:10.1086/657912

CHAPTER 11

Organizing an Evidence-Based Practice Implementation Plan

Alison H. Edie

After reading this chapter, learners should be able to:

1. Describe the process of implementing an evidence-based practice (EBP) project
2. Understand key EBP implementation concepts
3. Organize EPB implementation strategies
4. Create a poster for dissemination of an EBP project

EVIDENCE-BASED PRACTICE (EBP) SCENARIOS

Scenario 1

Anne attended a webinar session on the risk of smoking in pregnancy and the need for smoking cessation in women during reproductive years. She printed the screening handout and gave it to the nurses in her clinic to use during family planning visits. The smoking cessation educator provided a list of referral resources. The nurses believed the reason women came to the clinic was for birth control, not to make healthy lifestyle changes. Worrying that the flow of clinic traffic may be slowed, the nurse manager questioned why she was not consulted on an additional request for nurse workload. Practitioners were concerned that patients would not be seen efficiently. There were concerns that patients would be offended when challenged about smoking. The nurses believed they did not have additional patient education time because the primary purpose of their time with patients was to prevent unwanted pregnancy and sexually transmitted infections. Smoking cessation handouts were placed on the clinic counter for patients to pick up if they felt that they needed it.

Scenario 2

Kate, a nurse in a rural family planning clinic, recently attended a workshop on preventing tobacco use in women across the reproductive life span. Kate knew that premature births and low birth weights are reducible if women of childbearing age stop smoking before pregnancy. Kate learned that only 20% of women who are pregnant are able to quit smoking during pregnancy. Kate wanted to start screening women for tobacco use at every family planning visit and to inform women about associated risks of smoking to their health and the health of future children. The nurses would provide smoking cessation resources to all women who reported smoking.

Kate first discussed her idea with a nurse in the perinatal clinic who had successfully initiated an EBP project in the past year. In addition, Kate shared her idea for introducing smoking cessation as part of the women's health visit with the clinic's nurse manager. Kate asked if she could present what she learned at the workshop at the next clinic staff meeting. The manager agreed, and Kate prepared a presentation outlining the risk involved with smoking in women of reproductive age and the importance of smoking cessation before pregnancy. She asked if others would be interested in developing an EBP implementation plan to introduce smoking cessation counseling as part of the reproductive health visit. An EBP team of two nurses, a medical assistant, and a nurse-midwife formed with the support of the rest of the nursing staff and clinic manager. The team wrote a patient population, intervention, comparison, outcome, and time frame (PICOT) question, collaborated with the health science reference librarian, and created a table outlining the evidence supporting smoking cessation in women of reproductive age. The team continued to report their progress at monthly staff meetings and invited feedback from key stakeholders.

Once the project was ready to implement, the nurses added smoking cessation counseling for women during their reproductive health visit. The EBP implementation team met with the nursing staff after a trial period of 2 weeks. The nurses had concerns about the additional time needed for the visit and the availability of resources for referral in the community. The implementation team took these concerns to the nurse manager for support of the extra time needed for these visits. In collaboration with the smoking cessation health educator at the health department, they assembled a smoking cessation tool kit and referral process to a health educator. These activities reduced the amount of time needed for counseling by the individual nurses. In addition, the providers reviewed the plan for referrals with the women during the visit.

The implementation team presented "EBP Smoking Cessation in Women of Reproductive Age During a Family Planning Visit Project" during the poster session at the state meeting of public health nurses. They received an innovation award for their successful implementation of the EBP project.

Discussion

The preceding scenarios illustrate how implementation of EBP requires an interprofessional collaborative team approach and a well-designed *implementation plan*. Nurses are at the heart of implementing EBP, and when they do not have team support, collaboration, and a well-thought-out implementation plan, success of an EBP project is unlikely.

For over 20 years, many useful EBP models have been developed (see Appendix). The EBP models have provided nurses guidelines for translating research and other forms of evidence into clinical practice (White, Dudley-Brown, & Terhaar, 2016). The purpose of this chapter is not to detract from or replace current EBP models, but instead to provide a review of fundamental concepts and strategies that must be considered with any model when implementing EBP projects.

IMPLEMENTATION PLAN

Implementation means putting into effect. Implementation of EBP is the process of adopting EBP into clinical use to improve patient care and bridge the gap between relevant research findings and clinical practice. Without implementation, relevant research findings remain in scholarly journals, and interventions are not adapted and integrated into clinical settings (National Institutes of Health, 2016). Many contextual factors contribute to successful implementation of EBP. Positive organizational cultures, leadership value and support, nurses' readiness, and access to resources are factors that are critical in influencing successful integration of EBP into the healthcare setting (Gallagher-Ford, Fineout-Overholt, Melnyk, & Stillwell, 2011; Warren et al., 2016). Nurses have a central and irreplaceable role in the implementation of patient-centered EBP projects, and a working familiarity with basic EBP implantation concepts is necessary (see Box 11.1).

BOX 11.1 Implementation Concepts

Strategy: A strategy is a carefully developed plan or method designed to meet a goal.

Stakeholders: Persons with a concern in a process are stakeholders. Examples are administrative leaders and staff in the clinical setting, including nurses, medical assistants, providers, and patients (Wiseman, 2016). Stakeholders can be active participants in the project or indirectly associated. Both are critical in promoting or hindering a project, so care must be taken in identifying key stakeholders (Fineout-Overholt, Williamson, Gallagher-Ford, Melnyk, & Stillwell, 2011).

EBP Mentor: A clinician with expertise in EBP who provides knowledge and support. Successful implementation projects have EBP mentors. Lack of EBP mentors can pose a barrier to implementation and sustainability of a EBP change (Christenbery, Williamson, Sandlin, & Wells, 2016; Melnyk, Fineout-Overholt, Gallagher-Ford, & Stillwell, 2011).

EBP Team: Clinicians and key stakeholders who form a collaborative group whose purpose is to plan and implement an EBP project (Titler, 2008).

Nurse Readiness: Nurses' capabilities in EBP engagement and implementation. Factors include attitudes and beliefs in EBP, and knowledge and skills in implementation processes (Saunders, 2016; Warren et al., 2016).

Dissemination: Strategies to distribute and share information and knowledge from an EBP project with clinicians, leaders, and organizations to promote adaptation of intervention (Titler, 2008).

EBP, evidence-based practice.

Successful integration of EBP into a clinical setting requires careful development of implementation strategies and a well-constructed implementation plan. The *Implementation Strategies for Evidence-Based Practice Guide* (Cullen & Adams, 2012), based on four phases, helps nurses and nurse leaders organize strategies into an overarching plan. The four phases address the following implementation stages: (a) create awareness and interest, (b) build knowledge and commitment, (c) promote action and adoption, and (d) pursue integration and sustained use (see Figure 11.1). The four phases outline a logical mental

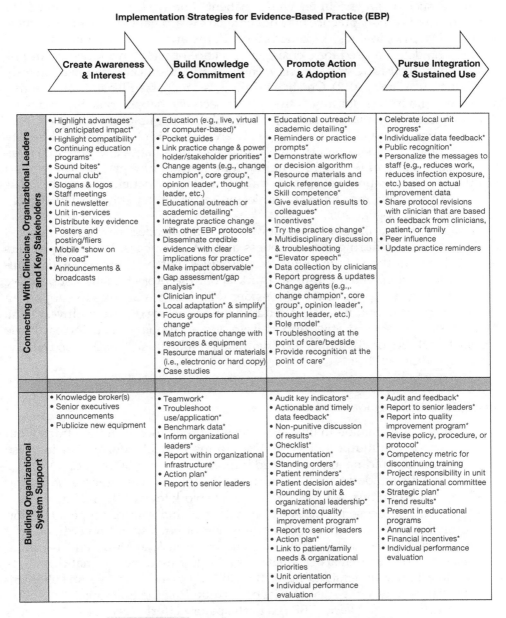

FIGURE 11.1 Implementation strategies for EBP

Source: Cullen and Adams (2012).
*Implementation strategy supported by some empirical evidence

schema that enables nurses to select appropriate implementation strategies along the EBP trajectory. The *Guide* is divided into two major sections. Section one targets EBP strategies for direct care nurses, healthcare organizational leaders, and stakeholders. The second section targets healthcare organization systems as entities of EBP support.

Phase I: Create Awareness and Interest

A trigger, such as an encounter with a patient concern, can lead an inquisitive nurse to reflect on how practice may be changed toward patient care improvement (Ciliska, DiCenso, Melnyk, & Stetler, 2005). In the awareness and interest phase, nurses who detect a need for a change in practice or who have ideas for an EBP project share their ideas and visions with peers and healthcare organization leaders (Cullen & Adams, 2012). Creative thinking is a valuable EBP skillset. Creating awareness and interest for innovative EBP projects can happen casually in day-to-day workplace conversations and more formally, for example, at a staff meeting.

Enthusiasm is catching. During the awareness and interest phase, it is critical to emphasize for stakeholders the anticipated advantages and potential positive outcomes of an EBP project. Highlighting how an EBP project will support healthcare organization norms and values related to patient-centered care is effective in arousing the interest of clinicians and other key stakeholders (Cullen & Adams, 2012; Rogers, 2003).

Healthcare organization managers and executive leaders need to be involved in the EBP project during the awareness and interest phase. Providing leaders with early notification of the EBP project provides them with time to gather sufficient information. Having time to think about the project enables supportive leaders to have an opportunity to consider the needed resources to support an EBP project and to outline anticipated returns on the organization's investment. Awareness and demonstrable support from organizational leaders increases use and sustainability of EBP projects (Hutchinson & Johnston, 2006; Moser, DeLuca, Bond, & Rollins, 2004).

Strategies for Building Awareness and Interest

- Post EBP information in unit areas such as break rooms and organizational electronic communications. Multiple forms of EBP information increase both understanding and perceived importance of an EBP project.
- Share EBP handouts and notes from professional conferences. A strong sense of group purpose helps all members work toward the EBP goal.
- Present EBP-focused articles at journal clubs and seminar-type education groups. A journal club consists of a group of nurses, and other interested healthcare professionals, who convene to discuss, analyze, and review a scholarly or research article related to a healthcare topic. Journal clubs promote a better understanding of the EBP topic and help key stakeholders critically analyze the state of science surrounding the EBP topic.
- Identify key *stakeholders*. EBP is a participatory effort. Keeping stakeholders informed helps to set participant expectations to achieve desired goals.
- Clearly articulate the EBP problem for all stakeholders.

- Be prepared to describe how the EBP project may improve patient care in a 30-second "elevator speech."
- Recruit members to be part of the *EBP Team* for an identified EBP project. Forming EBP teams of six to seven members helps to maintain the generation of creative ideas and build formidable collegial relationships.

Phase II: Build Knowledge and Commitment

The awareness and interest shared by stakeholders as described in phase I set the foundation for building knowledge and commitment for implementation of an EBP project. For example, connecting organizational cherished values and norms (e.g., patients should be free of pain) to a proposed EBP project (e.g., use of an opioid titration protocol for intractable cancer pain management) increases the likelihood of stakeholder commitment and associated knowledge development. Similar to stimulating awareness and interest, building EBP knowledge and commitment is a long-term responsibility that requires multiple and creative strategies.

As noted in Figure 11.1, education is a cardinal component of heightening knowledge and commitment; however, education must accompany other strategies to be of maximum effectiveness (Cullen & Adams, 2012; Davis, Tremblay, & Edwards, 2010). For example, a mentor (see Box 11.1) is important for enabling direct care nurses to have a complete understanding of EBP knowledge and to apply knowledge effectively to produce the best EBP outcomes (Christenbery, Williamson, Sandlin, & Wells, 2016; Fineout-Overholt, Levin, & Melnyk, 2004/2005). A healthcare organization that fosters knowledge and commitment for EBP constructs a foundation for fostering EBP *action and adoption*.

Strategies for Building Knowledge and Commitment

- Establish a relationship with an *EBP mentor*.
- *Collaborate* with a reference librarian for the literature review.
- Select a change agent to lead the team.
- Share the roll-out plan (see Figure 11.2).
- Fill out a gap analysis table (see Table 11.1). A gap analysis identifies the current state of practice to determine needed steps to be taken to move toward the desired state of practice.
- Fill out a SWOT Analysis Table (see Table 11.2). It identifies strengths, weaknesses, opportunities, and threats related to the EBP project.
- Create the *PICOT* question.
- Build an *EBP Analysis Table* to assess the strengths and limitations of relevant literature (see Table 11.3).
- Create an *Overall Analysis Table*, which compares current practice with recommendations, assesses gaps, sets desired outcomes, and synthesizes literature from the analysis table (see Table 11.4).
- Fill out the *EBP Implementation Table* (see Table 11.5). This enables the EBP team to review the strengths and limitations of the project.

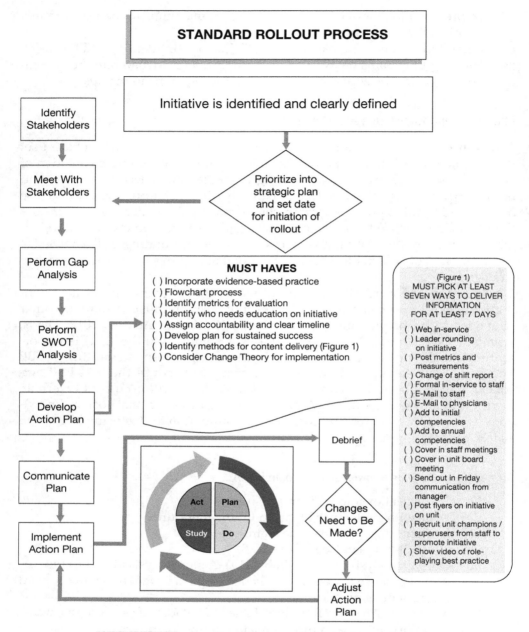

FIGURE 11.2 Roll-out plan for EBP implementation

EBP, evidence-based practice; SWOT, strengths, weaknesses, opportunities, and threats.
Source: Karin Skeen Wilson and Brent Lemmons, Vanderbilt University Medical Center.

- Provide *stakeholders* with continued updates.
- Share the results of searches and review key articles in journal clubs.
- Form a focus group to assess the proposed readiness of nurses to implement change in practice.

TABLE 11.1   EBP Analysis Table

Gap Analysis		
Consider the healthcare organization's mission, vision, strategy, and objectives.		
Current State	**Gap**	**Future State**
70% of patients discharged from medical pulmonary unit have a documented history of receiving the pneumococcal pneumonia vaccine.	30% of patients discharged from medical pulmonary unit are discharged without history of receiving pneumococcal pneumonia vaccine.	100% of patients over age 65 will receive pneumococcal pneumonia vaccine.

EBP, evidence-based practice.

TABLE 11.2   SWOT Analysis

Strengths	Weaknesses
1. What does the unit do well? 2. What are specific unit strengths? 3. What do others, external to the unit, see as its strengths? 4. What resources does the unit possess that will aid in implanting the EBP project?	1. In what areas does the unit need to improve before implementing the EBP project? 2. What do others external to the unit see as areas of weakness? 3. What resources does the unit need to successfully implement the EBP project?

Opportunities	Threats
1. What opportunities are available to the unit for improvement? 2. How might the unit turn opportunities into strengths to implement the EBP project? 3. How can the unit lessen or eliminate areas of weakness? 4. What can other units/organizations teach us about the proposed EBP project?	1. What barriers might the unit face in implementing the EBP project? 2. What individuals might impede the EBP project? 3. What could make the EBP project obsolete or unattainable?

EBP, evidence-based practice; SWOT, strengths, weaknesses, opportunities, and threats.

TABLE 11.3 Example of an Analysis Form

Team name:		**Team members:**			**Date:**	
PICOT question: For adolescents with chronic sickle cell disease pain, is remote monitoring of pain as effective as traditional clinic visits for pain management?						
Author/Year	**Question Hypotheses**	**Design/Sample and Sample Size**	**Intervention**	**Results/ Recommendations**	**Limitations**	**Level of Evidence**
Jacob, Duran, Stinson, Lewis, & Zelter, 2013	Examine pain in children with sickle cell disease who were participating in a wireless pain intervention program	Prospective longitudinal N = 67 (10–17 years)	Patients asked to use smartphone to access web-based pain diary twice a day for 9 months. Entries were monitored remotely by APRN. APRN contacted via text or phone for pain or symptoms requiring attention.	Positive ongoing communication with patient and APRN to better manage pain and other symptoms.	1. All participants were from an urban area. 2. Participants need wireless access to participate. 3. Participants were all older children, so this was not tested in a younger population or with parents completing the electronic diary. 4. Web-based diary only available in English.	Level IV

PICOT, patient population, intervention, comparison, outcome, time frame.

TABLE 11.4   Overall Body of Evidence Table

PICOT Question: For adolescents with chronic sickle cell anemia pain, is remote monitoring of pain as effective as traditional clinic visits for pain management?		
Level of Evidential Strength	**Number of Studies**	**Summary of Findings**
Level I Evidence from a systematic review or meta-analysis of all relevant randomized controlled trials (RCTs)	2	Both studies used two-group RCTs in large medical center clinics. Treatment groups showed significant improvement in pain management, and one group showed improvement in quality of life. Concern about generalizability (settings limited to large clinics).
Level II Evidence obtained from well-designed RCTs		
Level III Evidence obtained from well-designed controlled trials without randomization	1	Findings demonstrated improvement with pain management for patients who had an ongoing relationship with APRN. Ongoing remote communication seemed to have a positive impact on pain management.
Level IV Evidence from well-designed case control and cohort studies		
Level V Evidence from systematic reviews of descriptive and qualitative studies		
Level VI Evidence from descriptive or qualitative studies	1	Case report study. Patient had an overall positive experience with remote monitoring. Theme of feeling connected with APRN was noted in study.
Level VII Evidence from the opinion of authorities and/ or reports of expert committees		

Overall quality of evidence: Evidence is consistent in use of remote monitoring across several levels of studies. Will recommended remote monitoring intervention for use at our large medical center clinic.
APRN, advanced practice registered nurse; PICOT, patient population, intervention, comparison, outcome, time frame.
Source: Courtesy of Betsy Kennedy, Vanderbilt University, Nashville, Tennessee.

TABLE 11.5   EBP Implementation Plan Template

PICOT question:		
Team members:		
1.	What is the purpose of your EBP project, and why is it needed?	(Connect the purpose to the evidence.)
2.	Who are the stakeholders in implementing your project? Explain.	(Who needs to know, whom will it affect, why and when do they need to know?)
3.	What approvals may be needed before project implementation and information dissemination?	(Internal Review Board [IRB], unit managers?)
4.	What resources may be needed for project implementation and information dissemination?	(Financial resources, personnel, materials?)
5.	Identify potential barriers to project implementation and strategies to overcome them.	(Lack of knowledge, skills, motivators, mentors, time, autonomy, competing priorities, etc. How will you correct misconceptions and engage the staff/stakeholders, affect attitudes and/or unit culture?)
6.	Describe your action plan for project implementation.	(Particularly, what is your practice change and what will you do to implement it? What are your tools and timeline? How will you promote it—in-services, posters, other communication with staff? Is it a new protocol, procedure, or guideline for care? Provide a draft.)
7.	What baseline data might you need to collect to later determine outcomes?	(Thinking ahead to evaluation of outcomes, what information or indicators might you need to determine the success of the process and outcome?)

EBP, evidence-based practice; PICOT, patient population, intervention, comparison, outcome, time frame.

Phase III: Promote Action and Adoption

Following the promotion of awareness and positive attitudes and enhancing knowledge and a spirit of commitment, the next phase is promotion of action and adoption of EBP. Phase III involves changing behaviors, which is often the most challenging aspect of EBP implementation (Cullen & Adams, 2012). As discussed in Chapter 7, the process of arriving at stakeholder readiness to make practice changes and integrate new evidence into practice is multifactorial and must be addressed for successful action and adoption of proposed EBP interventions (Saunders, 2016).

Training and education to develop required skills and competencies for a recommended practice change are integral to Phase III (Hanrahan et al., 2015). Interventions to enhance action and adoption move from active learning to interactive demonstration (Cullen & Adams, 2012). In Phase III, direct care nurses need ongoing support from mentors, EPB champions, and healthcare organiza-tion leaders. Many practical strategies, such as practice prompts (e.g., electronic reminder that a urinary catheter is still in place), are necessary to sustain the momentum for action and adoption (Meddings et al., 2014).

It is important to be generous with time for the action and adoption phase to occur. Phase III requires direct care nurses to engage in many areas of criti-cal thinking, which require time for reflection, including (a) testing the prac-tice changes for efficacy and patient/user satisfaction, (b) exploring novel ways to integrate the change into practice, (c) adapting the practice change for unex-pected or unique circumstances, and (d) evaluating outcomes (Cullen & Adams, 2012). To provide ongoing input about the action and adoption of the EBP inter-vention, formative evaluation must occur throughout Phase III, and a summative evaluation needs to occur when Phase III is complete. Evaluation findings must be shared with key stakeholders so that appropriate adjustments to the interven-tion, if needed, can be made.

Nurses who are leading implementation of EBP projects need to be cogni-zant of late adopter or laggard responses to the intervention (see Chapter 7). It is sometimes helpful for late adopters to have opportunities to view early adopters using the intervention in real practice time.

Strategies for Action and Adoption

- Determine areas of support and resistance. Use focus groups to identify strengths and barriers.
- Engage in a communication plan with stakeholders.
- Introduce the plan for implementation at a "roll-out" event. Make it a cel-ebration with the focus on positive outcomes for patients and families.
- Provide training about the intervention at various shifts and times to include all who will be involved in the direct care of patients.
- Continue to have huddles (i.e., frequent, short briefings that allow team members to stay informed, make plans, and move forward) about the prog-ress of the intervention to identify potential stumbling blocks along the way.
- Continue to check in with the EBP mentor for guidance.
- Measure outcomes throughout the adoption phase to determine barriers and facilitators.
- Address barriers, and adjust the plan as needed.

Pursue Integration and Sustained Use

The final phase of the *Evidence-Based Practice Guide* integrates new practice inter-ventions into routine use and demonstrates positive outcomes of EBP interven-tions. In Phase IV, a culture of EBP becomes evident. EBP becomes normative as nurses demonstrate the positive impact of EBP change on patient care. To solidify the change, as part of normal operations, it is important for the change to be pub-licly recognized by healthcare organization leaders.

Posters, podcasts, practice reminders, and other methods used to help inte-grate the change into practice should not become stale but should be updated and refreshed to serve as pertinent reminders. It is important that evaluative data regarding EBP change be reported to key stakeholders. In addition, patient outcome successes should be celebrated, and plans to address relevant areas for change need to be noted. Sustained use of the intervention can be supported by integrating the change as part of policy and procedure updates. Reminders and reviews of patient outcomes will keep the clinical team invested in the continuation of the practice (Cullen & Adams, 2012).

Strategies for Integration and Sustained Use

- Disseminate the project to peers at the healthcare organization and at conferences through poster presentations.
- Track the results of interventions so that outcomes can be measured.
- Continue to check in with stakeholders to assess difficulties encountered.
- Assess patient satisfaction with the intervention.
- Share evaluation results with key stakeholders.
- Continue collaboration with the research librarian to keep up-to-date on the latest evidence related to intervention.
- Assess the readiness of direct care nurses to implement proposed changes in practice—analyze the time commitment and the buy-in.

DISSEMINATING EBP PROJECTS WITH POSTERS

Designing a Poster

EBP is a process of inquiry and creativity that systematically advances best practice. Engaging in EBP activities enables nurses to implement effective and sustainable changes in patient care decision making and patient outcomes. Upon completion of EBP projects, nurses are expected to disseminate project outcomes within the healthcare organization, healthcare community, and/or scientific groups. Poster sessions are frequently the initial opportunity nurses have to present EBP projects to other professionals. When members of an EBP team present EBP project posters to other professionals, discussion of patient-centered care ensues. Professional encounters at poster sessions often expand on the EBP project's usefulness to healthcare and patients (Christenbery & Latham, 2013; Ecoff & Stichler, 2015). The following are useful recommendations for poster development and presentation.

Planning

Time for reflection will include the following:

- Who is the target audience?
- What is the main point of the project?
- Which poster sections need to be emphasized?
- How should content be arranged?
- How will pictures or diagrams enhance the message?

Poster Headings

Organize headings into blocks. Most posters include the following:

- *Title with authors and institutional logos.* The title should emphasize the project's primary focus. A brief but informative title introduces the EBP project and indicates why the poster content is important to patient care. Preferably, titles are limited to 10 to 12 words.
- *Clinical problem.* Briefly discuss the clinical problem addressed by the EBP project, which may reference one or two relevant studies associated with the project's topic. The problem statement must be concise and state the need for the project. Often the project's PICOT question is placed in this section of the poster.
- *Goal and/or objectives of the project.* Key objectives should unambiguously state the project's aims. Limit the number of objectives to three or four for manageability. Organize the objectives in bullet format.
- *EBP intervention.* Include concise description of the protocol and rationale. Include intervention exposure, duration, and dose. Include a brief overview of clinical and/or demographic variables of sample and setting.
- *Methods description or design of project implementation plan.* Briefly outline the implementation plan. Emphasize components of the plan that made this particular project successful.
- *Outcomes or results.* Outcomes should focus on the clinical relevance. Outcomes are a primary section of the poster (see Figure 11.3) and need to be in a prominent location on the poster.
- *Recommendations.* Provide a concise summary of the project. Emphasize nursing implications and recommendations for practice. Simplicity and clarity of the take-home message will have a significant reader impact compared to an effusive conclusion.

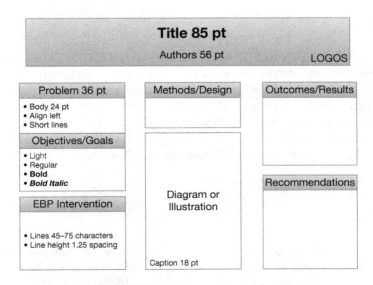

FIGURE 11.3   Poster design template

Organization

- **Template**—A template is useful in organizing content. Common design tools include PowerPoint, Keynote, Prezi, Adobe InDesign or Illustrator, QuarkXPress, Microsoft Publisher, and web-based designs.
- **Grid**—This keeps content organized and aligned, but element size may need to be varied.
- **Flow**—The most important content should be high and central. Readers follow from top to bottom and left to right.

Basic Guidelines for Design

- **Typography**
  - Limit use of font to one or two types, which can vary with bold, italics, and condensed.
  - Avoid using all capital letters.
  - Keep the text large enough to be able to read from 3 to 4 feet. Lettering in the title and headings should be 2 to 3 inches in height (i.e., 150 to 225 point), and lettering in the text should be minimally 48 point.
  - Align the text to the left margin.
  - Limit the entire text to no more than 500 words.

- **Color and Background**
  - Enhance with foreground/background contrast
  - No blue on black or yellow on white
  - Avoid background images that distract

(Christenbery & Latham, 2013; Ecoff & Stichler, 2015; Zoss, 2016)

SUMMARY

While not detracting from EBP models (see Appendix), this chapter provides suggestions and reminders for selecting key implementation strategies. EBP is becoming the standard for delivery of the best and most up-to-date patient-centered care. Undoubtedly, EBP implementation strategies are becoming a necessary component of the nurse's repertoire for the delivery of optimal care. This chapter outlines useful approaches to EBP implementation spanning from the inception of an EBP idea to the dissemination of the final EBP product.

REFERENCES

Christenbery, T. L., & Latham, T. G. (2013). Creating effective scholarly posters: A guide for DNP students. *Journal of the American Association of Nurse Practitioners, 25,* 16–23.

Christenbery, T. L., Williamson, A., Sandlin, V., & Wells, N. (2016). Immersion in evidence-based practice fellowship program. *Journal for Nurses in Professional Development, 32*(1), 15–20.

Ciliska, D., DiCenso, A., Melnyk, B. M., & Stetler, C. (2005). Using models and strategies for evidence-based practice. In B. M. Melnyk & E. Fineout-Overholt (Eds.), *Evidence-based practice in nursing & healthcare* (pp. 185–219). Philadelphia, PA: Lippincott Williams & Wilkins.

Cullen, L., & Adams, S. L. (2012). Planning for implementation of evidence-based practice. *Journal of Nursing Administration, 42*(4), 222–230. doi:10.1097/NNA.0b013e31824ccd0a

Davis, B., Tremblay, D., & Edwards, N. (2010). Sustaining evidence-based practice systems and measuring the impacts. In D. Bick & I. D. Graham (Eds.), *Evaluating the impact of implementing evidence-based practice* (pp. 166–188). London, England: Wiley-Blackwell.

Ecoff, L., & Stichler, J. F. (2015). Disseminating project outcomes in a scholarly poster. *HERD Health Environments Research & Design Journal, 8*(4), 131–138. doi:10.1177/1937586715583463

Fineout-Overholt, E., Levin, R. F., & Melnyk, B. M. (2004/2005). Strategies for advancing evidence-based practice in clinical settings. *Journal of the New York State Nurses Association, 35*(2), 28–32.

Fineout-Overholt, E., Williamson, K. M., Gallagher-Ford, L., Melnyk, B. M., & Stillwell, S. B. (2011). Evidence-based practice step by step: Following the evidence: Planning for sustainable change. *The American Journal of Nursing, 111*(1), 54–60. doi:10.1097/01.NAJ.0000393062.83761.c0

Gallagher-Ford, L., Fineout-Overholt, E., Melnyk, B. M., & Stillwell, S. B. (2011). Evidence-based practice, step by step: Implementing an evidence-based practice change. *American Journal of Nursing, 111*(3), 54–60. doi:10.1097/10.1097/01.NAJ.0000395243.14347.7e

Hanrahan, K., Wagner, M., Matthews, G., Stewart, S., Dawson, C., Greiner, J., . . . Williamson, A. (2015). Sacred cow gone to pasture: A systematic evaluation and integration of evidence-based practice. *Worldviews on Evidence-Based Nursing, 12*(1), 3–11. doi:10.1111/wvn.12072

Hutchinson, A. M., & Johnston, L. (2006). Beyond the BARRIERS scale: Commonly reported barriers to research use. *Journal of Nursing Administration, 36*(4), 189–199.

Jacob, E., Duran, J., Stinson, J., Lewis, M. A., & Zelter, L. (2013). Remote monitoring of pain and symptoms using wireless technology in children and adolescents with sickle cell disease. *Journal of the American Association of Nurse Practitioners, 25*(1), 42–54.

Meddings, J., Rogers, M. A. M., Krein, S. L., Fakih, M. G., Olmsted, R. N., & Saint, S. (2014). Reducing unnecessary catheter use and other strategies to prevent catheter-associated urinary tract infection: An integrative review. *BMJ Quality and Safety, 23,* 277–289. doi:10.1136/bmjqs-2012001774

Melnyk, B. M., Fineout-Overholt, E., Gallagher-Ford, L., & Stillwell, S. B. (2011). Evidence-based practice, step by step: Sustaining evidence-based practice through organizational policies and an innovative model. *American Journal of Nursing, 111*(9), 57–60. doi:10.1097/01.NAJ.0000405063.97774.0e

Moser, L., DeLuca, N., Bond, G., & Rollins, A. (2004). Implementing evidence-based psychosocial practices: Lessons learned from statewide implementation of two practices. *CNS Spectrum, 9*(12), 926–936.

National Institutes of Health. (2016). Dissemination and implementation research in health (R01), funding opportunity description. Retrieved from https://grants.nih.gov/grants/guide/pa-files/PAR-16-238.html

Rogers, E. M. (2003). *Diffusion of innovations* (5th ed.). New York, NY: Free Press.

Saunders, H. V. J. K. (2016). The state of readiness for evidence-based practice among nurses: An integrative review. *International Journal of Nursing Studies, 56,* 128–140.

Titler, M. (2008). The evidence for evidence-based practice implementation. In R. Hughes (Ed.), *Patient safety and quality: An evidence-based handbook for nurses*. Rockville, MD: Agency for Healthcare Research and Quality. Retrieved from https://www.ncbi.nlm.nih.gov/books/NBK2659

Warren, J. I., McLaughlin, M., Bardsley, J., Eich, J., Esche, C. A., Kropkowski, L., & Risch, S. (2016). The strengths and challenges of implementing EBP in healthcare systems. *Worldviews on Evidence-Based Nursing, 13*(1), 15–24. doi:10.1111/wvn.12149

White, K. M., Dudley-Brown, S., & Terhaar, M. F. (2016). *Translation of evidence into nursing and health care* (2nd ed.). New York, NY: Springer Publishing.

Wiseman, B. K. V. (2016). Patient safety – quality improvement. Retrieved from http://patientsafetyed.duhs.duke.edu/module_a/module_overview.html

Zoss, A. M. E. (2016, September 20). *Designing academic figures & posters*. Durham, NC: Duke University.

PART III

Science-Based Decisions and Evidence-Based Practice

CHAPTER 12

Translational Research

**Lianne Jeffs, Marianne Saragosa, and
Michelle Zahradnik**

Objectives

After reading this chapter, learners should be able to:

1. Define key translational research concepts
2. Describe the evolution of translational research and the translational science continuum
3. Use translational research methodologies in "real-world" settings
4. Identify barriers to translational research

EVIDENCE-BASED PRACTICE (EBP) SCENARIOS

Scenario 1

In attempts to improve the use of research, a community-based hospital implemented nursing education seminars. Hospital leadership invited nurses to participate in the seminars provided biweekly for 6 months. To promote participation, nurses received protected time and support by nursing management. The seminars provided an overview of biomedical and translational research in addition to translational research implementation strategies. Pre- and postevaluation surveys identified that the seminars were effective in improving understanding of translational research and furthering research comprehension. Nevertheless, the use of research findings in daily nursing practice remained static in all areas of the hospital. The lack of improvement prompted a research team to explore why the translational research strategy was not successful. The following is a summary of the team's findings. First, focusing solely on previous research outlining barriers in nursing research utilization did not provide an understanding of context-specific factors. Because the focus was on improving hospital-wide research utilization, hospital leadership overlooked unit-specific facilitators and barriers. Second, translational research is an interdisciplinary field requiring a cohesive team composed of a variety of health professionals. Focusing solely on the nurse's role without considering other key stakeholders negatively influenced the likelihood that education seminars would influence the use of biomedical and translational research.

Scenario 2

Prior to engaging in strategies aimed at reducing the gap between the use of evidence from biomedical and translational research, a research team targeted a single nursing unit at a hospital. As part of their efforts, the research team used the BARRIERS scale to evaluate barriers that impeded the translation of research into practice. The BARRIERS scale evaluates nurses' research attributes, the organization, the innovation, and communication of the research (Funk, Champagne, Wiese, & Tornquist, 1991). The research team was interested in the site-specific contextual factors that influence the implementation of evidence-based strategies. This examination suggested a number of barriers that required attention to enable successful translation of research. First, nurse-specific barriers included the inability to evaluate research and lack of research awareness. Second, the examination demonstrated the importance of working as a team by highlighting identified barriers, such as lack of physician compliance and being isolated from other knowledgeable colleagues. Third, the examination showed organizational barriers such as believing the facilities were inadequate for implementation. From this examination, the research team gained insight into the complexities involved with translational research. These insights helped tailor a learning strategy that was multidimensional, including education sessions in a series of monthly communities of practice meetings, ongoing mentorship, and protected time that enabled nurses to use evidence from biomedical and translational research in their daily clinical practice.

Discussion

In Scenario 1, the healthcare organization committed time and resources to implement best research into clinical practice. The organization had an unrealistic view of nurses as the sole consumers and users of research. This view is in contrast to the interdisciplinary view that must be taken to foster successful translational research endeavors. In addition, the organization relied on research about barriers and facilitators to translational research that may not have been generalizable to the organization. Overlooking an organizational assessment of potential barriers and facilitators to translational research was detrimental to the project. The organization is to be commended for pausing to evaluate what went wrong in order to determine how to best move forward in a positive direction as outlined in Scenario 2.

NEED FOR AND EVOLUTION OF TRANSLATIONAL RESEARCH

Scholarly literature reports that despite documented increases in discovery-oriented basic science and technology, delays in translating knowledge into practice in healthcare prevail (Baker, 2001). McGlynn et al. (2003) further reported that patients in the United States received only half of the recommended healthcare services. The gap surrounding the lack of research uptake into practice attracted the attention of practitioners, researchers, policy makers, and administrators (Baumbusch et al., 2008). To address this gap, the National Institutes of Health emphasized the importance of translational research in the 21st century research road map (Woolf, 2008). Similar efforts occurred in Canada with their national health research road map offering a strong translational research vision, which values increasing the uptake of research (Canadian Institutes of Health Research, 2009).

In translational research or science, often referred to as "from bench-to-bedside," "effective translation of the new knowledge, mechanisms, and techniques generated by advances in basic science research into new approaches for prevention, diagnosis, and treatment of disease is essential for improving health" (Fontanarosa & DeAngelis, 2002). A goal of translational research is to realize the clinical potential of new basic science and laboratory and biomedical knowledge (e.g., molecular biology, the genome, neuroscience, and immunology) in new therapeutic ways for clinical diagnosis, treatment, and prevention (Bell, Siobhan, Struber, & Davies, 2011; Ioannidis, 2004; Marincola, 2003). Translational research involves a bidirectional exchange, whereby there is a transfer of research into clinical practice and translation of clinical insights into research practice (Bell et al., 2011; Marincola, 2003), and this is then commercialized or "brought to market" (Woolf, 2008). Translational research focuses on ensuring that new treatments and research knowledge reach the intended patients or populations and are correctly implemented (Woolf, 2008). Goals of translational research include the following:

- Closing the gap to quality care by improving access
- Reorganizing and coordinating systems of care
- Assisting clinicians and patients to change behaviors to make better-informed healthcare choices
- Providing reminders and point-of-care decision support tools (see Table 12.1)
- Strengthening therapeutic relationships between patients and clinicians (Woolf, 2008)

Translational research and science continue to evolve as an interdisciplinary field of inquiry informed by the complexities of taking evidence "off the shelf" and into the practice setting (Bell et al., 2011; Ogbolu & Fitzpatrick, 2015). Over the last 15 years, several models for effective transfer of research findings into practice and how to best deliver, transfer, adapt, and make evidence-informed decisions have emerged in translational research and science (Baumbusch et al., 2008; Ogbolu & Fitzpatrick, 2015). These models receive further discussion in Chapter 13. Cumulative and collective efforts in translational research have resulted in advancing methods to improve the

TABLE 12.1   Point-of-Care Databases

Database	Description
ACP Journal Club (EBM reviews)	Articles from biomedical literature that report primary studies and systematic reviews that merit immediate attention to keep abreast of important advances in medicine. Clinical experts summarize articles in value-added abstracts with comments.
Clinical Key (available in mobile phone app)	Books, journals, practice guidelines, patient education material, medications, multimedia.
Cochrane Database of Systematic Reviews	Includes full-text Cochrane Collaborations, regularly updated systematic reviews of healthcare interventions.
Mosby's Consult	Features include patient education, drug calculators, drug monograph sections, and nursing care recommendations from evidence-based nursing monographs.
PEMSoft (mobile phone access)	Interactive clinical library for pediatric emergencies, critical care, and primary care. Categories include procedures, calculators, formularies, and toxicology.
PubMed Clinical Queries	Access to specialized PubMed searches that efficiently connect practitioners to EBP clinical literature. Not for use for comprehensive literature searches.
TRIP Database	Confluence of key evidence-based healthcare resources available on the Internet. TRIP searches major categories including (a) evidence-based journals, (b) specialty peer-reviewed journals, (c) general peer-reviewed journals, (d) query-answering services, (e) e-textbooks, (f) medical images, (g) patient information brochures, and (h) guidelines.
UpToDate	Evidence-based clinical decision support resource. Rigorous review and synthesis of the most recent healthcare information.

EBM, evidence-based medicine; EBP, evidence-based practice; TRIP, turning research into practice.

uptake, implementation, and translation of standards, public health policies, and evidence-based practices into expected standards of clinical practice (Brownson, Colditz, & Proctor, 2012).

THE TRANSLATIONAL SCIENCE CONTINUUM

Mitchell, Fisher, Hastings, Silverman, & Wallen (2010) developed the translational science continuum adapted from a variety of sources: the National Cancer Institute (www.cancer.gov), the National Institutes of Health (www.nih.gov), and the U.S. Department of Health and Human Resources (www.hhs.gov). The translational science continuum involves an iterative cycle to accelerate discovery, development, and delivery. The continuum generates, develops, and implements discoveries into effective and widely available clinical applications (see Figure 12.1). The translational science continuum involves moving across five phases: basic science discovery, early translation, late translation, dissemination, and adoption (Sussman, Valente, Rohrbach, Skara, & Pentz, 2006). The translational science continuum involves a wide variety of activities, including comparative effectiveness research, implementation research, dissemination, diffusion, knowledge transfer, uptake, research utilization, adoption, and sustainability (Mitchell et al., 2010).

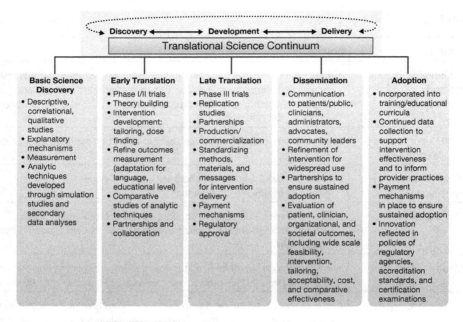

FIGURE 12.1   Translation science continuum

Source: From Mitchell et al. (2010).

CLINICAL AND TRANSLATIONAL SCIENCE AWARDS (CTSA) PROGRAM

The research road map mentioned earlier included a number of initiatives developed to address three main themes: *new pathways for discovery, research teams of the future,* and *reengineering the clinical research enterprise* (Zerhouni, 2007). The first two themes encompass the objectives of developing novel approaches of basic science methodology while developing unconventional research teams, which leads to a cohesive environment where diverse teams of scientists work together (Zerhouni, 2005b). The third theme focuses on emphasizing the importance of and redirecting resources to support clinical and translational research (Zerhouni, 2005b). Feedback provided by researchers across the spectrum of biomedical research, including basic, clinical, and translational scientists, has highlighted many challenges of working synergistically, which is required to translate biomedical advances into clinical research that leads to the adoption and delivery of effective healthcare practices (Zerhouni, 2005a, 2005b).

To date, the National Institutes of Health (NIH) has allotted significant attention and resources toward reducing the gap of applying scientific advances to real-world practice (Zerhouni, 2005a). For example, in response to the gap in biomedical research translation and goals of reengineering the clinical enterprise theme, the NIH developed the Clinical and Translational Science Awards (CTSA) program, which aims to accelerate translation from scientific innovation to health improvement (Drolet & Lorenzi, 2011). The program was developed to accelerate translation across the science continuum (see Figure 12.1) from basic to clinical science, involving human trials followed by translation from clinical science to the community (Zerhouni, 2007). The CTSA program provides funding to academic health centers (AHCs) to support the development of academic homes for clinical and translational science, which are often referred to as clinical and translational research institutes (CTRIs) (Zerhouni, 2005a). The CTRIs, designed by the AHCs, cite specific needs while providing the needed resources to conduct clinical and translational research (Zerhouni, 2005a).

Core components necessary to achieve accelerated translation into practice, incorporated into CTRIs, include the following:

- Trained clinical and translational researchers
- Interdisciplinary teams
- Integrated resources and informatics required to develop cost-effective research tools in a timely manner
- Inclusion of education
- Graduate and postgraduate programs in clinical and translational research
- Support for faculty positions aimed to influence the development of careers and expertise in this field (Zerhouni, 2007)

Initiated in 2006, the CTSA granted awards to 12 AHCs throughout the United States in addition to 52 planning grants to support application to the CTSA programs in the future (Zerhouni, 2007). Currently, the CTSA consortium includes over 50 AHCs interconnected to improve the efficiency of clinical studies, while supporting timely translation of basic science discoveries into clinical practice, influencing health outcomes (National Institute for Advancing Translational Sciences, 2016).

KEY CONCEPTS ASSOCIATED WITH TRANSLATIONAL RESEARCH

The evolution of translational research has resulted in the development of diverse models encompassing a variety of processes with the intent of improving the efficiency of translating basic science to the clinical level (Mitchell et al., 2010). Alongside advances in the field are many definitions used to describe translational research and associated key concepts (Graham et al., 2006; Mitchell et al., 2010; Straus, Tetroe, & Graham, 2013). The multidisciplinary nature of translational science and incorporation of diverse disciplines and organizations has influenced variation in translational research terminology (Mitchell et al., 2010). Furthermore, the lexicon used varies geographically and in response to the model applied (Straus et al., 2013). The lack of consistency and interchangeable use of terminology raises concerns for funding agencies. Developers of CTRI face challenges when outlining objectives, defining required knowledge and skill development of trainees, establishing program curricula, and evaluating outcomes (Rubio et al., 2010).

Developing a clear understanding of the terminology used despite inconsistencies is important for researchers and healthcare professionals in both research and practice settings (Mitchell et al., 2010). In attempts to provide conceptual clarity, Graham et al. (2006) and Mitchell et al. (2010) summarized key definitions for concepts and terms used during translational research (see Table 12.2).

TABLE 12.2   Translational Research Terminology

Term	Definition and Additional Comments
Translational research	Effective translation of new knowledge, mechanisms, and techniques generated by advances in basic science research into new approaches for prevention, diagnosis, and treatment of disease is essential for improving health (Fontanarosa & DeAngelis, 2002). Activities designed to transform ideas, insights, and discoveries generated through basic scientific inquiry and from clinical or population studies into effective and widely available clinical applications (Mitchell et al., 2010). <u>Additional Comments</u> Used interchangeably with the term *knowledge translation*. Both *translational research* and *knowledge translation* definitions identify the process of moving basic biomedical research from bench-to-bedside with the objective of improving health outcomes and the efficiency of the healthcare system (Graham et al., 2006).
Knowledge translation (KT)	The exchange, synthesis, and ethically sound application of knowledge within a complex system of interactions among researchers and users to improve health, provide more effective health services and products, and strengthen the healthcare system (Mitchell et al., 2010). <u>Additional Comments</u> Used interchangeably with the term *translational research*.
Knowledge transfer	Imparting research knowledge from producers to end users (Mitchell et al., 2010). <u>Additional Comments</u> Knowledge transfer differs from translational research and KT, because it represents the transfer of "all forms of knowing" rather than restricting the definition to the transfer of knowledge acquired through research (Graham et al., 2006). Knowledge transfer is often used to describe early stages in translational research (Graham et al., 2006).
Knowledge exchange	Knowledge exchange is collaborative problem solving between researchers and exchange decision makers that happens through linkage and exchange. Effective knowledge exchange involves interaction between decision makers and researchers, and results in mutual learning through the process of planning, producing, disseminating, and applying existing or new research in decision making (Graham et al., 2006). <u>Additional Comments</u> The Canadian Health Services Research Foundation has adopted *knowledge exchange* to describe processes formerly referred to as *knowledge transfer* (Canadian Foundation for Health Care Improvement, 2016).
Knowledge utilization	Research, scholarly, and programmatic interventions aimed at increasing the use of knowledge to solve human problems (Mitchell et al., 2010).
Research utilization	Process by which specific research-based knowledge (science) is implemented into practice (Graham et al., 2006). Process by which empirical findings from one or more studies are transformed into nursing interventions and/or into tools that support clinical decision making such as guidelines, protocols, or algorithms (Mitchell et al., 2010). <u>Additional Comments</u> Predominantly used in the nursing field (Graham et al., 2006). Research utilization differs from knowledge translation because the knowledge being transferred was generated through research (Graham et al., 2006).

(continued)

TABLE 12.2   Translational Research Terminology *(continued)*

Term	Definition and Additional Comments
Knowledge integration	The effective incorporation of knowledge into the decisions, practices, and policies of organizations and systems (Mitchell et al., 2010).
Dissemination research	Studies designed to evaluate the effectiveness of an intervention in a population and/or to evaluate a process of transferring to a target audience the knowledge, skills, and systems support needed to deliver an intervention (Mitchell et al., 2010).
Implementation science (also referred to as implementation)	Empirical study of the methods, strategies, and variables to influence the adoption of evidence-based healthcare practices by individuals and organizations to improve clinical and operational decision making (Mitchell et al., 2010). The execution of the adoption decision—that is, the innovation or the research is put into practice (Graham et al., 2006). Additional Comments Often used in the United Kingdom and Europe (Graham et al., 2006).
Dissemination	Passive and spontaneous (diffusion) and active and planned efforts to persuade target groups to adopt an innovation (Mitchell et al., 2010). The spreading of knowledge or research, such as is done in scientific journals and at scientific conferences (Graham et al., 2006). Additional Comments Both dissemination and diffusion are focused on enhancing stakeholder awareness of knowledge products rather than the generation and uptake of knowledge (Graham et al., 2006).
Diffusion	The process by which an innovation is communicated through certain channels over time among members of a social system (Graham, 2006).
Use	Acquisition of research knowledge and its utilization in action and decision making (Mitchell et al., 2010).
Adoption	Adoption is defined as having occurred when (a) individuals and systems possess and retain the necessary capacity for ongoing use of an innovation, and (b) when that innovation has become routine, and remains routine, until it reaches obsolescence (Mitchell et al., 2010).

Source: From Graham et al. (2006); Mitchell et al. (2010).

TRANSLATIONAL RESEARCH METHODS

Translational research involves systematic and innovative transdisciplinary research that both produces and translates research evidence for local contexts of clinical practice and policy (Bell et al., 2011). Translational research takes into account internal research validity and external or social validity (Bell et al., 2011). See Chapter 13 for more details on construct validity.

A hallmark of translational research is consensus building and enacting integrated knowledge translation (IKT) strategies to achieve change in communities of interest, consistent with best practice in the growing science of community engagement (Bell, 2010; Bell et al., 2011). IKT involves collaborative partnerships between those who produce research and those who use it with the aim of enhancing the relevance of the research and facilitating its use to optimize healthcare delivery system performance and outcomes (Gagliardi, Berta, Kothari, Boyko, & Urquhart, 2016; Lohr & Steinwachs, 2002; Van de Ven & Johnson, 2006). Specifically, decision makers can ensure that research questions are relevant to practice or policy, contribute to the research methods and data analysis, interpret results based on their contextual knowledge, and disseminate or translate findings or products (Keown, Van Eerd, & Irvin, 2008). Using an IKT approach, researchers can gain a nuanced understanding of the local context. They can thereby develop and pursue research questions that have real-world applicability and interpret results with a deeper understanding of contextual circumstances, which in turn enhances the usefulness of the research findings (Gagliardi et al., 2016).

Transdisciplinary research combines and synergizes new approaches using different methods from different disciplines beyond the "gold standard" of randomized clinical trials to keep pace with the complexity of healthcare interventions (Bell et al., 2011). Translational research uses both quantitative and qualitative methods for impact and process evaluation methods to examine barriers and facilitators (Straus et al., 2013). Quantitative designs involve a deductive process to investigate phenomena through the inquiry of specific questions or hypotheses; reliable and valid measurements that are objective, rigorous, and reductionist; and analysis that involves descriptive and inferential statistics (Yeh, 2014; see Table 12.3). Qualitative designs involve a naturalistic inquiry approach and inductive process to describe the phenomenon of interest in a narrative format; analysis involves developing themes and a coding schema (Yeh, 2014).

REAL-WORLD APPLICATIONS

Traditional evaluation designs that focus on determining the effectiveness of an intervention or program represent an oversimplification of the context, intervention,

TABLE 12.3   Quantitative Research Designs

Study Design	Description
Experimental	Compares treatment/intervention with a control group, involves randomization, estimates the probability of a causal link, and seeks to describe an association between the intervention and its outcomes.
Quasi-experimental	Compares treatment/intervention with a comparison group, not randomized, contributes to understanding the causal link, and seeks to describe an association between the intervention and its outcomes.
Nonexperimental	Aims to answer the etiology or related factors, involves descriptive design that measures the effect of an intervention after it has been implemented, and uses correlation, trend analysis, and descriptive statistics.
Systematic reviews	Aims to answer a specific research question through a review of relevant literature and involves identification, search, appraisal, and synthesis of high-quality research evidence relevant to the question at hand.

Source: From Higgins and Green (2008); Sidani and Braden (2011); Yeh (2014).

or program (Bell et al., 2011; Salter & Kothari, 2014). As such, methods in translational research have evolved beyond the traditional quantitative and qualitative designs to determine whether research findings work in "real-world" situations (Barnsteiner, Reeder, Palma, Preston, & Walton, 2010). Gaining traction are theory-driven evaluations that examine outcomes and possible causes (i.e., underlying causal mechanisms based on postulated associations between inputs, mediating factors, and outputs) and contextual factors associated with translating research evidence into practice and policy (Coryn, Noakes, Westine, & Schröter, 2011).

An example of a theory-driven evaluation is the realist evaluation developed by Pawson and Tilley (1997) that is used to identify which components of the intervention are most effective, and under what conditions, with a focus on contextual influences (Marchal, van Belle, van Olmen, Hoerée, & Kegels, 2012; Pawson & Tilley, 1997). The realist evaluation attempts to answer the question "what works, for whom, in what circumstances, and why?" Using a realist evaluation, researchers are able to understand how and why the implementation succeeds or fails. By identifying and examining underlying mechanisms associated with the intervention or program, a realist evaluation provides an explanatory framework for why study outcomes occur. The realist evaluation identifies conditions or contexts under which mechanisms operate, and the pattern of outcomes produced includes multimethods involving quantitative and qualitative approaches (Pawson, 2013; Pawson & Tilley, 1997; Salter & Kothari, 2014). For example, van Hooft, Been–Dahmen, Ista, van Staa, and Boeije (2016) conducted a realist evaluation to examine the effectiveness of nurse-led self-management interventions for patients with chronic conditions. The mechanisms resulting in the most successful outcomes were the patients' motivation and self-efficacy. Educational attempts to modify a patient's behavior were the least effective mechanisms. The influence of family involvement, peer support, type of condition, and when the patient diagnosis occurred were the most influential contexts leading to successful nurse-led self-management interventions (van Hooft et al., 2016).

Another example is the Consolidated Framework for Implementation Research (CFIR) that unifies published implementation theories into a comprehensive framework (Damschroder et al., 2009). The CFIR provides a consolidation of constructs found in published implementation theories with the objective of enhancing the understanding of the constructs and the application in specific contexts (Damschroder et al., 2009). The CFIR provides a standardized framework with consistent terminology used to evaluate the implementation process (Damschroder et al., 2009). Implementation of interventions receives evaluation through the selection of constructs from the CFIR, which directly apply to the setting under investigation.

The domains included in the framework encompass a variety of constructs. The following list outlines the five domains and examples of constructs within each:

- Intervention characteristics (intervention source, evidence strength and quality, adaptability)
- Outer setting (patient needs and resources, external policies, and incentives)
- Inner setting (structural characteristics, networks, and communications)

BOX 12.1   Consolidated Framework for Implementation Research: Evaluation

---

PATIENT Care CFIR Evaluation—Case Study (Breimaier, Heckemann, Halfens, & Lohrmann, 2015)

Background: Nursing management deemed the hospital-wide incidence of patient falls at a teaching hospital high. This influenced the implementation of a fall-prevention guideline (referred to as Falls CPG) with the objective of improving nursing practice with respect to fall prevention in two hospital departments. The CFIR, applied concurrently with the implementation of Falls CPG, evaluated the framework's usefulness.

Objective: The objective of the study was to evaluate the comprehensiveness, applicability, and usefulness of the CFIR during the implementation of an evidence-based guideline (i.e., research-based knowledge) for fall prevention in hospital-based nursing practice.

Methods: Comprehensiveness of CFIR evaluation aligns with the constructs included in the framework. The applicability and usefulness of the CFIR depended on the framework's ability to (a) guide the development of assessment questions and target influential factors, (b) act as a template for content analysis, and (c) serve as a method of interpreting study outcomes. Data sources collected and analyzed during the implementation process consisted of the principal investigator's research diary outlining decisions made, perceived facilitators, barriers and solutions, topics and results of meetings, and the observations/experiences of the comprehensiveness and applicability of the CFIR. Using quantitative questionnaires, qualitative interviews, and group discussion, evaluation of influential factors occurred at baseline, study midpoint, and postimplementation of the Falls CPG.

Outcomes: The CFIR is a beneficial framework throughout the stages of implementation (baseline, process, and final/outcome) of the Falls CPG. Constructs included in the CFIR provided a comprehensive overview of the context and implementation process. In addition to current constructs, the research team suggested the following constructs to enhance the comprehensiveness of the CFIR: stakeholders' aims, stakeholders' wishes/need when implementing an innovation, preestablished measures related to the intended innovation, and preestablished strategies for implementing an innovation. The CFIR is both useful and applicable.

CFIR, consolidated framework for implementation research; CPG, clinical practice guidelines.

- Characteristics of individuals (knowledge and beliefs about the intervention and self-efficacy)
- Implementation process (planning, engaging, and executing) (Damschroder et al., 2009)

The constructs support the assessment of the implementation context and progression while providing a framework in which additional theories can be developed (Damschroder et al., 2009). See Box 12.1 for a case example using the CFIR framework.

CHALLENGES ASSOCIATED WITH TRANSLATIONAL RESEARCH

Translating biomedical research into clinical settings continues to be met with challenges and behaviors experienced in clinical research, medical practice, nursing, and the public health (Payne, Johnson, Starren, Tilson, & Dowdy, 2005; Straus et al., 2013). These barriers have resulted in reduced interest, investment, and development of expertise in both clinical and translational research (Zerhouni, 2005a, 2005b).

A number of barriers have been classified as occurring during two specific *translational blocks* that describe the stages of translational research (Woolf,

2008). The first translational block describes the transfer of biomedical findings from basic science to clinical studies. The second translational block describes the translation from clinical studies to healthcare practice and decision making (Woolf, 2008).

The first translational block consists of the clinical research environment that ultimately influences the second translational block (Sung et al., 2003). The main challenges encountered in the clinical research environment include an increase in research costs, delayed results, inadequate funding, increased regulatory burden, fragmented infrastructure, incompatible databases, and insufficient numbers of qualified investigators (Sung et al., 2003). Additionally, with the current volume of findings produced during basic science research, it is difficult to achieve adequate participant recruitment (Straus et al., 2013). Study participants may be reluctant to participate because of privacy and safety concerns, potential adverse events, and prolonged time commitments (Sung et al., 2003).

Factors specific to the healthcare system (finances), healthcare organization (lack of equipment), healthcare teams (standards of care), healthcare professionals (knowledge, attitude, and skills), and patients (adherence) contribute to challenges faced during the second translational block (Damschroder et al., 2009; Straus et al., 2013). An increase in research-associated costs, securing time despite an increase in clinical service demands, difficulty obtaining complex resources, and a lack of funding have a negative impact on science translation (Sung et al., 2003; Zerhouni, 2005a). Additionally, the increased complexity of the translational research domains necessitates formal training over longer periods rather than the development of sufficient skills through work experience (Zerhouni, 2005a). Clinicians, who have a vital role in implementing new knowledge generated through research, often contend with poor access to research evidence, demanding schedules, difficulty understanding research, and a lack of research appraisal skills (Straus et al., 2013). Lastly, a shortage of information describing the process of implementation of research included in publications further increases the difficulty of replicating research findings (Straus et al., 2013).

Recognition and understanding of barriers are required to develop mitigating strategies. Both qualitative and quantitative methods are used in the identification of enablers and barriers (Straus et al., 2013). Qualitative methods include interviews and focus groups with healthcare professionals and end users, observation of facilitators and barriers, surveys, discussion between implementation researchers, and analysis of factors that enable or prevent translational research (Straus et al., 2013). Growing interest in translational research has also influenced the development of instruments designed to provide a structured assessment of facilitators and barriers (Straus et al., 2013).

The BARRIERS scale is an example of an instrument used in the nursing field to assess barriers involved in the translation of knowledge into practice (Straus et al., 2013). The four dimensions of focus used in the BARRIERS scale are the characteristics of the adopter (the nurse's research value, skills, and awareness), characteristics of the organization (setting barriers and limitations), characteristics of the innovation (qualities of the research), and characteristics of the communication (presentation and accessibility of the research) (Funk et al., 1991). These initiatives have led to the identification of a number of translational research barriers observed along the translational science continuum.

In attempts to mitigate the challenges and position translational research as a priority, NIH efforts, such as the CTSA program and the Institute of Medicine through the Clinical Research Roundtable, are showing promise (Sung et al., 2003; Woolf, 2008). Specific translational research programs related to health systems, hospitals, foundations, disease-related organizations, and industry are also succeeding (Sung et al., 2003; Woolf, 2008). Furthermore, two journals, *Translational Medicine* and the *Journal of Translational Medicine*, are focusing solely on translational research (Woolf, 2008).

SUMMARY

The gap in the translation of knowledge into practice and decision making coupled with the magnitude and pace of basic science discoveries highlight the importance of ongoing, dedicated interest in translational research. The evolving interdisciplinary field focuses on translation of knowledge from biomedical research to clinical studies and implementation of knowledge in real-world healthcare settings. Translational research aims to generate and translate research interactively with researchers and knowledge users using a variety of conceptual models. More recently, theory-driven evaluations, including the realist evaluation and the CFIR approaches, evaluate the outcomes, causes, and contextual factors involved in research translation. Despite advances in translational research, ongoing mitigating strategies (e.g., CTSA program development of CTRIs, additional research programs, and knowledge translation strategies) are required to address the barriers identified in both translational blocks to promote successful translation across the five phases of the translational science continuum.

REFERENCES

Baker, A. (2001). Crossing the quality chasm: A new health system for the 21st century. *British Medical Journal, 323*(7322), 1192.

Barnsteiner, J. H., Reeder, V. C., Palma, W. H., Preston, A. M., & Walton, M. K. (2010). Promoting evidence–based practice and translational research. *Nursing Administration Quarterly, 34*(3), 217–225.

Baumbusch, J. L., Kirkham, S. R., Khan, K. B., McDonald, H., Semeniuk, P., Tan, E., & Anderson, J. M. (2008). Pursuing common agendas: A collaborative model for knowledge translation between research and practice in clinical settings. *Research in Nursing & Health, 31*(2), 130–140.

Bell, E. (2010). *Research for health policy.* New York, NY: Oxford University Press.

Bell, E., Siobhan, H., Struber, J., & Davies, L. (2011). What is translational research? Background, concepts, and a definition. *International Public Health Journal, 3*(2), 133.

Breimaier, H. E., Heckemann, B., Halfens, R. J., & Lohrmann, C. (2015). The Consolidated Framework for Implementation Research (CFIR): A useful theoretical framework for guiding and evaluating a guideline implementation process in a hospital-based nursing practice. *BioMed Central Nursing, 14*, 43. doi:10.1186/s12912-015-0088-4

Brownson, R. C., Colditz, G. A., & Proctor, E. K. (2012). *Dissemination and implementation research in health: Translating science to practice*: New York, NY: Oxford University Press.

Canadian Foundation for Health Care Improvement. (2016). Glossary of knowledge exchange terms. Retrieved from http://www.cfhi-fcass.ca/Home.aspx

Canadian Institutes of Health Research. (2009). Health Research Roadmap: Creating innovative research for better health and health care. Retrieved from http://www.cihr-irsc.gc.ca/e/40490.html

Coryn, C. L., Noakes, L. A., Westine, C. D., & Schröter, D. C. (2011). A systematic review of theory-driven evaluation practice from 1990 to 2009. *American Journal of Evaluation, 32*(2), 199–226.

Damschroder, L. J., Aron, D. C., Keith, R. E., Kirsh, S. R., Alexander, J. A., & Lowery, J. C. (2009). Fostering implementation of health services research findings into practice: A consolidated framework for advancing implementation science. *Implementation Science, 4*(1), 1.

Drolet, B. C., & Lorenzi, N. M. (2011). Translational research: Understanding the continuum from bench to bedside. *Translational Research, 157*(1), 1–5.

Fontanarosa, P. B., & DeAngelis, C. D. (2002). Basic science and translational research in JAMA. *Journal of the American Medical Association, 287*(13), 1728.

Funk, S. G., Champagne, M. T., Wiese, R. A., & Tornquist, E. M. (1991). BARRIERS: The barriers to research utilization scale. *Applied Nursing Research, 4*(1), 39–45.

Gagliardi, A. R., Berta, W., Kothari, A., Boyko, J., & Urquhart, R. (2016). Integrated knowledge translation (IKT) in health care: A scoping review. *Implementation Science, 11*(1), 1.

Graham, I. D., Logan, J., Harrison, M. B., Straus, S. E., Tetroe, J., Caswell, W., & Robinson, N. (2006). Lost in knowledge translation: Time for a map? *Journal of Continuing Education in the Health Professions, 26*(1), 13–24.

Higgins, J. P., & Green, S. (2008). *Cochrane handbook for systematic reviews of interventions* (Vol. 5). Hoboken, NJ: Wiley Online Library.

Ioannidis, J. P. (2004). Materializing research promises: Opportunities, priorities and conflicts in translational medicine. *Journal of Translational Medicine, 2*(1), 1.

Keown, K., Van Eerd, D., & Irvin, E. (2008). Stakeholder engagement opportunities in systematic reviews: Knowledge transfer for policy and practice. *Journal of Continuing Education in the Health Professions, 28*(2), 67–72.

Lohr, K. N., & Steinwachs, D. M. (2002). Health services research: An evolving definition of the field. *Health Services Research, 37*(1), 15.

Marchal, B., van Belle, S., van Olmen, J., Hoerée, T., & Kegels, G. (2012). Is realist evaluation keeping its promise? A review of published empirical studies in the field of health systems research. *Evaluation, 18*(2), 192–212.

Marincola, F. M. (2003). Translational medicine: A two-way road. *Journal of Translational Medicine, 1*(1) 1.

McGlynn, E. A., Asch, S. M., Adams, J., Keesey, J., Hicks, J., DeCristofaro, A., & Kerr, E. A. (2003). The quality of health care delivered to adults in the United States. *New England Journal of Medicine, 348*(26), 2635–2645.

Mitchell, S. A., Fisher, C. A., Hastings, C. E., Silverman, L. B., & Wallen, G. R. (2010). A thematic analysis of theoretical models for translational science in nursing: Mapping the field. *Nursing Outlook, 58*(6), 287–300.

National Institute for Advancing Translational Sciences. (2016). CTSA Program hubs. Retrieved from https://ncats.nih.gov/ctsa/about/hubs

Ogbolu, Y., & Fitzpatrick, G. A. (2015). Advancing organizational cultural competency with dissemination and implementation frameworks: Towards translating standards into clinical practice. *Advances in Nursing Science, 38*(3), 203–214.

Pawson, R. (2013). *The science of evaluation: A realist manifesto.* New York, NY: Sage.

Pawson, R., & Tilley, N. (1997). *Realistic evaluation.* New York, NY: Sage.

Payne, P. R., Johnson, S. B., Starren, J. B., Tilson, H. H., & Dowdy, D. (2005). Breaking the translational barriers: The value of integrating biomedical informatics and translational research. *Journal of Investigative Medicine, 53*(4), 192–201.

Rubio, D. M., Schoenbaum, E. E., Lee, L. S., Schteingart, D. E., Marantz, P. R., Anderson, K. E., . . . Esposito, K. (2010). Defining translational research: Implications for training. *Academic Medicine, 85*(3), 470–475.

Salter, K. L., & Kothari, A. (2014). Using realist evaluation to open the black box of knowledge translation: A state-of-the-art review. *Implementation Science, 9*, 115.

Sidani, S., & Braden, C. J. (2011). *Design, evaluation, and translation of nursing interventions.* Hoboken, NJ: Wiley.

Straus, S. E., Tetroe, J., & Graham, I. D. (2013). *Knowledge translation in health care: Moving from evidence to practice* (Vol. 2): Hoboken, NJ: Wiley.

Sung, N. S., Crowley Jr., W. F., Genel, M., Salber, P., Sandy, L., Sherwood, L. M., . . . Getz, K. (2003). Central challenges facing the national clinical research enterprise. *Journal of the American Medical Association, 289*(10), 1278–1287.

Sussman, S., Valente, T. W., Rohrbach, L. A., Skara, S., & Pentz, M. A. (2006). Translation in the health professions: Converting science into action. *Evaluation & the Health Professions, 29*(1), 7–32.

van Hooft, S. M., Been-Dahmen, J. M., Ista, E., van Staa, A., & Boeije, H. R. (2016). A realist review: What do nurse led self-management interventions achieve for outpatients with a chronic condition? *Journal of Advanced Nursing, 73*(6), 1255–1271. doi:10.1111/jan.13189

Van de Ven, A. H., & Johnson, P. E. (2006). Knowledge for theory and practice. *Academy of Management Review, 31*(4), 802–821.

Woolf, S. H. (2008). The meaning of translational research and why it matters. *Journal of the American Medical Association, 299*(2), 211–213.

Yeh, M.-L. (2014). Message from the editor: Achieving knowledge translation in nursing care: The need for greater rigor in applying evidence to practice. *Journal of Nursing Research, 22*(4). doi:10.1097/JNR.0000000000000065

Zerhouni, E. A. (2005a). Translational and clinical science: Time for a new vision. *The New England Journal of Medicine, 353*(15), 1621–1623.

Zerhouni, E. A. (2005b). US biomedical research: Basic, translational, and clinical sciences. *Journal of the American Medical Association, 294*, 1352–1358.

Zerhouni, E. A. (2007). Translational research: Moving discovery to practice. *Clinical Pharmacology Therapeutics, 81*(1), 126–128.

CHAPTER 13

Translational Science: Bridging the Gap Between Science and Application

Lianne Jeffs, Marianne Saragosa, and Michelle Zahradnik

Objectives

After reading this chapter, learners should be able to:

1. Describe nursing's historical involvement in translational science
2. Differentiate between translational science models
3. Apply translational science in the clinical setting
4. Describe construct validity in intervention research
5. Identify key elements of program evaluation in translational science

EVIDENCE-BASED PRACTICE (EBP) SCENARIOS

Scenario 1

For those living in residential care, advanced age and multiple comorbid conditions put them at increased risk of pressure ulcer development. Pressure ulcers affect a patient's physical functioning and general well-being. Organizational leaders at a 400-bed nursing home decided to focus on reducing pressure ulcers among residents as part of a quality improvement strategy. The chief nursing officer (CNO) and three physicians associated with the nursing home met to discuss the pressure ulcer problem. The meeting did not include any nursing staff, allied health professionals, residents, or residents' family members. The small leadership group formed a pressure ulcer subcommittee and identified a newly released nursing best practice guideline on pressure ulcers for adoption. Implementing the guideline was not considered to be a complex project, and a member of the nursing department, with experience in wound care, was chosen to "champion" the guideline implementation. With minimal feedback from nursing personnel at the nursing home, the champion attempted to implement new practices, including weekly rounding with the charge nurse on each unit to assess residents' pressure ulcers and to provide pressure ulcer education for family members. After 6 months of trialing the guidelines, routine resident assessments found no change in pressure ulcer occurrence. Consequently, the subcommittee was dissolved, and the "champion" returned to her normal assignment.

Failure to see any clinical difference may have been the result of a number of factors. First, the nurse asked to take on the project had no formal experience in leading a quality improvement project or specific leadership coaching. Second, resources, including clinician education, policy on pressure ulcer reduction, or risk management plan, were not used as a way of building capacity for all healthcare providers. Third, strategies to support practice change, such as documentation and raising awareness about the project, were not fully considered.

Scenario 2

A project team at an academic medical center in the Midwest was interested in increasing the rate of newborns fed breast milk exclusively during the birth hospitalization. To guide the breastfeeding program, the project team selected two integrated implementation models: the Six Sigma Define, Measure, Analyze, Improve, and Control (DMAIC) quality improvement methodology and the Translational Research Model developed by Titler (2010). The project team included a broad range of stakeholders (e.g., physicians, nurses, and lactation consultants) who analyzed factors associated with the lack of exclusive breastfeeding. From this analysis, the project team identified, planned, implemented, and evaluated interventions aimed at improving rates of exclusive breastfeeding. Interventions to support exclusive breastfeeding included a policy stating supplemental feedings had to be ordered by a medical provider only when clinically indicated. In addition, the project team selected skin-to-skin contact at birth, an intervention known to be associated with increased rates of exclusive breastfeeding. Understanding the importance of both exclusive breastfeeding and skin-to-skin practices is critical to the acceptance of the practice. Consequently, the nursing staff received communication including e-mails, web resources, and related research material; participated in discussions at the unit level; interacted with a lactation consultant; and had supportive opinion leaders. To sustain the practice change, nurses were involved in audit and feedback opportunities, whereby they received direct feedback on the practice of skin-to-skin contact. Nursing documentation was also assessed for evidence of nurses indicating that the newborn was placed skin-to-skin with the mother and not removed until the first breastfeeding episode occurred. The outcome of this project, which used EBP and translational models, was a significant increase in the rate of exclusive newborn breastfeeding within the hospitalization period.

Discussion

Scenario 1 emphasizes negative outcomes of failing to use a translational research model to help bridge the gap between science and application to patient care. In Scenario 1, the healthcare organization used scarce resources in an ineffective effort to translate clinical practice guidelines into practice. The results of this endeavor were frustrated staff, wasted time and resources, and continuation of undesirable patient outcomes. These problems would likely have been averted if the healthcare organization had used EBP and translational models, which were used to produce positive outcomes in Scenario 2.

NURSING'S HISTORICAL INVOLVEMENT IN TRANSLATIONAL SCIENCE

Nurses are the largest group of health professionals in the healthcare workforce; therefore, nurses' ability to efficiently and effectively translate credible research evidence into nursing practice is necessary for optimal patient and population care (World Health Organization, 2011; Yost et al., 2014). The nursing profession has a long history with translating research findings into practice, beginning with Nightingale, who used mortality data to optimize environmental conditions and the health of soldiers during the Crimean War (Kirchhoff, 2004; McDonald, 2001).

Currently, nurses are expected to engage in translating research evidence into practice with critical input related to patient preferences, clinical context and resources, and clinical expertise in decision making (Yost et al., 2014) and healthcare policy (Doane, Reimer-Kirkham, Antifeau, & Stajduhar, 2015). As a practice-based profession, informed by a sound knowledge base, nursing focuses on providing care and therapeutics in the form of nursing interventions that assist in meeting patient needs across a broad spectrum of healthcare environments (Lockwood & Hopp, 2016).

Nurses are accountable in leading efforts to advance translational science, particularly in the development of clinical practices and care delivery systems that result in quality patient care and improved outcomes (Doane et al., 2015). However, nurses continue to be challenged with the efficient and effective translation of research into clinical practice (Baumbusch et al., 2008). Thus, a better understanding of methods used to accelerate knowledge translation into clinical nursing care and healthcare policy is necessary (Baumbusch et al., 2008; Yeh, 2014). To provide nurses a foundation for integrating science into practice and policy, this chapter provides a useful review and critique of current translational science models, implementation of intervention research, program evaluation, and translational science in the practice setting.

TRANSLATIONAL MODELS

Translating research findings to influence clinical practice and patient care is enhanced when informed by translational models (Kitson & Harvey, 2016). Translational models provide implementation strategies, elucidate contextual variables, and contribute to the scientific knowledge base of translational research (Titler, 2010). Historically, translational models have depicted a *linear* approach with unidirectional movement of research-generated evidence into practice or policy (Doane et al., 2015). Linear models, often described as "knowledge transfer" and "research utilization," emphasize a one-way process. In linear models, researchers generate new knowledge, which becomes disseminated to users (e.g., nurses) and integrated into healthcare practice and policy (Best & Holmes, 2010). Examples of linear thinking are well represented in biomedical research. For example, Crowley et al. (2004) illustrate the linear approach in traditional "bench-to-bedside" translation of basic research into patient care. An example of linear translational research into clinical applicability is molecular targeted therapy, in which cancer cell growth is inhibited by interference with selected molecules that are required for tumor growth (Saiio, Nishio, & Tamura, 2003).

More recent translational models depict an *iterative cycle* or exchange of translating evidence and new knowledge into practice settings (Kitson & Harvey, 2016). Iterative cycle models are more reflective of healthcare systems, which are constantly adapting to change and driven by interactions between system components that produce unexpected changes (Best & Holmes, 2010). The following translational models represent frequently used approaches to translating research knowledge into practice:

- Translation Research Model
- Knowledge-To-Action (KTA) Cycle
- Integrated-Promoting Action on Research Implementation in Health Services (i-PARIHS)
- Ottawa Model of Research Use (OMRU)
- Agency for Healthcare Research and Quality (AHRQ) Care Model (Toolkit)

Table 13.1 provides a definition, strengths, and limitations of each model and toolkit.

Translation Research Model

The Translation Research Model, built on Rogers' seminal Diffusion of Innovations model (discussed in Chapter 7), provides a conceptual map for designing studies that test effects of interventions on the rate and extent of adopting innovations into practice (Aebersold, 2010; Titler, 2010). According to the Translation Research Model, diffusion is influenced by the interaction among the nature (e.g., type and strength of evidence or clinical topic) of the innovation and the manner in which the innovation is communicated and disseminated to users of a social system (e.g., healthcare organization or nursing profession; Titler, 2010; Tschannen, Talsma, Gombert, & Mowry, 2011). According to Titler (2010), the Translation Research Model has four key elements: (a) nature of innovation, (b) dissemination process, (c) users of the innovation, and (d) social systems. Each element must be assessed for appropriate strategies that promote EBP within the context of the participatory change (i.e., healthcare organization) to promote effective adoption of an innovation (Titler, 2010; see Figure 13.1).

TABLE 13.1 **Review of Translational Models**

Model	Description	Strengths	Limitations
Translation Research Model	Provides a framework for testing and/or identifying strategies to promote the adoption of evidence-based practices.	Framework targets context defined as the social system of care delivery in translational science. Framework engages point-of-care healthcare providers.	Limited empirical evidence of the model's utility.
Knowledge-to-Action Cycle	Composed of two components: (a) knowledge creation and (b) action, each of which consists of several phases. The phases may occur either sequentially or simultaneously, and may also have reciprocal influence.	Represents a comprehensive depiction of translational research, because the model includes both knowledge-generation processes and the tailoring of new knowledge to diverse users. Focuses on adapting knowledge to the local context.	Lends better to the hospital and clinical setting than policy context. Complexities that need to be considered when changing practices are not portrayed.
i-PARIHS	Proposes that successful implementation occurs from the facilitation of an innovation with the users of the innovation in their local context. Depicts the central role of human agency in defining and shaping knowledge utilization, and context that spans the micro, meso, and micro levels of implementation.	Explicitly details the role of the facilitator, areas the facilitator must focus on, and key facilitator skills for successful use. It is underpinned by relevant theories of innovation, behavioral and organizational change, and improvement.	There is limited evaluation of the framework in prospective implementation studies.
Ottawa Model of Research Use	Composed of six core elements: (a) practice environment, (b) potential adopters, (c) evidence-based innovation, (d) dissemination strategies, (e) adoption, and (f) health outcome of the process.	Defines key elements in the process of research use. Claims to be applicable to all levels of health system (i.e., clinicians, policy makers, and researchers).	Focused on clinical setting rather than healthcare organization systems. Requires validated instruments to support the model.
Agency for Healthcare Research and Quality Care Model Toolkit	The Care Model Toolkit describes the specific steps involved in the Care Model implementation. Clinical settings are expected to go through each of the four phases of Care Model implementation.	A targeted model of care is being implemented.	Lack of empirical evidence to support the step-wise approach to change. Model does not consider contextual variances in the practice setting. Lack of a visual representation of the model.

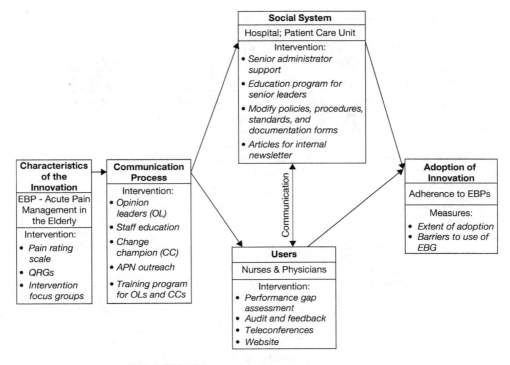

FIGURE 13.1   **Translational Research Model**

Source: From Titler (2010).
EBG, evidence-based guideline; EBP, evidence-based practice.

Knowledge-to-Action Cycle

The KTA cycle is composed of knowledge creation and action components (see Figure 13.2). Knowledge creation, such as advances in genetic testing, is represented by a funnel at the center of the KTA cycle (Straus & Holroyd-Leduc, 2008). As new knowledge travels through the funnel, the knowledge is refined and becomes appropriate for patient application. The funnel represents types of research or knowledge that can be used in healthcare, including knowledge inquiry, knowledge synthesis, and knowledge tools and products (I. D. Graham et al., 2006). The knowledge producers and researchers tailor their activities, including customized messages and methods of dissemination, to the needs of end users (e.g., nurses, patients; I. D. Graham et al., 2006). The action cycle represents activities undertaken to facilitate implementation or application of knowledge.

The KTA cycle is a dynamic model and allows for seven action phases to be influenced by the preceding phases, and for feedback to occur between phases (I. D. Graham et al., 2006). The seven action cycle phases are as follows:

1. Identifying a problem to be addressed and identifying, reviewing, and selecting knowledge or research relevant to the identified problem
2. Adapting the identified knowledge or research to a local context
3. Assessing barriers to knowledge use

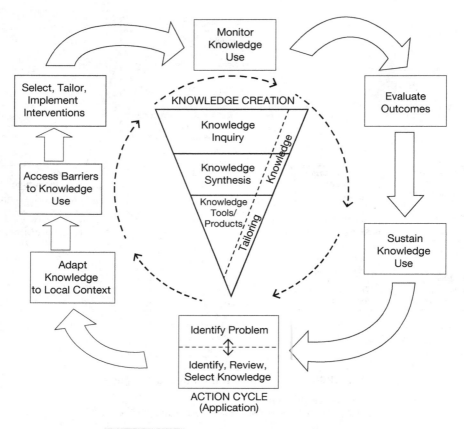

FIGURE 13.2   Knowledge-To-Action Cycle

Source: From Straus and Holroyd-Leduc (2008).

4. Selecting, tailoring, and implementing interventions that promote the use of the knowledge
5. Monitoring knowledge use
6. Evaluating outcomes of knowledge application
7. Sustaining ongoing knowledge use

The action phase is underpinned by planned-action theories, frameworks, and models, which represent deliberate change happening in groups that vary according to size and setting (I. D. Graham et al., 2006; Straus & Holroyd-Leduc, 2008; see Figure 13.3).

Integrated-Promoting Action on Research Implementation in Health Services (i-PARIHS) Framework

The original PARIHS model was built on the understanding that successful implementation of knowledge into practice is a function of three components: (a) quality and type of evidence, (b) characteristics of the setting (context), and (c) how evidence (knowledge) was introduced into practice (facilitation; Harvey & Kitson, 2016). The revised version, i-PARIHS, includes a refined description of

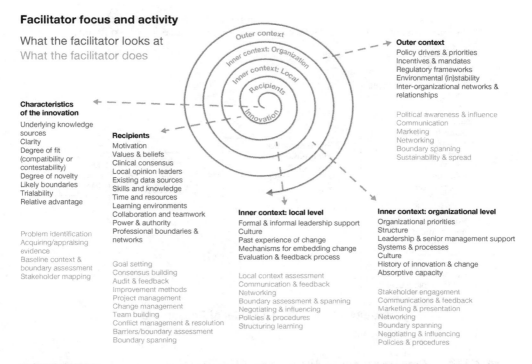

Facilitator focus and activity

What the facilitator looks at
What the facilitator does

Outer context
Policy drivers & priorities
Incentives & mandates
Regulatory frameworks
Environmental (in)stability
Inter-organizational networks & relationships

Political awareness & influence
Communication
Marketing
Networking
Boundary spanning
Sustainability & spread

Characteristics of the innovation
Underlying knowledge sources
Clarity
Degree of fit (compatibility or contestability)
Degree of novelty
Likely boundaries
Trialability
Relative advantage

Problem identification
Acquiring/appraising evidence
Baseline context & boundary assessment
Stakeholder mapping

Recipients
Motivation
Values & beliefs
Clinical consensus
Local opinion leaders
Existing data sources
Skills and knowledge
Time and resources
Learning environments
Collaboration and teamwork
Power & authority
Professional boundaries & networks

Goal setting
Consensus building
Audit & feedback
Improvement methods
Project management
Change management
Team building
Conflict management & resolution
Barriers/boundary assessment
Boundary spanning

Inner context: local level
Formal & informal leadership support
Culture
Past experience of change
Mechanisms for embedding change
Evaluation & feedback process

Local context assessment
Communication & feedback
Networking
Boundary assessment & spanning
Negotiating & influencing
Policies & procedures
Structuring learning

Inner context: organizational level
Organizational priorities
Structure
Leadership & senior management support
Systems & processes
Culture
History of innovation & change
Absorptive capacity

Stakeholder engagement
Communications & feedback
Marketing & presentation
Networking
Boundary spanning
Negotiating & influencing
Policies & procedures

FIGURE 13.3   Integrated-promoting action on research implementation in health services (i-PARIHS) framework

Source: From Harvey and Kitson (2016).

the contextual elements and a new component to assist users in deciding how they want to use new evidence. The core constructs of the i-PARIHS model are facilitation, innovation, recipients, and context. Facilitation is defined as an active element to help navigate users through complex change processes and contextual barriers that challenge evidence adoption (Harvey & Kitson, 2016). Key to the i-PARIHS model is the improved usability of the framework in a structured approach represented by a Facilitator's Toolkit, which uses quality improvement, audit, and feedback methods (Harvey & Kitson, 2015; see Figure 13.3).

Ottawa Model of Research Use

The OMRU was initially developed for policy makers seeking to increase the use of health research by direct care clinicians and for researchers who were interested in how evidence was integrated into practice (Logan & Graham, 1998). The following elements address the components of research implementation: (a) practice environment, (b) potential adopters (see Table 13.2), (c) evidence-based innovation, (d) dissemination strategies, (e) adoption, and (f) health outcomes of the process (Logan & Graham, 1998). Each of the six OMRU components is interconnected through a process of evaluation (Logan & Graham, 1998). In the OMRU, research use is based on interconnected decisions and actions by different stakeholders at each component (Logan & Graham, 1998). The first step in the OMRU is to assess each element for barriers and facilitators. The OMRU is considered an

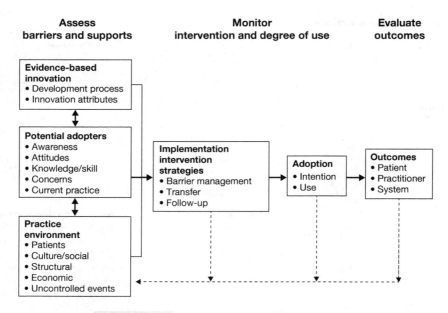

Assess
barriers and supports

Monitor
intervention and degree of use

Evaluate
outcomes

FIGURE 13.4   **Ottawa Model of Research Use**

Source: From Logan and Graham (1998).

TABLE 13.2   **Categorizations of Adopters**

Adopter Category	Definition	Innovativeness Degree
Innovators	Interest in innovation leads them out of their social circle to try new ideas	2.5%
Early adopters	Are considered the opinion leaders in most systems	13.5%
Early majority	Will adopt new ideas just before the average member of a social system	34%
Late majority	Skeptical group, adopting new ideas just after the average member of a social system	34%
Laggards	Will only accept a new idea when surrounded by peers satisfied with the new idea	16%

interactive model of research development and use representing the multifaceted nature of translational research (K. Graham & Logan, 2004; see Figure 13.4).

Agency for Healthcare Research and Quality Care Model Toolkit

The AHRQ commissioned the development of a Care Model toolkit to promote dissemination of the Care Model, originally titled the Chronic Care Model (AHRQ, 2013a). The Care Model has been expanded to include the concept of patient-centered medical home that emphasizes an organized and planned approach to improving patient health outcomes. The toolkit contains recommended processes for implementing the Care Model and connections to important strategies that clinicians use to support changes (AHRQ, 2013b; see Box 13.1).

BOX 13.1   Toolkit Phases and Key Changes in the Care Model

Phase 1: Getting Started

   1.1   Organize the quality improvement team

   1.2   Familiarize the entire team with key improvement strategies

Phase 2: Assess Data and Set Priorities for Improvement

   2.1   Use data to set priorities

   2.2   Select performance measures based on the needs assessment

Phase 3: Redesign Care and Business Systems

   3.1   Organize the care team

   3.2   Clearly define patient panels

   3.3   Create infrastructure to support patients at every visit

   3.4   Plan care

   3.5   Ensure support for self-management

Phase 4: Continuously Improve Performance and Sustain Changes

   4.1   Reexamine the outcomes and make adjustments for continued improvement

   4.2   Capture incentives based on quality of care

BUILDING THE SCIENTIFIC KNOWLEDGE BASE AND TRANSLATIONAL SCIENCE IN THE PRACTICE SETTING

The intent of translational research is to promote the adoption of optimal healthcare interventions; however, unsubstantiated research is often used to support translational interventions in emerging nursing practices (Bhattacharyya, Estey, & Zwarenstein, 2011; Straus, Tetroe, & Graham, 2013). Specifically, minimal evidence exists to support how interventions work and under what circumstances the interventions might work best (Grimshaw et al., 2004). Pressure to improve the quality of care delivery often, inadvertently, leads to dissemination of interventions that fail to produce expected outcomes. Table 13.3 depicts rationale and counterpoints for the rapid dissemination and evaluation of quality improvement interventions (Auerbach, Landefeld, & Shojania, 2007). Further research is needed to gain a perspective on critical processes and elements for successful change associated with translating evidence and new knowledge into practice (Grol & Grimshaw, 2003).

Translational research evaluation requires the appraisal of multiple and complex levels of interaction among patients, healthcare providers, multidisciplinary teams, healthcare facilities, and local and national healthcare systems (Bhattacharyya et al., 2011). Certain methods exist to facilitate the translation of science into practice. As an initial step to evaluating the impact of an intervention, nurses need to discern whether the intervention generates local or generalizable knowledge (Straus et al., 2013). Local knowledge concerns a nurse's responsibility for quality improvement within an institution, while the

TABLE 13.3   Arguments for and Against Rapid Dissemination of Quality-Improvement Interventions

Argument	Why Proceeding Quickly Is Critical	Why Evaluation Is Critical
We cannot wait—the need to improve the quality of care is urgent.	Thousands of patients are injured or killed each year by medical errors.	The need to improve the treatment of many diseases is equally urgent, and we demand rigorous evidence that a therapy works before recommending it widely.
Any effort to improve quality is better than the current state of affairs.	On balance, the harms of quality improvement are likely to be far less than those of the status quo.	Knowledge of the harms and opportunity costs of quality improvement is important for an understanding of the net benefit to patients and the healthcare system, which is often small.
Emulating successful organizations can speed effective improvement.	Emulation and collaboration provide an efficient means of disseminating potentially effective solutions.	Emulation and collaboration can incorrectly promote or even replicate interventions that have not worked.
The effectiveness of some quality-improvement strategies is obvious.	Insistence on evidence may lead us to the underuse of interventions that are obviously effective.	Even though many quality-improvement practices have a simple rationale, they may be less effective than expected and can be difficult to implement fully.
Innovation can be catalyzed by dissemination of strategies that have promise but are unproven.	Preliminary data provide an important opportunity to speed innovation and improve care rapidly.	Flawed, biased, or incomplete data may lead to adoption of interventions that are ineffective or harmful.
The framework of evidence-based medicine does not apply to quality improvement.	The nature of quality improvement exempts improvement from the usual strategies of assessment.	Given the complexity of quality and safety problems, the complexity of their causes, and how little we understand them, we should use rigorous study designs to evaluate quality and safety.
Developing evidence in quality improvement is too costly.	The resources and expertise required to evaluate quality and safety interventions rigorously make trials impractical, particularly when the field is moving so quickly.	As compared with the large opportunity costs incurred by wide implementation of ineffective quality and safety strategies, investments in better evaluation would be small.

latter, generalizable knowledge, is of interest to knowledge translation for nurse researchers (Bhattacharyya et al., 2011). Local knowledge development is gaining insight into whether an intervention worked and in what healthcare context it worked. An example of local knowledge is a nurse manager evaluating the implementation of a new diabetes management guideline in a single outpatient clinic. Through the evaluation effort, data can be used in quality improvement efforts to increase the utilization of the diabetes management guideline by local clinicians and ultimately improve patient outcomes. In contrast, researchers engaged in a multisite translational study evaluating the implementation of new diabetes management guidelines produce knowledge that is generalizable to multiple, far-reaching clinics engaged in diabetes management.

A research study underpinned by a theory of change, such as *Lewin's Theory of Change* (e.g., unfreezing, transitioning, and refreezing), helps investigators identify possible mechanisms of change they are seeking to facilitate. The theory also enables researchers to describe how best to enact changes to achieve a proposed outcome, as well as ensure the right outcomes are operationalized and appropriately measured (French et al., 2012; Straus et al., 2013). See Chapter 7 for a more detailed description of Lewin's Theory of Planned Change.

A study design should be selected based on available resources (e.g., data management or statistical analysis) and whether the study goal is to generate local or generalizable knowledge. An initial parameter in choosing a study design should focus on internal validity. Internal validity is the degree to which an observed effect can, without bias, be attributed to the study's intervention (Straus et al., 2013). A second parameter is external validity, or generalizability, which is the extent to which a study's results can be applied to other settings (Eldridge, Ashby, Bennett, Wakelin, & Feder, 2008).

VALIDITY IN INTERVENTION RESEARCH

Assuring construct validity (i.e., accuracy of study results) is an important component of intervention research (Creswell & Clark, 2007). Validity in quantitative research is assessed by credibility of (a) the scores from the instruments chosen and (b) the soundness of conclusions drawn from the results of the analyses (Creswell & Clark, 2007). Construct study validity is defined by the degree to which inferences can be made from study activities to the theoretical constructs (Sidani & Braden, 2011). A construct is an attribute, proficiency, ability, and/or skill and is schematically represented by established theories (Brown, 2000). For example, "stress" is considered an important construct in the nursing profession as it helps in understanding patients' responses to illness (Clarke, 1984).

Several potential threats exist in relation to construct validity of an intervention. For example, inappropriate operationalization or description of how study concepts and/or variables will be measured (Sidani & Braden, 2011) and false-positive or false-negative conclusions are threats to construct validity (Bagozzi, Yi, & Phillips, 1991). To minimize the possibility of these threats, clear conceptualization of the concepts, variables, and outcomes is required. Further, it is advisable to select outcome measurements/instruments that demonstrate content and construct validity and reliability and that have been used with a target population (Sidani & Braden, 2011). Sidani and Braden (2011) warn against "method bias," or the use of a single instrument to measure each study outcome, or one method of data collection referred to as mono-operation and mono-method biases, respectively. By using multiple measures and/or different methods for data collection, the possibility of introducing "systematic errors" in outcome responses is minimized (Bagozzi et al., 1991; Sidani & Braden, 2011).

PICOT questions provide a structured, systematic approach to identifying key conceptual components to a clinical issue (Stillwell, Fineout-Overholt, Melnyk, &

Williamson, 2010). PICOT is an acronym that represents elements of the clinical question: patient population (P), intervention or issue of interest (I), comparison group or issue of interest (C), outcome(s) of interest (O), and time it takes for the intervention to achieve the outcome(s) (T) (Stillwell et al., 2010). See Table 13.4 for PICOT definition and example. Because PICOT questions require identification of concepts and variables, they help form the foundation for a study's construct validity.

ROLE OF PROGRAM EVALUATION AND PROJECT MANAGEMENT IN TRANSLATIONAL SCIENCE

Program evaluation is a systematic collection, analysis, and reporting of information about a program to assist in decision making (Van Marris & King, 2006). Program evaluation is used to determine program effectiveness and the extent to which a program or initiative is meeting expected outcomes to inform potential program actions or changes (Fraser Health Authority, 2009). Program evaluation should be used to evaluate translational science activities and the translation of evidence into practice. Optimal program evaluation involves both formative and summative evaluations. Formative evaluations examine and explore the *ongoing delivery* of a program or intervention, the quality of implementation, and the assessment of the organizational context, personnel, and procedures (e.g., needs assessment and process evaluation). Summative evaluations examine the *terminal impact,* effect, and outcomes of a program or intervention (e.g., cost-effectiveness; Posavac & Carey, 2007).

Program translational research frequently involves the implementation of complex interventions in *project management* (Loo, 2003). Best practices for project management for translational research include enacting the project management

TABLE 13.4   PICOT Question: Definition and Example

Research question: *In cardiac surgery patients, how does the use of chlorhexidine bath wipes compared with soap and water affect postoperative sternal wound infection rates?*		
P Patient population	What is the patient or group of patients of interest?	Cardiac surgery patients
I Intervention of interest	What is the main intervention or treatment you wish to consider?	Chlorhexidine bath wipes
C Comparison intervention	Is there an alternative intervention or treatment to compare?	Soap and water as comparison intervention
O Outcome(s)	What is the clinical outcome(s)?	Sternal wound infection rates are the outcome
T Time*	How much time does it take to demonstrate the clinical outcome(s)?	Postoperative period
*Note that the time (T) component of the PICOT question is not always required. *Source:* Echevarria and Walker (2014).		

life cycle that consists of five phases: (a) initiating, (b) planning, (c) executing, (d) monitoring and controlling, and (e) closing (Loo, 2003; Project Management Institute, 2013; Wild, Hastings, Gubernick, Ross, & Fehrenbach, 2004). The nature and scope of a research project are determined in the initiating phase. The initiating phase is followed by the planning phase that determines what is to be accomplished in the study, starting with a generalized plan and moving to detailed planning (Loo, 2003). The main purpose of the planning phase is to establish deliverables, study milestones (timeline), budget, team accountabilities, and resources needed to effectively manage a research project (Kerzner, 2010; Loo, 2003). The third phase, executing, helps to ensure a project's deliverables are achieved according to the study design and in a timely manner. The executing phase involves having adequate resources, such as human resources and supplies, services, technology, and equipment (Kerzner, 2010). The fourth phase, monitoring, includes ongoing monitoring and controlling of the project and ongoing monitoring of study activities, budget, and management of emergent risks that might impede deliverables and milestones (Lewis, 2006; Loo, 2003). The fifth phase, closing, includes acceptance of the study's ending that involves the writing of a formal report, presentations to the funding agency and other key stakeholders, and peer-reviewed manuscripts.

Engagement of key stakeholders, such as patients, clinicians and service providers, managers and decision makers, and policy makers, is important through all project management phases. The involvement of key stakeholders is important because stakeholder engagement helps to ensure that interventions and programs have a greater likelihood of meeting the needs and preferences of those they are targeted toward. It is well documented that stakeholder engagement leads to desirable outcomes, experiences, and consumer satisfaction (Gagliardi, Berta, Kothari, Boyko, & Urquhart, 2016; Loo, 2003).

SUMMARY

The nursing profession has a long history with translating research findings into practice and is increasingly expected to engage in translating research evidence into clinical practice and healthcare policy. Several translational models have emerged from a linear movement of research-generated evidence into practice or policy to iterative cycles of translating evidence into practice settings. The models have assisted in identifying facilitators and barriers to translating evidence in the clinical settings. Translational research evaluation is necessary to assess the impact of new evidence in practice. Although there may be ongoing pressure to rapidly implement evidence without proper evaluation, such an approach can lead to dissemination of interventions that fail to meet patient healthcare needs. Therefore, careful thought is needed when selecting a translational theory to underpin translational research. Translational theory may effectively guide the design of the intervention study to evaluate the effects of the intervention, interpret study results, and help translate the intervention to real-world settings. Key to these efforts is ensuring the presence of construct validity and having a structured project management approach to the planning, implementation, and program evaluation activities of translational research efforts.

REFERENCES

Aebersold, M. (2010). Using simulation to improve the use of evidence-based practice guidelines. *Western Journal of Nursing Research, 33,* 296–305.

Agency for Healthcare Research and Quality. (2013a). Module 16: Introduction to the care model. Retrieved from http://www.ahrq.gov/professionals/prevention-chronic-care/improve/system/pfhandbook/mod16.html

Agency for Healthcare Research and Quality. (2013b). Module 18 trainer's guide: Using the AHRQ care model toolkit with practices. Retrieved from http://www.ahrq.gov/professionals/prevention-chronic-care/improve/system/pfhandbook/mod18.html

Auerbach, A. D., Landefeld, C. S., & Shojania, K. G. (2007). The tension between needing to improve care and knowing how to do it. *New England Journal of Medicine, 357*(6), 608–613.

Bagozzi, R. P., Yi, Y., & Phillips, L. W. (1991). Assessing construct validity in organizational research. *Administrative Science Quarterly, 36,* 421–458.

Baumbusch, J. L., Kirkham, S. R., Khan, K. B., McDonald, H., Semeniuk, P., Tan, E., & Anderson, J. M. (2008). Pursuing common agendas: A collaborative model for knowledge translation between research and practice in clinical settings. *Research in Nursing & Health, 31*(2), 130–140.

Best, A., & Holmes, B. (2010). Systems thinking, knowledge and action: Towards better models and methods. *Evidence & Policy: A Journal of Research, Debate and Practice, 6*(2), 145–159.

Bhattacharyya, O. K., Estey, E. A., & Zwarenstein, M. (2011). Methodologies to evaluate the effectiveness of knowledge translation interventions: A primer for researchers and health care managers. *Journal of Clinical Epidemiology, 64*(1), 32–40.

Brown, J. D. (2000). What is construct validity? Retrieved from https://jalt.org/test/PDF/Brown8.pdf

Clarke, M. (1984). Stress and coping: Constructs for nursing. *Journal of Advanced Nursing, 9*(1), 3–13.

Creswell, J. W., & Clark, V. L. P. (2007). *Designing and conducting mixed methods research.* Thousand Oaks, CA: Sage.

Crowley Jr, W. F., Sherwood, L., Salber, P., Scheinberg, D., Slavkin, H., Tilson, H., … Dobs, A. (2004). Clinical research in the United States at a crossroads: Proposal for a novel public-private partnership to establish a national clinical research enterprise. *Journal of the American Medical Association, 291*(9), 1120–1126.

Doane, G. H., Reimer-Kirkham, S., Antifeau, E., & Stajduhar, K. (2015). (Re)theorizing integrated knowledge translation: A heuristic for knowledge-as-action. *Advances in Nursing Science, 38*(3), 175–186.

Echevarria, I. M., & Walker, S. (2014). To make your case, start with a PICOT question. *Nursing, 44*(2), 18–19.

Eldridge, S., Ashby, D., Bennett, C., Wakelin, M., & Feder, G. (2008). Internal and external validity of cluster randomised trials: Systematic review of recent trials. *British Medical Journal, 336*(7649), 876–880.

Fraser Health Authority. (2009). A guide to planning and conducting program evaluation. Retrieved from http://research.fraserhealth.ca/media/2009-05-11-A-Guide-to-Planning-and-Conducting-Program-Evaluation-v2.pdf

French, S. D., Green, S. E., O'Connor, D. A., McKenzie, J. E., Francis, J. J., Michie, S., … Grimshaw, J. M. (2012). Developing theory-informed behaviour change interventions to implement evidence into practice: A systematic approach using the Theoretical Domains Framework. *Implementation Science, 7,* 38. doi:10.1186/1748-5908-7-38

Gagliardi, A. R., Berta, W., Kothari, A., Boyko, J., & Urquhart, R. (2016). Integrated knowledge translation (IKT) in health care: A scoping review. *Implementation Science, 11*(1), 1.

Graham, I. D., Logan, J., Harrison, M. B., Straus, S. E., Tetroe, J., Caswell, W., & Robinson, N. (2006). Lost in knowledge translation: Time for a map? *Journal of Continuing Education in the Health Professions, 26*(1), 13–24.

Graham, K., & Logan, J. (2004). Using the Ottawa Model of Research Use to implement a skin care program. *Journal of Nursing Care Quality, 19*(1), 18–26.

Grimshaw, J., Thomas, R., MacLennan, G., Fraser, C., Ramsay, C., Vale, L. E., … Shirran, L. (2004). Effectiveness and efficiency of guideline dissemination and implementation strategies. *Health Technology Assessment, 8*(6), 1–72.

Grol, R., & Grimshaw, J. (2003). From best evidence to best practice: Effective implementation of change in patients' care. *The Lancet, 362*(9391), 1225–1230.

Harvey, G., & Kitson, A. (2015). *Implementing evidence-based practice in healthcare: A facilitation guide*: New York, NY: Routledge Taylor & Francis Group.

Harvey, G., & Kitson, A. (2016). PARIHS revisited: From heuristic to integrated framework for the successful implementation of knowledge into practice. *Implementation Science, 11*(1), 1.

Kerzner, H. R. (2010). *Project management-best practices: Achieving global excellence* (Vol. 14). Hoboken, NJ: John Wiley & Sons.

Kirchhoff, K. T. (2004). State of the science of translational research: From demonstration projects to intervention testing. *Worldviews on Evidence-Based Nursing, 1*, S6-S12. doi: 10.1111/j.1524-475X.2004.04039.x

Kitson, A. L., & Harvey, G. (2016). Methods to succeed in effective knowledge translation in clinical practice. *Journal of Nursing Scholarship, 48*(3), 294–302. doi:10.1111/jnu.12206

Lewis, J. P. (2006). *The project manager's desk reference* (3rd ed.). New York, NY: McGraw-Hill.

Lockwood, C., & Hopp, L. (2016). Knowledge translation: What it is and the relevance to evidence-based healthcare and nursing. *International Journal of Nursing Practice, 22*(4), 319–321.

Logan, J., & Graham, I. D. (1998). Toward a comprehensive interdisciplinary model of health care research use. *Science Communication, 20*(2), 227–246.

Loo, R. (2003). Project management: A core competency for professional nurses and nurse managers. *Journal for Nurses in Professional Development, 19*(4), 187–193.

McDonald, L. (2001). Florence Nightingale and the early origins of evidence-based nursing. *Evidence Based Nursing, 4*(3), 68–69.

Posavac, E., & Carey, R. (2007). *Program evaluation: Designing and case studies.* Upper Saddle River, NJ: Prentice Hall.

Project Management Institute. (2013). *A guide to the project management body of knowledge* (5th ed.). Newtown Square, PA: Author.

Saiio, N., Nishio, K., & Tamura, T. (2003). Translational and clinical studies of target-based cancer therapy. *International Journal of Clinical Oncology, 8*(4), 187–192.

Sidani, S., & Braden, C. J. (2011). *Design, evaluation, and translation of nursing interventions.* Hoboken, NJ: John Wiley & Sons.

Stillwell, S. B., Fineout-Overholt, E., Melnyk, B. M., & Williamson, K. M. (2010). Evidence-based practice, step by step: Asking the clinical question: A key step in evidence-based practice. *The American Journal of Nursing, 110*(3), 58–61.

Straus, S. E., & Holroyd-Leduc, J. (2008). Knowledge-to-action cycle. *Evidence Based Medicine, 13*(4), 98–100.

Straus, S. E., Tetroe, J., & Graham, I. D. (2013). *Knowledge translation in health care: Moving from evidence to practice.* Hoboken, NJ: John Wiley.

Titler, M. G. (2010). Translation science and context. *Research and Theory for Nursing Practice, 24*(1), 35–55.

Tschannen, D., Talsma, A., Gombert, J., & Mowry, J. (2011). Using the TRIP model to disseminate an IT-based pressure ulcer intervention. *Western Journal of Nursing Research, 33,* 427–442.

Van Marris, B., & King, B. (2006). *Evaluating health promotion programs.* Toronto, Canada: Health Communication Unit, Centre for Health Promotion, University of Toronto.

Wild, E. L., Hastings, T. M., Gubernick, R., Ross, D. A., & Fehrenbach, S. N. (2004). Key elements for successful integrated health information systems: Lessons from the states. *Journal of Public Health Management and Practice, 10,* S36–S47.

World Health Organization. (2011). *World health statistics 2011.* Geneva, Switzerland: Author.

Yeh, M.-L. (2014). Achieving knowledge translation in nursing care: The need for greater rigor in applying evidence to practice. *The Journal of Nursing Research, 22*(4), 1–221.

Yost, J., Thompson, D., Ganann, R., Aloweni, F., Newman, K., McKibbon, A., ... Ciliska, D. (2014). Knowledge translation strategies for enhancing nurses' evidence-informed decision making: A scoping review. *Worldviews on Evidence-Based Nursing, 11*(3), 156–167. doi: 10.1111/wvn.12043

CHAPTER 14

Quality Improvement Processes and Evidence-Based Practice

Susie Leming-Lee and Richard Watters

Objectives

After reading this chapter, learners should be able to:

1. Describe the relevance of quality improvement (QI) for healthcare
2. Outline the history of QI
3. Articulate the relationship between QI and evidence-based practice (EBP)
4. Compare and contrast QI systems
5. Analyze ethics of conducting QI projects

EVIDENCE-BASED PRACTICE (EBP) SCENARIOS

Scenario 1

To address the national problem of healthcare-associated infections, administrators at a medical center organized a multidisciplinary leadership committee to advance and sustain hand hygiene adherence. The administrators established a committee to design and implement an organization-wide hand hygiene program, which included hand hygiene observation process training. Thousands of hospital services' hand hygiene observations were collected for 1 year. The findings indicated that operating room (OR) staff were not meeting the hand hygiene adherence target goal despite intervention strategies used to improve hand hygiene compliance.

OR staff nonadherence to hand hygiene best practice was perplexing to the committee. The aim of the hospital committee's work was to protect patients and surgical team members by reducing surgical site infections and exposure to contaminants by improving hand hygiene adherence from 74% to 90%. How might the organization achieve this aim? A goal of this chapter is to provide readers with requisite knowledge, skills, and beliefs about QI to determine appropriate steps to take to improve quality of care and meet QI target goals in healthcare settings.

Scenario 2

The Toyota Production System (TPS) Lean 5S Project was conducted in a tertiary care hospital to reduce craniotomy infection rates. The TPS's Lean 5S process identifies work practice distractions and interruptions in work flow. Literature indicates there is a high level of distractions and interruptions in surgical flow processes that increase the occurrence of surgical errors and infections (Wiegmann, ElBardissi, Dearani, Daly, & Sundt, 2007).

As part of the TPS Lean 5S Project, a multidisciplinary task force of care providers close to the delivery of care to patients requiring neurosurgery was used to address the increase in craniotomy infections and OR foot traffic. The Model for Improvement (MFI) was used to guide the TPS 5S project work, which was to decrease neurosurgery infection rates by 90%. The literature indicated that when TPS's Lean 5S tool was used to reorganize an operating room to prevent the circulating nurse and other members of the OR team from leaving the OR during surgery to search for items needed for the surgery, the number of times the OR door was opened and closed was reduced, leading to decreased foot traffic in the OR. Too much OR traffic can compromise airflow systems. The studies revealed that enough door openings can defeat the safety effects of positive pressure systems meant to keep germ-contaminated air out of sterile operating rooms (Mears, Blanding, & Belkoff, 2015).

The team began a plan-do-study-act (PDSA) cycle by *planning* the 5S project. This included conducting an OR staff needs assessment and performing a spaghetti diagram of the designated OR to determine the number of times the circulating nurse left the room in search of supplies and equipment. Then, the design of a new floor plan for the OR was initiated using 5S principles. The *do* phase involved 5S *just-in-time training* for the OR staff, applying visual management principles in the designated OR, arranging the OR according to a new floor plan, and standardizing the supplies and equipment needed and used in the OR where the majority of craniotomies are performed. During the *study* phase, the team gathered and analyzed weekly craniotomy infection rates. During the first 2 months, the craniotomy infection rate decreased from 10 per 100 cases to 1 per 100 cases, meeting the aim of reducing craniotomy infection rates by 90%. The team, during the *act* phase of the project, presented the results of the project to the Perioperative Executive Committee. The committee decided the new 5S process should remain in place and that the new 5S process should be disseminated to other neurosurgery ORs.

The application of the Lean 5S QI tools and techniques along with the application of EBP provided the team with needed information and resources to meet the aim of the project and improve surgical outcomes for neurosurgery patients undergoing a craniotomy. The integration of QI methodology and EBP made a positive difference to patients and the healthcare system.

Discussion

Scenarios 1 and 2 both focus on a major patient care problem, hospital-associated infections. Both hospitals were committed to helping reduce or eliminate hospital-associated infections. In Scenario 1 the hospital began its journey without a reliable road map and after a year ended up where they started. In Scenario 2 the hospital used a well-thought-out quality improvement plan with stakeholder approval. The hospital in Scenario 2, understandably, made significant progress in lowering infection rates.

QUALITY IMPROVEMENT AND EBP

Healthcare QI is the systematic and continuous action that leads to quantifiable improvement in healthcare services and the health status of identified patient groups (Health Resources and Services Administration, 2017). Nurses can no longer be *only* clinical experts, but must also be change agents for improving healthcare services. The U.S. healthcare system presents a fundamental paradox. For the past 50 years, there has been an increase in biomedical knowledge, improved surgical procedures, and innovation in therapies and management of conditions that previously were fatal (American Society for Quality [ASQ], 2012). Nevertheless, the U.S. healthcare system is failing on basic dimensions of quality, outcomes, costs, and equity (ASQ, 2012). To eradicate these failings, nurses must understand the application of QI and the unique and important ways QI links to EBP.

There is a growing interest in promoting EBP and QI in clinical settings to foster high-quality care and maximize patient and family satisfaction with the care experience. EBP is a problem-solving approach in which best evidence, clinical expertise, and values are integrated to improve health outcomes (Sackett, Rosenberg, Gray, Haynes, & Richardson, 1996). QI is a systematic, data-driven activity to improve healthcare delivery; thus, QI provides an important context for EBP.

Unarguably, EBP and QI are distinct yet related areas of inquiry (Newhouse, 2007; Shirey et al., 2011). Possessing the abilities to implement both QI and EBP endeavors is recognized as a core essential for nurses (American Association of Colleges of Nursing, 2016; Institute of Medicine [IOM], 2003). Knowledge of EBP is positively associated with quality of patient care (Shuval et al., 2010). Nurses who engage in both QI and EBP activities prevent and reduce incorrect and unnecessary acts and errors of omission by using the best evidence and improving the process of healthcare delivery (Batalden & Davidoff, 2007; Hwang & Park, 2015; Rosenthal, 2007). QI provides an indispensable framework that supports EBP in creating a more predictable, effective, efficient, equitable, and patient-centered healthcare system.

HISTORICAL PERSPECTIVE OF QUALITY IMPROVEMENT AND PATIENT SAFETY

QI initiatives are driving significant changes in the U.S. healthcare system. These changes have been shaped by the historical confluence of QI activities in manufacturing, medicine, and nursing. The history of QI is rich and global, and an appreciation of this history is beneficial to nurses who engage in healthcare QI activities (Perla, Provost, & Parry, 2013). QI did not originate in healthcare; many current QI models and tools used in healthcare QI were created for improvement in the manufacturing sector (Cantiello, Panagiota, Moncada, & Abdul, 2016). This section reviews salient QI contributions from manufacturing, healthcare, and nursing.

Concerted efforts to improve quality of manufactured products began in the early 20th century (Handfield, 1989). In the mid-1920s, Shewhart developed the *control chart* or Shewhart Cycle. The Shewhart Cycle interconnected QI and *statistics* to manage and improve manufacturing processes (Best & Neuhauser, 2006; Handfield, 1989). The Shewhart Cycle consists of four primary elements: *plan, do, check/study,* and *act* (PDSA). The Shewhart Cycle, discussed in detail later in this chapter, is used widely in both manufacturing and healthcare to improve final products or patient outcomes, respectively (Bisgaard & de Mast, 2006; Gupta, 2006; Tague, 2005). In fact, PDSA is a prominent QI feature of many DNP (doctor of nursing practice) projects (White, Dudley-Brown, & Terhaar, 2016).

Using Shewhart's foundational QI work, Deming brought QI initiatives to the broader business world. In the 1940s, when the Japanese economy was severely depreciated, Japanese business leaders requested Deming's help to generate QI initiatives. Deming stressed that work environments must foster the concept of continuous improvement. Deming's QI philosophy emphasized that employees from frontline positions must be as involved in QI efforts as those in leadership positions. Using Deming's QI techniques, Japanese businesses became world leaders in manufacturing high-quality products at competitive costs, which inspired international adoption of many of Deming's QI principles (Handfield, 1989; M. L. Lynn & Osborn, 1991). In the 1980s, U.S. healthcare organizations began to incorporate QI principles from the business sector in the delivery of healthcare (Luce, Bindman, & Lee, 1994).

Prior to the 1980s, several important QI efforts were initiated specifically for healthcare. In the early 20th century (circa 1910), Codman pioneered improving patient care by following up with patients to ensure that healthcare treatments had desired outcomes. Codman's initiative provided a framework for the American College of Surgeons to develop minimum standards of care (Luce et al., 1994). In the mid-20th century, the Joint Commission on Accreditation of Healthcare Organizations was formed to advocate for quality healthcare (Luce et al., 1994). In the early 21st century, the IOM published several reports about the failing U.S. healthcare system and made several important recommendations for healthcare improvement (Table 14.1).

Nursing has made significant contributions to QI. Nightingale is credited with being the first person to document healthcare QI activities and outcomes (Nightingale, 1863). Clara Barton established the Sanitary Commission, which inspected and upgraded hospitals and Union Army living conditions (Lewis, 2013; Oats, 1994). In the late 20th century, the American Nurses Association evaluated healthcare quality and developed nursing-sensitive indicators, which

TABLE 14.1   Summary of Institute of Medicine (IOM) Reports

Institute of Medicine Report	Purpose of Report
To Err Is Human: Building a Safer Health System (2000)	To report widespread system errors and adverse events in U.S. healthcare organizations
Crossing the Quality Chasm: A New Health System for the 21st Century (2001a)	To identify critical gaps in the delivery of patient care services
Envisioning a National Health Care Quality Report (2001b)	To address the collection, analysis, and reporting of quality data
Leadership by Example: Coordinating Government Roles in Improving Health Care Quality (2002)	To address the duplication and disparate approaches to performance measures by government agencies
Priority Areas for National Action: Transforming Health Care Quality (2003a)	To identify priorities from earlier IOM reports and suggest a framework for action

led to mandates for safe nurse-to-patient ratios in hospitals (American Nurses Association, 1999). At the close of the 20th century, Magnet® Recognition Programs were initiated to align nurses' professional values (e.g., EBP) and expertise with QI in healthcare (Aiken, Havens, & Sloane, 2000).

The development of QI in healthcare has been a multidisciplinary effort. The evolution of QI science enables nurses to provide safer and higher-quality healthcare. This historical outline provides nurses a framework for reflecting on nursing's important role in the continuing evolution of healthcare safety and quality.

Clinical Microsystem and Quality Improvement

The IOM report (2001a) underscores that current healthcare systems are failing and are not providing safe patient care. The U.S. healthcare system is often severely flawed and dysfunctional and trying harder will not fix the system, but changing systems of care may lead to healthcare improvement (Nelson et al., 2002). The healthcare system in the United States, under specific conditions, can deliver high-quality state-of-the-art care.

To improve patient care, nurses rely on contextual understandings of healthcare organizations. One approach to contextually understanding healthcare organizations is through the conceptualization of *microsystems* and *macrosystems*. A clinical microsystem is a small, functional, front-line unit composed of nurses and other healthcare personnel who work together to provide care for identified groups of patients. Microsystems comprise discrete units of care, such as surgical intensive care units or ophthalmology centers, which provide direct healthcare to consumers (Barach & Johnson, 2006). Clinical microsystems are often embedded in larger organizations (i.e., macrosystems), such as medical centers. Microsystems are the essential building blocks of healthcare organizations and the clinical environments where patients and practitioners intersect. The quality and value of care produced by healthcare organizations or macrosystems can be no better than the quality of services generated at the microsystem level (Nelson et al., 2002).

Microsystems are healthcare units that provide the most healthcare to the most people; therefore, they require ongoing evaluation. Nurses comprise the largest workforce within microsystems and have important evaluative roles concerning the work within microsystems. The Institute for Healthcare Improvement (IHI) provides a framework for assessing six distinct microsystem areas:

1. Describe the *Purpose* of the microsystem.
2. Describe *Patients* who receive care in the microsystem.
3. Describe the microsystem's *Personnel*.
4. Describe the microsystem's *Processes* of care delivery.
5. Describe *Patterns* of the system.
6. Describe areas that need improvement within the microsystem (IHI, 2017a).

Defining and understanding quality, QI, healthcare quality, and how healthcare systems function is essential knowledge for nurses who are involved in leading and/or participating in QI initiatives. QI knowledge, skills, and abilities provide the foundation to enact change that leads to patient-centered, safe, efficient, effective, timely, and equitable healthcare delivery.

The Science of Improvement

The science of QI is an applied science (i.e., application of scientific knowledge to practical problems) that emphasizes innovation, rapid-cycle testing in the field, and dissemination of outcomes to generate knowledge about what changes, in which contexts, produce desired improvements (IHI, 2017e). The science of improvement is multidisciplinary (e.g., nursing, medicine, and sociology) and draws on diverse areas of content, such as clinical science, systems theory, statistics, and psychology (IHI, 2017b; Table 14.2).

QUALITY IMPROVEMENT MANAGEMENT SYSTEMS

A *quality management system* (QMS) is a formalized method of documenting processes, procedures, and responsibilities for achieving organizational goals (ASQ, 2016a). A QMS serves several purposes, such as improving processes, lowering cost, identifying and facilitating training opportunities, reducing waste, engaging staff, and setting organization-wide direction (ASQ, 2016a). Quality management has moved beyond manufacturing into service, healthcare, education, and government sectors (ASQ, 2016a). Four of the most frequently used QMS models are (a) the Toyota Production System (TPS), (b) the Six Sigma System, (c) the Baldrige Criteria System, and (d) the ISO 9000 System. Each model is described in the following sections.

The Toyota Production System

The TPS was developed by Toyota's chief production engineer Taiichi Ohno. Ohno adapted Deming's philosophy of flawless quality and the PDSA model to Japanese automobile manufacturing and included a requisite component of eliminating waste. Organizational efficiency is the cornerstone of the *Toyota Lean Production Model* methodology. Efficiency is defined as the relationship between

TABLE 14.2   Seven Propositions of the Science of Improvement

Propositions	Brief Summary Description of Proposition	What Proposition Means to Applying or Teaching Improvement Methods
1. The science of improvement is grounded in testing and learning cycles.	Leads to the justification of the Plan-Do-Study-Act (PDSA) cycles of improvement as an approach that is aligned with the scientific method.	The PDSA approach requires that a predication (hypothesis) is described, the data are collected to test the prediction, the analysis of the data is used to determine whether the prediction is correct or not, and the results generate learning and form the basis for the next improvement cycle test.
2. The philosophical foundation of the science of improvement is conceptualistic pragmatism.	Leads to the importance of using prior and existing knowledge to form theories, develop changes, and make predictions as to what will happen when these changes are applied. This proposition also supports the use of the Shewhart control charts as tools to measure existing system performance and to guide future prediction of the system performance.	Conceptualistic pragmatism states that everyone's observations are informed by their past experience (conceptualistic). In turn, these experiences are used to predict a range of possible futures that can be acted on (pragmatic). Inferring from these underlines the importance of forming theories from existing knowledge and then predicting what will happen as these theories are applied in the form of change concepts. Studying data over time through Shewhart's control chart methodology and theory of variation is central to improvement methods and reflects Lewis' pragmatism.
3. The science of improvement embraces a combination of psychology and logic (e.g., a weak form of "*psychologism*").	Provides the basis for multidisciplinary collaboration addressing problems from different perspectives, which is one psychology attribute of Deming's System of Profound Knowledge. This proposition underlines why it is important to use social sciences approaches in the improvement methods and activities.	Psychologism is a view that acknowledges that both psychology and formal ways of knowing, such as analytical philosophy, logic, and mathematics, are essential to understanding human behavior and decision making. This idea was once rejected by Western philosophers but is now considered a critical component to the science of improvement focusing on understanding the multiple dimensions of thought and action.
4. The science of improvement considers the contexts of justification and discovery.	Reinforces the notion that improvement efforts always involve a component of discovery and creativity in problem solving. These activities must be balanced by some form of justification such as using data to know if the tests of change worked, how well the change worked, and what will be the next steps in the improvement process.	The context of justification answers the questions "What do we know?" and "How do we know?" while the context of discovery is focused on the processes of discovery and innovation, which are fluid and dynamic. Both justification and discovery are core quality improvement concepts, and there is a focus on rapidly testing ideas to determine if and to what degree the concepts work.

(continued)

TABLE 14.2   Seven Propositions of the Science of Improvement (*continued*)

Propositions	Brief Summary Description of Proposition	What Proposition Means to Applying or Teaching Improvement Methods
5. The science of improvement requires the use of operational definitions.	Emphasizes the need for improvers to develop consistent, clear definitions of the terms they use. The improvers must also ensure that others involved in improvement understand those definitions to have a shared understanding.	Operational definitions provide a method for developing a shared meaning and understanding of concepts, ideas, goals/ aim, and measures. Without operational definitions, the meaning and intent of words and actions are only known by the individuals who use them. Collective action and effective communication require that all involved in the improvement initiative be on the same page; operational definitions are designed to minimize confusion and move those involved toward a shared understanding.
6. The science of improvement employs Shewhart's theory of cause systems.	Stresses understanding variation using improvement tools (such as Shewhart's control charts). These tools allow us to understand whether a process is stable or in control and to distinguish between process special and common cause variation.	Shewhart's control chart method is more than a statistical tool; it is a theory of variation and the voice of the process. The focus of the control chart is on learning whether a process is stable, in control, and can be used to determine whether the implemented changes result in improvement. The idea of a "chance-cause" system indicates that a process will behave within certain normal (random) limits based on the system; this is the voice of the process. If there is a failure to recognize this chance-cause system, this leads to the risk of tampering with a stable system, the effect of which can often be increased variation and poorer performance.
7. Systems theory directly informs the science of improvement.	Provides the basis for Deming's System of Profound Knowledge component, Appreciation for a System. This component focuses on system thinking, which means viewing the organization as dynamic and adapting to the customer's needs; it is composed of interdependent people, departments, processes, equipment, products, and facilities, all working toward a common purpose or aim.	The thought processes, the language, and the systems theory methods of understanding are critical to leading to improvement. Systems thinking linked with the pragmatism of proposition two (2) and Shewhart's theory of variation in proposition three (3) leads to Deming's concept of analytic studies. Systems thinking provides a focus on how the components relate to each other as a whole to create a system. Systems thinking is not a natural act, so it is essential to become comfortable with systems thinking to keep the focus on how the parts of a system are connected, rather than the performance of the parts of the system.

Source: Adapted from Perla et al. (2013).

inputs and outputs. The fewer inputs (resources) used to obtain a given output, the greater is the efficiency (Langley, Nolan, Nolan, Norman, & Provost, 1996). Lean methodology provides an organization with a systematic process and tools to improve efficiency through the elimination of eight types of waste: (a) defects/

rework, (b) overproduction, (c) waiting, (d) confusion—not clear, (e) transporting, (f) inventory, (g) motion, and (h) excess processing (Liker, 2004).

The TPS's Lean methodology is a rigorous improvement system designed to transform waste into value from the consumer's perspective (Kim, Spahlinger, Kin, & Billi, 2006). Lean methodology's primary underpinnings are *respect for people* and *continuous improvement*. These underpinnings have five key elements: (a) challenge, (b) continuous improvement, (c) observe, (d) respect, and (e) teamwork (Liker & Hoseus, 2008). The respect for people underpinning addresses a need for developing leaders who understand the work, developing exceptional people and teams that follow the organization's philosophy, and respecting the suppliers by challenging them and helping them to improve (Hoseus & Liker, 2008).

The continuous improvement underpinning suggests five stages of improvement: (a) value to the customer, created by the producer and defined in terms of specific products with specific capability offered at specific prices; (b) value stream mapping, which identifies the end-to-end process; (c) flow, which stipulates that products move smoothly and directly from process to process without waiting or waste; (d) customer pull, which creates a new production dynamic away from batches and queues; and (e) perfection, which is the reminder that Lean methodology embraces a continuous improvement mentality and attempts to remove nonvalue activity, simplify processes, and satisfy the customer's delivery needs (Nave, 2002; Young & McClean, 2006).

The tactical knowledge that underscores Toyota Lean Production methodology is captured in four basic rules:

1. Work shall be highly specified as to content, sequence, timing, and outcome.
2. Customer-supplier connections must be direct, and there must be an unambiguous yes-or-no way to send requests and receive responses.
3. Pathways for every product and service must be simple and direct.
4. Improvement must be in accordance with the scientific method and under the guidance of a teacher throughout the organization (Spear & Bowen, 1999).

The Lean methodology tool includes the basic seven quality improvement tools along with tools such as value-added analysis, value stream mapping, mistake proofing, and a tool unique to Lean, 5S (i.e., five steps). The five steps that go into this system for workplace organization and standardization begin with the letter "S" in Japanese: seiri, seiton, seiso, seiketsu, and shitsuke. These five terms are loosely translated into English as sort, set in order, shine, standardize, and sustain (Nave, 2002). The 5S technique is seen as the first step in implementing Lean methodology into an organization.

Six Sigma

Since its inception at Motorola in the early 1980s, Six Sigma has enabled organizations to solve problems, improve processes, increase profits, and improve customer satisfaction (Rudisill & Druley, 2004). Six Sigma is a data-driven process improvement methodology designed to identify and eliminate defects and reduce variation over time through the use of statistical rigor (Vest & Gamm, 2009). *Sigma* is a statistical measurement that reflects how well a product or process is performing. Higher sigma values indicate better performance, while lower values indicate a greater number of defects per unit. Six Sigma defects are limited to 3.4 defects per one million opportunities. Organizations aim for the 3.4 per million target by carefully applying Six Sigma methodology to every aspect of a specific product or process. Six Sigma allows for redirection of resources, time, and energy toward activities that bring desired value to customers (Seecof, 2016).

Six Sigma provides organizations with tools to improve the capability of their business processes. Experts in Six Sigma use both qualitative and quantitative techniques to drive process improvement. Tools such as statistical process control (SPC), control charts, process mapping, and failure mode and effects analysis are used in managing and improving systems (ASQ, 2016b). Six Sigma uses the rigorous methodology known as DMAIC (i.e., define, measure, analyze, improve, and control) to guide improvement work. DMAIC defines the process steps a Six Sigma practitioner is expected to follow, which begin with identifying the problem and end with implementing long-lasting solutions. To develop new processes or products in need of a total redesign, Six Sigma recognizes DMADV (i.e., define, measure, analyze, design, and verify). While DMAIC/DMADV are not the only Six Sigma methodologies in use today, they are the most widely adopted and recognized (ASQ, 2016b; Tague, 2005).

Six Sigma has been revolutionizing a diverse range of business organizations. The Six Sigma approach is relatively new to healthcare organizations. Given the widely reported incidence of healthcare errors (IOM, 2000), it is evident that healthcare organizations provide ample opportunities for the application of Six Sigma methodology to reduce errors at the clinical process or project level.

Malcolm Baldrige Criteria

The Malcolm Baldrige Criteria framework uses *performance excellence* as an integrated approach to organizational performance management. Performance excellence results in delivery of value to customers and stakeholders, and it contributes to organizational sustainability, improvement of organizational effectiveness, and organizational and personal learning (NIST, 2016). The Malcolm Baldrige Criteria framework provides a systems approach to managing an organization's processes and systems. The foundation of the Malcolm Baldrige Criteria framework is a set of core values and concepts that are embedded beliefs and behaviors found in high-performing organizations. The performance system consists of seven categories: (a) leadership; (b) strategic planning; (c) customer and market share; (d) measurement, analysis, and knowledge management; (e) human resource focus; (f) process management; and (g) business results (NIST, 2016).

International Organization for Standardization

The International Organization for Standardization (ISO) is an international agency composed of the national standards bodies of more than 160 countries. This set of international quality management standards has been adopted by organizations worldwide to facilitate international trade and act as a foundation to standardize and improve work processes and the service provided to consumers. ISO is the most recognized and implemented quality management system standard in the world (ASQ, 2016c). In 2015, The ISO 9000 standards were revised to reflect three primary standards: (a) ISO 9000, Quality Management Systems: Fundamentals and Vocabulary; (b) ISO 9001, Quality Management Systems: Requirements; and (c) ISO 9004, Quality Management Systems: Guidelines for Performance Improvement (Mitra, 2016). The revised ISO 9000 standards follow a high-level structure and a uniform use of core texts and terms. The revision includes a process-oriented approach and includes knowledge management, change management, and risk management (Mitra, 2016).

QUALITY IMPROVEMENT PROCESSES: A NEED FOR A FRAMEWORK/MODEL

Frameworks or models are needed to design, develop, implement, and evaluate QI initiatives. Without a model, it is difficult to assess causal linkages between structure and care processes and/or the impact of causal linkages on outcomes. Models provide a systematic approach to QI by guiding the design of an improvement project and the data collection, analysis, and interpretation of results (El-Jardali & Lagacé, 2005; Vincent, Taylor-Adams, & Stanhope, 1998). A model helps ensure that critical improvement project steps are present and systematic; however, no single model addresses all situations in need of QI initiatives (Duke University, 2016a).

Numerous QI models are used to guide improvement projects. Planning, implementation, analysis, and review are common elements found in credible QI models or frameworks. One of the most frequently used QI frameworks is based on Deming's work—that is, the Model for Improvement (MFI), created by Associates for Process Improvement (API). This MFI is a straightforward, effective, and reliable framework used to foster successful process or system changes (IHI, 2017c).

The MFI provides a framework for developing, testing, and implementing changes that lead to improvement. The MFI supports a full range of improvement efforts from the informal to the complex (Moen & Norman, 2006). The MFI consists of two parts of equal importance. Part 1, the "thinking part," involves the following three questions:

1. What is the QI team trying to accomplish?
   This question is intended to provide a clear understanding of improvements the team would like to make. Having a clear, measurable aim is critical for a successful improvement initiative (Ogrinc et al., 2012).
2. How will the QI team know a change is an improvement?
   This question helps QI team members determine the best outcome measures for the QI project.
3. What changes can the QI team make that lead to improvements?
   This question stimulates change ideas. Using this question, the QI team incorporates knowledge and experience to guide changes that might be adapted to best fit the improvement initiative.

Part 2 of the MFI is the "doing part"—that is, the tactics included in the PDSA cycle of change (Figure 14.1). Quality improvement initiatives test change through the systematic improvement science of the PDSA cycle part of the improvement model (Langley et al., 1996). The PDSA model emphasizes the role of learning in improvement (Westcott, 2006). Action is initiated by developing a hypothesis or prediction, a data collection plan, and a plan (P) for evaluation, which is followed by putting the plan into action and data collection (D). In the next stage, study (S), the results of the action are examined critically and then compared with the prediction, and what was learned is summarized. Did the action produce the desired results? Were any new problems created? Was the action worthwhile in terms of cost and other impacts? The knowledge gained in the third step is then acted on. Act (A) includes changing the plan by amplifying or reducing its scope, adopting the plan, or abandoning the plan, then determining a need to develop further PDSA cycles to move the work forward (Westcott, 2006).

Quality improvement frameworks or models contribute valuable concepts and technique; however, selection of a quality improvement model is dependent on the culture of an organization. As a change agent, it is essential to understand the organizational culture and use whatever strengths the model possesses to guide improvement efforts (Nave, 2002).

MEASUREMENT AND THE SCIENTIFIC METHOD

In the current healthcare system, there is a need for improved quality measures. Quality measures are used to (a) document the quality of care using clinical indicators, (b) support quality improvement initiatives, (c) make comparisons through benchmarking, (d) make judgments, (e) determine priorities, (f) support accountability, and (g) provide transparency in healthcare (Mainz, 2003b). During the mid-1800s and early 1900s, healthcare pioneers, such as Nightingale and Codman,

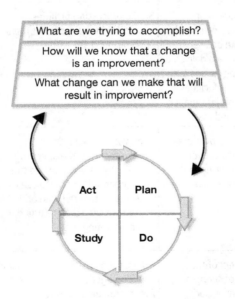

FIGURE 14.1   **Model for Improvement**

Source: From Langley et al. (2009); developed by Associates in Process Improvement (Copyright © 2016 Associates in Process Improvement).

advocated for healthcare reform by using quantifiable data to measure quality outcomes. Identifying outcomes of healthcare leads to methods that improve care (Ogrinc et al., 2012). Donabedian, another pioneer of quality measurement, followed Nightingale's and Codman's beliefs about the need to measure quality by introducing a model of healthcare quality designed to focus measurement using the categories of *structure*, *process*, and *outcome* (Varkey, Reller, & Resar, 2007).

Structure criteria include the environment in which healthcare is delivered. *Process* criteria consider how care is delivered. *Outcome* criteria are focused on recovery, restoration of function, and survival (Romano & Mutter, 2004). The outcome quality indicators are the most frequently reported and most widely understood. The criteria of structure, process, and outcomes must be addressed collectively to achieve optimal quality of care (Prathibha, Reller, & Resar, 2007). Table 14.3 defines each of the measurement criteria and provides an example of each measurement criterion and the corresponding measurement criterion indicator.

The Donabedian Model provides a systems-based framework for examining health services and evaluating quality of care for both quality assurance (QA) and QI paradigms. QA is concerned with inspection, thresholds, problems, and assurance. QI is concerned with systems and processes, constant effort, information flow and communication, and assessment and improvement (Romano & Mutter, 2004). QI has

TABLE 14.3   Measurement Criteria

Measurement Criteria	Definition of Measurement Criteria	Example of Measurement Criteria	Example of Measurement Criteria Indicators
Structure	The environment or infrastructure in which healthcare or a service or services are delivered, which may include such elements as facilities, equipment, information systems, and staff.	Sterile processing facilities, surgical instruments, washers, sterilizers, case carts	100% of sterile processing equipment will be operational daily.
Process	The steps or procedures required to deliver care or services to the customer/patient.	Removal and replacement of instruments in the operating room. Items are removed from the operating room in case cart, cleaned, sterilized, and added to the case cart, then returned to the operating room.	100% of all surgical case instruments will be counted and placed in the case cart prior to leaving the operating room at the end of each surgical case daily.
Outcome	The net effect of the delivery of services, which may include recovery, restoration of function, and survival.	Are instruments clean, sterile, and undamaged? Are instruments in correct case cart? Are instruments returned to correct operating room?	100% of all surgical instruments in the instrument tray will be sterile for use for each surgical case daily.

Source: Adapted from Lighter (2011).

become the quality paradigm of choice for QI practitioners and regulatory agencies such as The Joint Commission and the Centers for Medicaid and Medicare. Significant differences exist between the components of the QA and QI paradigms. Table 14.4 compares the two paradigms and illustrates a comparison of why quality improvement has become the paradigm of choice for quality improvement practitioners and regulatory agencies responsible for quality of care in healthcare organizations.

Defining Clinical Indicators

A clinical indicator for performance and outcome measures is a method for monitoring and assessing the quality of care and services provided to a consumer (Romano & Mutter, 2004). A clinical indicator quantitatively assesses selected healthcare processes or outcomes (Mainz, 2003a). Clinical indicators are categorized according to the Donabedian Model of measurement, as structures, processes, and outcomes, and they assess aspects of these criteria (Donabedian, 2005). Clinical indicators can be recorded as either rate or mean based to provide a quantitative basis for quality improvement. Clinical indicators may also be sentinel incidents of care that prompt further investigation (Mainz, 2003a). Examples of clinical indicators include blood cultures before administration of antibiotics, antibiotic prophylaxis within 1 hour of surgery, falls reported, urinary catheter–associated urinary tract infections, in-hospital mortality rate, and 30-day readmission rate. Furthermore, indicators can be generic measures that are relevant for most patients, or they can be disease-specific and express the quality of care for patients with specific diagnoses (Mainz, 2003a).

Monitoring healthcare quality is especially challenging without the use of clinical indicators. Clinical indicators create the basis for quality improvement and prioritization within a healthcare system. To ensure clinical indicators are reliable and valid, they must be designed, defined, and implemented with scientific rigor (Mainz, 2003b). Evidence-based indicators are true measures of quality and are used to predict the probability of patient outcomes. However, indicators based on professional consensus without evidence may be feasible for select patient populations, certain conditions, or certain treatments. A major factor of clinical indicators is risk adjusting. Failing to adjust for risk may create variable bias and result in incorrect inferences regarding the effects of a healthcare organization's quality of care (Romano & Mutter, 2004).

TABLE 14.4   Comparison of Quality Assurance and Quality Improvement

Quality Assurance	Quality Improvement
What went wrong?	What can we do to improve?
Reactive	Proactive
Often punitive, policing	Avoids blame
Tries to find who was at fault	Fosters system change
Focuses on the specific incident	Focuses on the entire system

Source: Adapted from Duke University School of Medicine (2016a).

Operational Definitions of Clinical Indicators

An operational definition of an indicator is a clearly specified, detailed description that explains how to measure a variable. Operational definitions should include where the data will be generated and gathered, such as the healthcare record, administrative and financial records, or patient reports (Ogrinc et al., 2012). Operational definitions are a method for developing a shared meaning and understanding of measures, goals, ideas, and concepts. Without operational definitions, the meaning and intent of words and actions are known only by the individuals who will use them. Operational definitions are designed to minimize confusion and promote shared understanding of outcome measurements (Perla, Provost, & Parry, 2013).

An operational definition needs to include the numerator (e.g., number of medication errors) and denominator (e.g., number of medications administered). For example, if a healthcare team wants to decrease medication errors, the numerator would be the number of reported medication errors, and the denominator would be the number of all administered medications. When developing operational definitions for indicators, there is a final consideration, which is understanding the context for measurements. Operational definitions must be consistent across all those participating in improvement initiatives (Hintch, 2016).

Benchmarking

Benchmarking, developed by Xerox in the 1980s, is the process of comparing one's performance to that of others. Benchmarking begins with standardized, comparative measurement and is also used to understand why there are performance differences between what appear to be similar processes (Plsek, 1999). Benchmarking is often associated with "best practice." Benchmarking is not a rigorous research methodology, but instead is a practical and action-oriented approach to analyzing performance (Plsek, 1999).

Clinical Value Compass: Balanced Measures

The Clinical Value Compass Model is an excellent resource to help identify and evaluate the effectiveness and efficiency of a QI initiative using clinical indicators. The model provides a balanced approach to measurement. The Clinical Value Compass consists of the following domains: (a) clinical, (b) functional, (c) satisfaction, and (d) costs (Nelson, Batalden, Lazar, & Brin, 2007). The Clinical Value Compass is useful in evaluating the outcome measures of clinical setting improvement projects, because the model allows for a balanced and meaningful profile of care given processes and outcomes (Nelson et al., 2007; Figure 14.2).

BASIC AND ADVANCED QUALITY IMPROVEMENT TECHNIQUES AND TOOL BOX

QI tools help predict conditions, performance, and process behavior. QI tools allow for efficient collection and analysis of data, which is important when there is an urgency to resolve a problem. Although there are many quality improvement

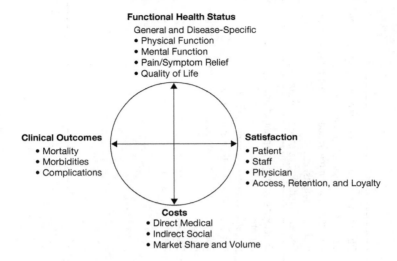

Measurement of Health Outcome

Functional Health Status
General and Disease-Specific
• Physical Function
• Mental Function
• Pain/Symptom Relief
• Quality of Life

Clinical Outcomes
• Mortality
• Morbidities
• Complications

Satisfaction
• Patient
• Staff
• Physician
• Access, Retention, and Loyalty

Costs
• Direct Medical
• Indirect Social
• Market Share and Volume

FIGURE 14.2   **Clinical Value Compass**

Source: From Langley et al. (2009).

tools, seven tools are most frequently used by quality improvement practitioners: (a) check sheet, (b) process flow diagram or chart, (c) cause-and-effect diagram (Ishikawa Diagram or fishbone), (d) Pareto chart, (e) scatter diagram, (f) histogram, and (g) control chart. Table 14.5 lists the frequently used tools, briefly describes the tools, and identifies when to use the tools.

Data Collection and Analysis

When implementing QI programs, it is mission critical to understand the importance of data collection for QI initiatives. Successful change cannot be initiated without data. Effective data collection helps provide informed decisions by reducing uncertainty. Data collection and comparison with desired performance levels enable practitioners to learn about the causes of a problem, what should be measured, and how the outcomes should be measured (Revelle, 2016). The following steps need to be followed to determine an appropriate data collection strategy:

- Determine:
  - The purpose of the data to be collected
  - The nature of the data to be collected
  - The characteristics of the data to be collected
  - Whether the data can be expressed to invite comparison with similar processes
  - Whether data place priority on the most important quality influences and whether the data are economical and easy to collect
  - The best type of data-gathering check sheet to use (e.g., tally sheet or check sheet)
  - Whether it will be possible to use random sampling (Revelle, 2016)

TABLE 14.5 Quality Improvement Techniques and Tool Box

Tool or Technique Category	Tool Name	Description	Use the Tool When
Basic Tools	Check sheet	• A simple check sheet is a structured, prepared form for collecting and analyzing data. This is a generic tool that can be adapted for a wide variety of purposes.	• Observing and collecting data repeatedly by the same person or at the same location • Collecting data on the frequency or patterns of events, problems, defects, etc. • Collecting data from a production process
	Process flow diagram, also called process flowchart or process flow map	• Variations: micro flowchart; macro flowchart; top-down flowchart; detailed flowchart (also called process map, micro map, macro map, service map, or symbolic flowchart); deployment flowchart (also called down-across or cross-functional flowchart, swimlanes); several-leveled flowchart. • A process flow diagram or flowchart is a picture of the separate steps of a process in sequential order. • Elements may include sequence of actions or steps, materials or services entering or leaving the process (inputs and outputs), decisions that must be made, people involved in the process, time involved at each step, and/or process measurements. • The process can be anything: a manufacturing process, an administrative or service process, a project plan. This is a generic tool that can be adapted for a wide variety of purposes.	• Developing an understanding of how a process is performed • Studying a process for improvement • Communicating to others how a process is performed • Communicating between people involved with the same process • Documenting a process • Planning a project

(continued)

TABLE 14.5 Quality Improvement Techniques and Tool Box *(continued)*

Fishbone diagram, also called cause-and-effect diagram, or ishikawa diagram or root cause analysis using *5 whys*	• A fishbone diagram identifies many possible causes for an effect or problem. It can be used to structure a brainstorming session. It immediately sorts ideas into useful categories. • *5 Whys:* When a problem, error, or defect occurs, it is critical to ask why. Asking why five times for each problem or defect identified allows you to get to the root cause of the problem, defect, or error. If the root cause is not identified you may not find the right solution to the problem, defect, or error.	• Identifying possible causes for a problem, which is especially helpful if team's thinking becomes unproductive, dead end, or in a rut
Run chart	A run chart is a line graph showing a process measurement on the vertical axis and the time on the horizontal axis. It is the simplest statistical tool. Often a reference line shows the average of the data. • A graphical tool to monitor important process variables over time • A helpful tool in identifying trends and cycles over time • One of the most important tools for assessing the effectiveness of change	• Monitoring a continuous variable over time • Examining patterns, such as trends, cycles • Conducting preliminary analysis to find obvious problems • Collecting insufficient points of data to draw a control chart
Brainstorming	• Brainstorming is a method for generating many creative ideas in a short period of time that is free of criticism and judgment.	• Selecting multiple options • Collecting innovative, creative, original ideas is desired • Engaging the entire group is desired
Advanced Statistical Tools and Techniques	Pareto chart, also called Pareto diagram, Pareto analysis	• A Pareto chart is a bar graph. The lengths of the bars represent frequency or cost (time or money), and are arranged with the longest bars on the left and the shortest to the right. In this way, the chart visually depicts which situations are more significant.	• Analyzing data about the frequency of problems or causes in a process • Focusing on the most significant problem or cause; however, there are many problems or causes • Analyzing broad causes by looking at their specific components • Communicating about the data with others

(continued)

Control chart also shewhart chart	"A control chart is simply a run chart with statistically determined upper and lower limits drawn on either side of the process average…. The upper and lower control limits are determined by allowing a process to run untouched and then analyzing the results using a mathematical formula" (Walton, 1986, p. 114). Data are plotted in time order. A control chart always has a central line for the average, an upper line for the upper control limit, and a lower line for the lower control limit. These lines are determined from historical data. By comparing current data to these lines, you can draw conclusions about whether the process variation is consistent (in control) or is unpredictable (out of control, affected by special causes of variation).	<ul><li>Studying how a process changes over time</li><li>Analyzing patterns of process variation from special causes (nonroutine events) or common causes (built into the process)</li><li>Controlling ongoing processes by finding and correcting problems as they occur</li><li>Predicting the expected range of outcomes from a process</li><li>Determining whether a process is stable (in statistical control)</li><li>Determining whether the quality improvement project should aim to prevent specific process problems or to make fundamental changes to the process</li></ul>
Scatter diagram	"A scatter diagram is a method of charting the relationship between two variables" (Walton, 1986, p. 111).	<ul><li>Pairing numerical data</li><li>Determining if the dependent variable may have multiple values for each value of your independent variable</li><li>Determining whether the two variables are related</li><li>Identifying potential root causes of problems</li><li>Determining objectively whether a particular cause and effect are related after brainstorming causes and effects using a fishbone diagram</li><li>Determining whether two effects that appear to be related both occur with the same cause</li><li>Testing for autocorrelation before constructing a control chart</li></ul>

(continued)

TABLE 14.5 Quality Improvement Techniques and Tool Box *(continued)*

Histogram	A histogram displays a frequency distribution of how often each different value in a set of data occurs. It is the most commonly used graph to show frequency distributions. Histograms look like a bar chart, but there are important differences between them.	• Examining that data are numerical • Examining the shape of the data's distribution, especially when determining whether the output of a process is distributed approximately normally • Analyzing whether a process can meet the customer's requirements • Determining whether a process change has occurred from one time period to another • Determining whether the outputs of two or more processes are different • Communicating the distribution of data quickly and easily to others
Failure modes and effect analysis (FMEA), also known as failure modes, effects, and criticality analysis (FMECA)	A FMEA is a step-by-step approach for identifying all possible failures in a design, a manufacturing or assembly process, or a product or service. "*Failure modes*" means the ways or modes in which something might fail. Failures are any errors or defects, especially ones that affect the customer, and can be potential or actual. "*Effects analysis*" refers to studying the consequences of those failures. Failures are prioritized according to how serious their consequences are, how frequently they occur, and how easily they can be detected. The purpose of the FMEA is to take actions to eliminate or reduce failures, starting with the highest-priority ones. FMEA also documents current knowledge and actions about the risks of failures, for use in continuous improvement. FMEA is used during design to prevent failures. Later it is used for control, before and during ongoing operation of the process. Ideally, FMEA begins during the earliest conceptual stages of design and continues throughout the life of the product or service.	• Designing or redesigning a process, product, or service after quality function deployment • Applying an existing process, product, or service in a new way • Developing control plans before designing a new or modified process • Planning improvement goals for an existing process, product, or service • Analyzing failures of an existing process, product, or service • Evaluating, periodically, throughout the life of the process, product, or service

(continued)

	Microsystem analysis	A microsystem analysis is an approach or methodology used to improve the quality and value of patient care as well as the work-life of personnel providing the care. The analysis involves an assessment, diagnoses, and action/treatment plan using improvement methods and tools (The Dartmouth Institute for Health Policy and Clinical Practice, 2015).	● Assessing how your clinical microsystem compares to the 10 key "success" characteristics of high-performing clinical microsystems ● Leadership ● Organizational support ● Staff focus ● Education and training ● Interdependence ● Patient focus ● Community and market focus ● Performance results ● Process improvement ● Information and information technology (IHI, 2017e)
Lean	Gemba walk	"Gemba walks are typically defined as going to where the action is. They are a key element of the Toyota Production System. Every Gemba walk is also a teaching exercise." If knowledge seeking questions are asked to the employees and then responses are given, this interaction, showing respect for the employees' knowledge of the system, can have a positive impact on the quality of the service or product (Bremer, 2015).	● Identifying waste in the process or system; is standardized work occurring; is there interruption in the work flow (Liker & Hoseus, 2008) ● Communicating with employees ● Investigating facts to make correct decisions ● Building consensus ● Understanding the process or system problem
	Kanban system	● A method of using cards as visual signals for triggering or controlling the flow of materials or parts during a production system (e.g., medical supplies).	● Identifying employees need to know their work production priorities ● Eliminating unnecessary paper ● Increasing employee skill levels ● Empowering employees to perform work when and where it is needed, ensuring there is no need to wait to be assigned a work task (Macinnes & Kingery, 2002)

(continued)

TABLE 14.5 Quality Improvement Techniques and Tool Box (continued)

Standard work	A process to gather the relevant information to document the best practice of producing work unit or providing a service (Hadfield, Holmes, Kozlowski, & Sperl, 2008).	• Establishing best practices or best sequence of activities
Kaizen and kaizen event	Kaizen is a Japanese term that means change (Kai) for the better (zen)—gradual unending improvement by doing little things better and setting and achieving increasingly higher standards. A Kaizen event is a method for accelerating the pace of quality improvement in a setting (George, Rolands, Price, & Maxey, 2005).	• Identifying waste in the process or system through such methods as value stream mapping, Gemba walks, or data collection • Identifying when results are immediately needed • Determining if there is a minimal implementation risk (George et al., 2005)
5S	5S, which stands for sort, set in order, shine, standardize, and sustain, is based on the Japanese concept for housekeeping (seiri, seiton, seiso, seiketsu, and shitsuke). This process supports Lean in its most basic form. Maintaining a simplified and streamlined work environment helps eliminate waste on organizational and personal levels. This is the foundation for spreading Lean to all at process and organizational levels (Zidel, 2006).	• Determining a need to give order to a space • Determining a need to prevent searching for items • Identifying a need to reduce probability of errors • Identifying a need to increase productivity • Identifying a need to increase response time • Identifying a need to modify the appearance of the area, conveying a more professional appearance (Zidel, 2006)
Spaghetti diagram	Spaghetti diagram is a visual representation using a continuous flow line tracing the path of an item or activity through a process. This diagram of a work area shows the actual path taken by a worker, patient, or product as it moves through a process (Chalice, 2007). The continuous flow line enables process teams to identify redundancies in the work flow and opportunities to expedite process flow.	• Depicting the flow of people, information, or materials • Reducing process time waste
Value stream mapping	Value stream mapping (VSM) is a pencil-and-paper tool used in two stages. First, follow a service or product's production path from beginning to end and draw a visual representation, current state map, of every process in the material and information flows. Second, draw a future state map of how value should flow. The most important map is the future state map.	• Determining employees need to be able to easily identify and eliminate areas of waste (Macinnes & Kingery, 2002) • Identifying a need to highlight the connection among activities and information and material flow • Helping employees to understand the entire value system rather than just a single function of that system

(continued)

A3	A3 reports, created by Toyota, is a simple and concise, high-level means of identifying and solving problems. This report, printed on a single sheet of paper, 11 × 17, is an effective tool because in addition to text, the tool contains visuals such as pictures, diagrams, and charts to improve communication.	• Providing a report to leadership • Communicating project results
Heijunka—smoothing the process	A method of leveling production by assigning work to match the outputs to reduce idle time, usually at the final assembly line. It involves averaging both the volume and sequence of different model types on a mixed model production line. Using this method avoids excessive batching of different types of product and volume fluctuations in the same product.	• Balancing appropriate workloads and duties of staff • Identifying a visual system if work is behind schedule • Reducing wait times • Achieving continuous work flow (Hadfield, Holmes, Kozlowski, & Sperl)
Poka Yoke—mistake proofing	*Poka Yoke* or "mistake proofing" is the use of any automatic device or method that either makes it impossible for an error to occur or makes the error immediately obvious once it has occurred. Derived from two Japanese words: *Yokeru* meaning "to avoid" and *Poka* which means "errors" (Zidel, 2006).	• Identifying defects • Preventing future defects
Jidoka—Just-in-time production	Stopping a line automatically when a defective part is detected. Any necessary improvements can then be made by directing attention to the stopped equipment and the worker who stopped the operation. The Jidoka system puts faith in the worker as a thinker and allows all workers the right to stop the line on which they are working.	• Allowing employees to raise nonconformances when defects have occurred and to become involved in their solution
Trystorming	A process for generating and quickly trying ideas rather than simply discussing those ideas, similar to brainstorming; however, action is taken at the time ideas are generated (Chalice, 2007).	• Identifying quick, effective solutions to problems

Source: Adapted from Tague (2005).

Teams

A team is not typically described as a QI tool; however, some quality improvement practitioners maintain that teams are the most powerful tool in the QI tool box (Grigsby & Magrane, 2016). Teams are the engine that propels the QI process. A team is a group of people working together to achieve a common purpose for which they hold themselves collectively accountable (Scholtes, Joiner, & Streibel, 2010). For a QI project to be successful, it is critical for an organization to use the knowledge, skills, experiences, and perspectives of a wide range of people to solve multifaceted problems, make appropriate decisions, and deliver effective, efficient solutions (Health Resources and Services Administration [HRSA], 2016; Scholtes, Joiner, & Streibel, 2010). In establishing a quality improvement team, thoughtful attention should be given to selection of team members. A team should be multidisciplinary when

- The task is complex
- Efficient use of resources is required
- Creativity is necessary
- Cooperation is essential for implementation
- The path to improvement is unclear
- Fast learning is necessary
- High commitment is desired
- The process involved is cross-functional
- Members have a stake in the outcome (Scholtes, Joiner, & Streibel, 2010)

Team members closest to the work often know the "how-to" solutions to the problem (Langley et al., 2009). A shared vision that is clearly and frequently communicated to team members is essential to keep the team focused on the aim and objectives of the improvement initiative.

Although there is no official how-to guide for selecting team members, the following questions are helpful to guide the team member selection process:

- Is the member committed to the success of the improvement initiative or project?
- Is the member willing to assume individual responsibility to complete the task?
- Is the member willing to learn from other team members?
- Is the member willing to maintain open communications with team members and leadership?
- Does the member work directly with the process or system targeted for improvement (HRSA, 2016)?

THE ETHICS OF CONDUCTING QUALITY IMPROVEMENT PROJECTS

The principal investigator of a research study, who is responsible for the proper conduct of the research, is easily identifiable, but this is often not the case with QI initiatives. There is no regulatory or ethical oversight or a need for informed consent in the quality improvement initiatives, which is unlike clinical research where it is necessary to protect the human subjects involved in the research (Bellin & Dubler, 2001). J. Lynn et al. (2007) note that ethical issues arise in QI because attempts to improve quality may inadvertently cause harm, waste scarce resources, or affect some patients unfairly. In addition, some activities using QI methods have been categorized as research that uses patients as subjects, which brings the activities under the ethical and regulatory requirements governing human subjects research, including review by institutional review boards (IRBs) (J. Lynn et al., 2007). Substantial delays, costs, and conflicts can occur when quality improvement activities fall under research regulations. This often leads to federal agencies disagreeing about the boundaries between research and QI. In addition, QI practitioners, healthcare organizations, agencies that fund research, policy makers, and IRBs may also experience uncertainty about ethical and legal requirements. As a result, these types of situations have generated disincentives to engage in QI (J. Lynn et al., 2007).

In light of the differing opinions and views related to the ethical oversight of quality improvement activities in healthcare, how should QI practitioners be held accountable for their work in improvement? Baily, Bottrell, Lynn, and Jennings (2006) maintain that protection of human participants in QI belongs in the clinical accountability system because ethical decision making is an intrinsic part of everyday clinical management. However, some argue that change in healthcare is inherently biased toward making the patient worse off for the sake of the "bottom line." QI might be considered a cover for change motivated by concern for profits rather than concern for patients. In response to this argument, Baily et al. (2006) suggest that in today's healthcare system, it is often possible to make changes that improve quality and lower cost at the same time (Baily et al., 2006). The reallocation of resources devoted to removing this waste is beneficial to improving patient care without increasing cost (Baily et al., 2006).

As change agents, QI practitioners need to be vigilant regarding the ethics of issues related to the practice of conducting QI initiatives. There is also a need to be knowledgeable and responsive to questions regarding ethics and QI as ethics experts continue to seek a solution to address the blurred line between ethics and quality improvement (Faden et al., 2013).

SUMMARY

This chapter briefly describes a historical perspective of QI and patient safety. The concept of QI and the science supporting QI are discussed. Theories and models for planned change and QI management systems are introduced. The chapter concludes with a brief discussion about ethics in conducting quality improvement initiatives.

REFERENCES

Aiken, L. H., Havens, D. S., & Sloane, D. M. (2000). The Magnet Nursing Service Recognition Program: A comparison of two groups of hospitals. *American Journal of Nursing, 100*(3), 26–36.

American Association of Colleges of Nursing. (2016). AACN essentials. Retrieved from http://www.aacnnursing.org/Education-Resources/AACN-Essentials

American Nurses Association. (1999). American Nurses Association (ANA) indicator history. Retrieved from http://www.nursingworld.org/MainMenuCategories/ThePracticeofProfessionalNursing/PatientSafetyQuality/Research-Measurement/Nursing-and-Quality.pdf

American Society for Quality. (2012). Keeping current. Health care report: U.S. healthcare system sorely needs quality. Retrieved from http://asq.org/quality-progress/2012/10/keeping-current.html

American Society for Quality. (2016a). History of quality. Retrieved from http://asq.org/learn-about-quality/history-of-quality/overview/overview.html

American Society for Quality. (2016b.) History of quality: The industrial revolution. Retrieved from http://asq.org/learn-about-quality/history-of-quality/overview/industrial-revolution.html

American Society for Quality (ASQ). (2016c). The early 20th century. Retrieved from http://asq.org/learn-about-quality/history-of-quality/overview/20th-century.html

Baily, M. A., Bottrell, M., Lynn, J., & Jennings, B. (2006). The ethics of using QI methods to improve health care quality and safety. *Hastings Center Report, 36*(4), S1–40.

Barach, P., & Johnson, J. K. (2006). Understanding the complexity of redesigning the clinical microsystem. *Quality and Safety in Health Care, 15*(1), i10–i16. doi:10.1136/qshc.2005.015859

Batalden, P. B., & Davidoff, F. (2007). What is quality improvement and how can it transform healthcare? *Quality and Safety in Heath Care, 16*(1), 2–3.

Bellin, E. & Dubler, N. N. (2001). The quality improvement-research divide and the need for external oversight. *American Journal of Public Health, 91*(9), 1512–1517.

Best, M., & Neuhauser, D. (2006). Walter A Shewart, 1924, and the Hawthorne factory. *Quality and Safety in Health Care, 15*(2), 142–143. doi:10.1136/qshc.2006.018093

Bisgaard, S., & de Mast, J. (2006). After Six Sigma: What's next? *Quality Progress, 39*(1), 30–36.

Bremer, M. (2015). Walk the line: The effective way to do a Gemba walk. Retrieved from http://asq.org/quality-progress/2015/03/lean/walk-the-line.html

Cantiello, J., Panagiota, K., Moncada, S., & Abdul, S. (2016). The evolution of quality in healthcare: Patient-centered care and health information technology applications. *Journal of Hospital Administration, 5*(2), 62–68.

Chalice, R. (2007). *Improving healthcare using Toyota Lean Production Methods* (2nd ed.). Milwaukee, WI: ASQ Quality Press.

The Dartmouth Institute for Health Policy and Clinical Practice. (2017). Retrieved from http://tdi.dartmouth.edu

Donabedian, A. (2005). Evaluating the quality of medical care. *Milbank Quarterly, 83*(4), 691–729.

Duke University School of Medicine. (2016a). Contrasting QI and QA. Retrieved from http://patientsafetyed.duhs.duke.edu/module_a/introduction/contrasting_qi_qa.html

Duke University School of Medicine. (2016b). FADE. Retrieved from http://patientsafetyed.duhs.duke.edu/module_a/methods/fade.html

El-Jardali, F., & Lagacé, M. (2005). Making hospital care safer and better: the structure-process connection leading to adverse events. *Healthcare Quarterly, 8*(2), 40-48.

Faden, R. R., Kass, N. E., Goodman, S. N., Pronovost, P., Tunis, S., & Beauchamp, T. L. (2013). An ethics framework for a learning health care system: A departure from traditional research ethics and clinical ethics. *Hastings Center Report, 43*(s1), S16–S27.

George, M., Rowlands, D., Price, M., & Maxey, J. (2005). *The Lean Six Sigma pocket toolbook*. New York, NY: McGraw-Hill.

Grigsby, R. K., & Magrane, D. (2016). Feature: Teams as tools for changing the culture of academic medicine. Retrieved from https://www.aamc.org/members/gfa/faculty_vitae/176006/teams_as_tools_for_changing.html

Gupta, P. (2006). Beyond PDCA: A new process management model. *Quality Progress, 39*(7), 45–52.

Hadfield, D., Holmes, S., Kozlowski, S., & Sperl, T. (2008). *The lean healthcare pocket guide XL.* Chelsea, MI: MCS Media.

Handfield, R. (1989). Quality management in Japan versus the United States: An overview. *Production and Management Inventory Journal, 30*(2), 79–85.

Health Resources and Services Administration (2016). Improvement teams. Retrieved from http://www.hrsa.gov/quality/toolbox/508pdfs/improvementteams.pdf

Health Resources and Services Administration. (2017). HRSA quality toolkit. Retrieved from https://www.hrsa.gov/sites/default/files/quality/toolbox/508pdfs/qualityimprovement.pdf

Hintch, B. (2016). Milestones in quality improvement measurement. Retrieved from http://www.hfma.org/Leadership/E-Bulletins/2016/March/Milestones_in_Quality_Improvement_Measurement/?utm_source=Real%20Magnet&utm_medium=Email&utm_campaign=93370132

Hwang, J. I., & Park, H. A. (2015). Relationships between evidence-based practice quality improvement and clinical error experience of nurses in Korean hospitals. *Journal of Nursing Management, 23,* 651–660.

Institute for Healthcare Improvement. (2017a). Clinical microsystem assessment tool. Retrieved from http://www.ihi.org/resources/pages/tools/clinicalmicrosystemassessmenttool.aspx

Institute for Healthcare Improvement. (2017b). Like magic? ("Every system is perfectly designed…"). Retrieved from http://www.ihi.org/communities/blogs/_layouts/ihi/community/blog/itemview.aspx?List=7d1126ec-8f63-4a3b-9926-c44ea3036813&ID=159

Institute for Healthcare Improvement. (2017c). Science of improvement. Retrieved from http://www.ihi.org/about/Pages/ScienceofImprovement.aspx

Institute for Healthcare Improvement. (2017d). Science of improvement: Establishing measures. Retrieved from http://www.ihi.org/resources/Pages/HowtoImprove/ScienceofImprovementEstablishingMeasures.aspx

Institute for Healthcare Improvement. (2017e). Whole system measures. Retrieved from http://www.ihi.org/resources/Pages/IHIWhitePapers/WholeSystemMeasuresWhitePaper.aspx

Institute of Medicine. (2000). *To err is human: Building a safer health system* (L. T. Kohn, J. M. Corrigan, & M. S. Donaldson, Eds.). Washington, DC: National Academies Press.

Institute of Medicine. (2001a). *Crossing the quality chasm: A new health system for the 21st century.* Washington, DC: National Academies Press.

Institute of Medicine (2001b). *Envisioning a national health care quality report* (J. M. Corrigan, M. P. Hurtado, & E. K. Swift, Eds.). Washington, DC: National Academies Press.

Institute of Medicine. (2003a). *Priority areas for national action: Transforming health care quality* (K. Adams & J. M. Corrigan, Eds.). Washington, DC: National Academies Press.

Institute of Medicine. (2003b). *Health professions education: A bridge to quality* (A. C. Greiner & E. Knebel, Eds.). Washington, DC: National Academies Press.

Institute of Medicine. (2011). *The future of nursing. Leading change, advancing health.* Washington, DC: National Academies Press.

Kim, C. S., Spahlinger, D. A., Kin, J. M., & Billi, J. E. (2006). Lean health care: What can hospitals learn from a world class automaker? *Journal of Hospital Medicine, 1*(3), 191–199.

Langley, G. J., Moen, R. D., Nolan, K. M., Nolan, T. W., Norman, C. L., & Provost, L. P. (2009). *The improvement guide: A practical approach to enhancing organizational performance.* San Francisco, CA: Jossey-Bass.

Langley, G. J., Nolan, K. M., Nolan, T. W., Norman, C. L., & Provost, L. P. (1996). *The improvement guide: A practical approach to enhancing organizational performance* (2nd ed.). San Francisco, CA: Jossey-Bass.

Lewis, J. J. (2013). The United States Sanitary Commission. Retrieved from https://www.thoughtco.com/sanitary-commission-ussc-3528670

Lighter, D. E. (2011). *Advanced performance improvement in health care: Principles and methods.* Sudbury, MA: Jones & Bartlett.

Liker, J. K. (2004). *The Toyota Way: 14 management principles from the world's greatest manufacturer.* New York, NY: McGraw-Hill.

Liker, J. K., & Hoseus, M. (2008). *Toyota culture: The heart and soul of the Toyota Way.* New York, NY: McGraw-Hill.

Luce, J. M., Bindman, A., & Lee, P. R. (1994). A brief history of health care quality assessment and improvement in the United States. *Western Journal of Medicine, 160*(3), 263–268.

Lynn, J., Baily, M. A., Bottrell, M., Jennings, B., Levine, R. J., Davidoff, F., . . . Agich, G. J. (2007). The ethics of using quality improvement methods in health care. *Annals of Internal Medicine, 146*(9), 666–673.

Lynn, M. L., & Osborn, D. P. (1991). Deming's quality principles: A health care application. *Hospital and Health Services Administration, 36*(1), 111–120.

Macinnes, R. L., & Kingery, C. (2002). *The lean memory enterprise jogger™.* Salem, NH: GOAL,OPQ

Mainz, J. (2003a). Defining and classifying clinical indicators for quality improvement. *International Journal for Quality in Health Care, 15*(6), 523–530.

Mainz, J. (2003b). Developing evidence-based clinical indicators: A state of the art methods primer. *International Journal for Quality in Health Care, 15*(Suppl. 1), i5–i11.

Mears, S. C., Blanding, R., & Belkoff, S. M. (2015). Door opening affects operating room pressure during joint arthroplasty. *Orthopedics, 38*(11), e991–e994. doi:10.3928/01477447-20151020-07

Mitra, A. (2016). *Fundamentals of quality control and improvement* (4th ed.). Hoboken, NJ: John Wiley.

Moen, R., & Norman, C. (2006). Evolution of the PDSA cycle. Retrieved from http://www.westga.edu/~dturner/PDCA.pdf

National Institute of Standards and Technology. (2016). Baldrige performance excellence program. Retrieved from https://www.nist.gov/baldrige/how-baldrige-works

Nave, D. (2002). How to compare Six Sigma, Lean and the theory of constraints. *Quality Progress, 35*(3), 73.

Nelson, E. C., Batalden, P. B., Godfrey, M. M., & Lazar, J. S. (2011). *Value by design: Developing clinical microsystems to achieve organizational excellence.* San Francisco, CA: Jossey-Bass.

Nelson, E. C., Batalden, P. B., Huber, T. P., Mohr, J. J., Godfrey, M. M., Headrick, L. A., & Wasson, J. H. (2002). Microsystems in health care: Part 1. Learning from high-performing front-line clinical units. *The Joint Commission Journal on Quality Improvement, 28*(9), 472–493.

Nelson, E. C., Batalden, P. B., Lazar, J. S., & Brin, K. P. (2007). Understanding clinical improvement: Foundations of knowledge for change in health care systems. In E. C. Nelson, P. B. Batalden, & J. S. Lazar (Eds.), *Practice-based learning and improvement: A clinical improvement action guide* (pp. 1–12). Oakbrook Terrace, IL: Joint Commission Resources.

Newhouse, R. P. (2007). Diffusing confusion among evidence-based practice quality improvement and research. *Journal of Nursing Administration, 37*(10), 432–435.

Nightingale, F. (1863). *Notes on Hospitals.* London, UK: Longman, Greene, Longman, Roberts, and Green.

Oats, S. (1994). *Woman of valor: Clara Barton and the CIVIL WAR.* New York, NY: Simon & Schuster.

Ogrinc, G. S., Headrick, L. A., Moore, S. M., Barton, A. J., Dolansky, M. A., & Madigosky, W. S. (2012). *Fundamentals of health care improvement: A guide to improving your patient's care* (2nd ed.). Oak Terrace, IL: Joint Commission Resources.

Perla, R. J., Provost, L. P., & Parry, G. J. (2013). Seven propositions of the science of improvement: Exploring foundations. *Quality Management in Healthcare, 22*(3), 170–186.

Plsek, P. (1999). Section 1: Evidenced-based quality improvement, principles, and perspectives. Quality improvement methods in clinical. Retrieved from http://www.directedcreativity.com/pages/PlsekPeds.pdf

Revelle, J. B. (2016). All about data. Retrieved from http://asq.org/quality-progress/2016/01/best-of-back-to-basics-problem-solving/all-about-data.pdf

Romano, P. S., & Mutter, R. (2004). The evolving science of quality measurement for hospitals: Implications for studies of competition and consolidation. *International Journal of Health Care Finance and Economics, 4*(2), 131–157.

Rosenthal, M. B. (2007). Nonpayment for performance: Medicine's new reimbursement rule. *New England Journal of Medicine, 367*(16), 1573–1575.

Rudisill, F., & Druley, S. (2004). Which Six Sigma metric should I use? *Quality Progress, 37*(3), 104.

Sackett, D. L., Rosenberg, W. M., Gray, J. A., Haynes, R. B., & Richardson, W. S. (1996). Evidence based medicine: What it is and what it isn't. *British Medical Journal, 312*(7023), 71–72.

Scholtes, P. R., Joiner, B. L., & Streibel, B. J. (2010). *Team handbook* (3rd ed.). Middleton, WI: Advertisers Press.

Seecof, D. (2016). Applying Six Sigma to patient care. Retrieved from https://www.isixsigma.com/industries/healthcare/applying-six-sigma-patient-care

Shirey, M. R., Hauck, S. L., Embree, J. L., Kinner, T. J., Schaar, G. L., Phillips, L. A., . . . McCool, I. A. (2011). Showcasing differences between quality improvement, evidence-based practice, and research. *The Journal of Continuing Education in Nursing, 42*(2), 57–68.

Shuval, K., Linn, L., Brezis, M., Shadmi, E., Green, M. L., & Reis, S. (2010). Association between primary care physicians evidence-based medicine knowledge and quality of care. *International Journal for Quality in Health Care, 22*(1), 16–23.

Spear, S., & Bowen, H. K. (1999). Decoding the DNA of the Toyota Production System. *Harvard Business Review, 77*(5), 95–106.

Tague, N. R. (2005). *The Quality Toolbox* (Vol. 600). Milwaukee, WI: ASQ Quality Press.

Varkey, P., Reller, M. K., & Resar, R. K. (2007). Basics of quality improvement in health care. *Mayo Clinic Proceedings, 82*(6), 735–739.

Vest, J. R., & Gamm, L. D. (2009). A critical review of the research literature of Six Sigma, Lean and StuderGroup's Hardwiring Excellence in the United States: The need to demonstrate and communicate the effectiveness of transformation strategies in healthcare. *Implementation Science, 4*, 35. doi:10.1186/1748-5908-4-35

Vincent, C., Taylor-Adams, S., & Stanhope, N. (1998). Framework for analysing risk and safety in clinical medicine. *British Medical Journal, 316*(7138), 1154–1157.

Walton, M. (1986). *The Deming management method.* New York, NY: Berkley Publishing Group.

Westcott, R. T. (Ed.). (2006). *The certified manager of quality/organizational excellence handbook* (3rd ed.). Milwaukee, WI: ASQ Quality Press.

Wiegmann, D. A., ElBardissi, A. W., Dearani, J. A., Daly, R. C., & Sundt, T. M. (2007). Disruptions in surgical flow and their relationship to surgical errors: An exploratory investigation. *Surgery, 142*(5) 658–656

Young, T. P., & McClean, S. I. (2006). A critical look at Lean thinking in healthcare. *Quality Safe Health Care, 17*(17), 382–386.

Zidel, T. G. (2006). *A Lean guide to transforming healthcare.* Milwaukee, WI: ASQ Quality Press.

PART IV

Evidence-Based Practice: Empowering Nurses

CHAPTER 15

Evidence-Based Practice: A Culture of Organizational Empowerment

Thomas L. Christenbery

Objectives

After reading this chapter, learners should be able to:

1. Recall the Institute of Medicine's (IOM) standards regarding evidence-based practice (EBP)
2. Describe the components of structural empowerment
3. Make inferences about linkages among structural empowerment, nurse empowerment, and EBP

EVIDENCE-BASED PRACTICE (EBP) SCENARIOS

Scenario 1

A team of inner-city community health nurses noted the number of elderly clients was growing, and, in general, they were failing to take medications as prescribed. The nurses wondered what perceptions and beliefs multiethnic, elderly inner-city clients might have about medication adherence. The nurses thought a focus group, consisting of elderly clients, might help them better understand clients' medication adherence issues. The clinic nurses approached two advanced practice registered nurses (APRNs) about this idea. One APRN said the idea already had been studied exhaustively and suggested a review of recent research. The other APRN said maybe clinicians were ordering too many medications and perhaps clinicians should limit the number of medications prescribed as an approach to resolving the problem. The nurses were not deterred but consulted with the clinic's manager who said, "Not with your workload. Just keep doing the basic nursing care that is needed of you. I'm sure the APRNs and physicians will be on top of this problem."

Scenario 2

A team of inner-city community health nurses noted the number of elderly clients was growing, and, in general, they were failing to take medications as prescribed. The nurses wondered what perceptions and beliefs multiethnic, elderly inner-city clients might have about medication adherence. The nurses thought a focus group, consisting of elderly clients, might help them better understand clients' medication adherence issues. The nurses mentioned the focus group idea to two of the clinic's APRNs who told them that although this phenomenon had been explored elsewhere, their clinic population was different, and they should pursue their idea as an EBP project. One of the APRN's DNP (doctor of nursing practice) projects had used a focus group to help answer an EBP question, and she said she would mentor the clinic nurses through the EBP process. The other APRN had just written a manuscript for publication and found that a city librarian, although not a medical librarian, was helpful in locating appropriate scholarly resources for EBP projects. The clinic nurses consulted with the health center's director about pursuing the focus group as an EBP project. The director indicated that space was tight at the clinic; however, she agreed their idea for an EBP project might be helpful for the clinic's clients, so she would attempt to allocate space to accommodate the focus group.

Discussion

The preceding scenarios depict the same clinical concern but with different organizational responses. The first scenario may lead to positive client-centered care outcomes, while the second scenario holds no promise of positive outcomes. An aim of this chapter is to introduce organizational characteristics that help determine a nurse's success in the use of EBP.

An IOM aim is that 90% of nurses' clinical decisions will be evidence-based by 2020 (Institute of Medicine [IOM], 2010). In keeping with the IOM's vision for 21st-century healthcare, nurses must use the best evidence to provide the most appropriate care for patients (McClellan, McGinnis, Nabel, & Olsen, 2008). Consequently, healthcare organizations have a commitment to increase nurse engagement in EBP (Wilson et al., 2015). As nursing students and nurses consider their career trajectories, they need to be mindful of organizations that endorse EBP as a means to provide the best opportunities to learn, progress, and contribute to optimal care. Considerable research has identified characteristics of organizations that foster a culture of EBP (Laschinger & Havens, 1996; Melnyk, 2012). Schools of nursing have an obligation to help students recognize organizational characteristics that both foster nurse readiness for engagement in EBP and sustain enthusiasm for EBP as a foundation for positive patient outcomes.

Organizations in which nurses are empowered to fully engage in EBP, and thereby optimally practice their profession, are organizations with specific structural characteristics or determinants (Laschinger, Almost, & Tuer-Hodes, 2003). *Empowered* is a widely used concept with multiple and various meanings (Rodwell, 1996). Within organizational literature, empowered means having the ability to "get things done." More explicitly, participants (e.g., nurses, physicians, and social workers) in organizations who are empowered have abilities to mobilize resources and achieve professional goals (Kanter, 1993; Wilson et al., 2015). Conversely, participants in organizations who are not empowered often sense they are entrapped in traditional hierarchal contexts in which their perceived and/or actual autonomy and control over a work environment are stifled. In healthcare settings, professional goal achievement and project completion are problems for participants who do not perceive a sense of empowerment (Kuokkanen & Leino-Kilpi, 2000).

Theoretical descriptions and research evidence indicate that participant empowerment in organizations is associated with the presence of four key structural determinants: (a) information, (b) support, (c) resources, and (d) opportunity (Kanter, 1993). The mediating effects of information, support, resources, and opportunity form an organizational structure that enables nurses to achieve a sense of professional empowerment (Christenbery, Williamson, Sandlin, & Wells, 2016; Laschinger & Havens, 1996; see Figure 15.1). Several articles discuss information, support, resources, and opportunity as essential structural determinants that promote incorporating best evidence into practice (Dunning, 2013; Hagen & Walden, 2015; Scala, Price, & Day, 2016). Healthcare organizations that foster information, support, resources, and opportunity, as structural determinants, tend to engage nurses in the process of incorporating new evidence into practice (Christenbery et al., 2016; Laschinger et al., 2003). Each determinant of structural empowerment is important and, therefore, worthy of introductory discussion.

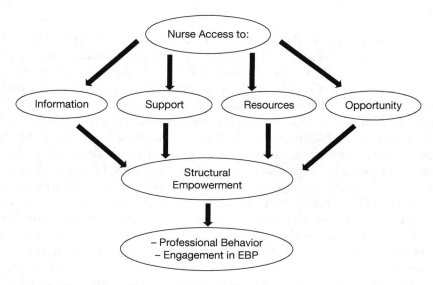

FIGURE 15.1 Model of structural empowerment

EBP, evidence-based practice.

INFORMATION

Information, as a structural determinant, refers to possessing knowledge that is necessary to be effective within an organization and having technical knowledge and skillsets to manage the knowledge (Orgambidez-Ramos & Borrego-Ales, 2014). Empowerment is facilitated when nurses have unimpaired access to critical healthcare organizational information. Critical information includes relevant knowledge about an organization's mission, goals, and values; it also includes having active roles in the management and decision-making processes related to the mission, goals, and values. Engagement in EBP frequently provides nurses greater access to organizational information through contacts (e.g., librarians, physicians, and researchers) made during the EBP process, thereby enhancing a deeper understanding and appreciation of the organization's goals and expectations.

SUPPORT

Organizational support is indispensable for accomplishing job responsibilities and fueling decision-making energies associated with those responsibilities (Kanter, 1993). Organizational support in healthcare enables nurses to effectively participate in the process and delivery of EBP. Organizational support includes both guidance for solving EBP problems and constructive feedback from other organizational participants such as nurse colleagues, physicians, and supervisors. Reassurance from organizational participants is a source of inspiration to fully engage in and sustain the EBP process. Successful initiation of EBP and long-term engagement with EBP are contingent on organizational support (Laschinger & Havens, 1996).

RESOURCES

Access to organizational resources refers to the ability to secure material, money, time, equipment, and human resources (i.e., organizational personnel; Kanter, 1993). Resources are needed to accomplish organizational goals and support organizational values. Nurses who have access to suitable resources and the requisite skills to use those resources have the freedom to be increasingly self-directed and intellectually inspired to use EBP as a means to approach and solve patient care or systems problems (Christenbery et al., 2016). Access to resources is identified as the most strongly related empowerment structure for nurses' control over their clinical practice (Laschinger et al., 2003).

OPPORTUNITY

Organizational opportunity, related to structural empowerment, refers to the potential for growth and upward mobility within the organization as well as the opportunity to enhance work-related knowledge and skills (Kanter, 1993).

Nurses who are not provided the opportunity to develop and advance receive an unspoken message that they do not mean much to the healthcare organization (Kanter, 1993; Patrick & Laschinger, 2006). Organizational opportunity allows nurses to demonstrate out-of-the-ordinary creativity and ability and be perceived as successful and promotable participants. Organizations that encourage engagement in EBP typically provide nurses a wide variety of opportunities to use discipline-specific knowledge and skills, with intellect and ingenuity, to accomplish meaningful patient-centered goals (Melnyk, Fineout-Overholt, Gallagher-Ford, & Kaplan, 2012).

Information, support, resources, and opportunity in healthcare organizations are established precursors for structural empowerment (Laschinger & Havens, 1996). In the 21st century, many nurses report they do not feel empowered (Fletcher, 2006; Manojlovich, 2007). Nurses who perceive a lack of professional empowerment tend to be less effective in "getting things done" and in influencing others to engage in the delivery of optimal patient care. Thus, it is vital to discuss, especially in terms of EBP, the importance of structural empowerment.

STRUCTURAL EMPOWERMENT

Research demonstrates that empowered nurses are decidedly motivated and inspire others by sharing their sources of empowerment (Laschinger & Havens, 1996). Empowered nurses are less likely to experience professional role strain (Laschinger, Finegan, & Shamian, 2001) and career fatigue (Laschinger, Finegan, Shamian, & Wilk, 2001). In contrast, nurses who lack a sense of empowerment often express feelings of frustration and failure, even though they are still accountable for comparable work-related outcomes as nurses who possess a sense of empowerment (Laschinger & Havens, 1996).

There are alternative conceptualizations of organizational empowerment. Kanter (1993) contends that empowerment is derived from social structures in the workplace that enable participants to be more satisfied and productive in work-related activities. Chandler (1992) proposed that empowerment is a product formed from work-related relationships. Ryles (1999) maintained that a sense of empowerment arises from within one's own psychological constitution.

When considering potential work environments that support nurse empowerment, it would be difficult for nurses to select empowering organizational environments based on assessment of group relationships or the psychological makeup of the organization's participants. However, nurses can select empowering work environments that endorse EBP based on the representation of organizational social structures (i.e., information, support, resources, and opportunity). By asking questions and making observations directly related to the four components of structural empowerment, nurses can detect if organizations have an empowerment infrastructure in place to support their use of EBP (Table 15.1).

Structural empowerment is held on a continuum from less to more empowerment, depending on the degree of absence or presence of the four structural components. Structural empowerment fosters nurses' creativity and allows that creativity to be fully expressed (Clavelle, Porter O'Grady, Weston, & Verran, 2016). In the presence of the structural empowerment components, nurses' engagement

TABLE 15.1   Organizational Characteristics That Indicate Endorsement of EBP

To assess organizations that empower nurses to engage fully in EBP, ask questions and make observations regarding the various structural empowerment characteristics.

Information	Support	Resources	Opportunity
● Access to information (e.g., librarian on staff, immediate connection to electronic literature, technical and informatics support) ● Clearinghouse of evidence-based information (online)	● Leadership awareness of EBP ● Organization values and supports spirit of inquiry ● Managerial support ● Availability of EBP mentors ● Peer support ● MD support and collaboration	● Education (e.g., EBP Fellowship Program, journal clubs, EBP website) ● Written organizational EBP expectations and standards ● Staff awareness of EBP ● Continuing education resources ● Organizational education offerings related to EBP and skill development to engage in EBP ● Financial backing for EBP initiatives	● Time specifically allocated for EBP activity ● Organization supports internal and external dissemination of EBP projects ● History of supporting EBP project ● Organizational recognition for EBP projects

EBP, evidence-based practice.

in EBP becomes more evident with deliverables related to quality of patient care and safety. Nurses have identified engagement in EBP as an empowering experience by giving them "voice" and allowing them to improve the quality of care provided to patients (Melnyk et al., 2012).

Many healthcare organizations promote the structural determinants of information, support, resources, and opportunity as a means to empower nurses and encourage nurse participation in EBP. Examples of dissemination of EBP projects from such organizations include changing NPO practice in the emergency department (Denton, 2015), implementing skin-skin contact in the operating room following caesarean section (Grassley & Jones, 2014), and monitoring delirium in the postanesthesia care unit (Card et al., 2012).

EXEMPLAR: STRUCTURAL EMPOWERMENT AND EBP

A major metropolitan medical center operates a pediatric satellite clinic in a rural community where a number of children have chronic heart conditions and receive follow-up care at the satellite clinic. Because these patients' parents often seemed stressed, clinic nurses wondered if parents of children with long-term, and often disabling, heart conditions might benefit from peer support groups.

The nurses heard clinic physicians and APRNs talk about the importance of always using current and best evidence to guide practice. Although unfamiliar with the EBP process, the nurses decided to approach the parent peer support group idea as an EBP project. First, the nurses sought permission from the clinic manager who believed the EBP approach for this concern was worthy of exploring (*support*). The manager directed the nurses to one of the APRNs who had experience with EBP (*information, support*). The APRN encouraged pursuit of the project and suggested the nurses contact the nurse researcher who coordinated EBP projects at the medical center (*support*).

The nurse researcher agreed to meet with the clinic nurses via Skype (*resource*). The nurse researcher thought the project had merit and discussed the steps of the EBP process with the nurses. The nurse researcher sent the nurses three relevant nursing journal articles on conducting an EBP project and provided them access to the medical center's EBP website (*support, information*). The nurse researcher agreed to serve as a consultant for the EBP project and agreed to meet with the nurses via Skype every 2 weeks for an update on the project's process (*information, support*). With the nurse researcher's help, the clinic nurses developed a patient population, intervention, comparison, outcome, and time frame (PICOT) question for their project (*support, resource*). In addition, the nurse researcher made initial contact with the medical center librarian who oriented the nurses to use of appropriate databases for locating research articles. Only a limited number of relevant primary studies (i.e., original research) were found indicating a possible gap in knowledge related to parent peer support groups.

In subsequent biweekly meetings, the nurse researcher assisted the clinic nurses to evaluate and synthesize research literature for both methodological quality and level of evidence. In addition, studies were evaluated for type, duration, long-term effects, and cost benefits of parent peer support groups. The review and analysis of literature found that parent peer support groups have the potential to improve parents' perceptions of quality of life; however, findings across studies were inconsistent, inconclusive, and weak. In addition, the research articles were primarily qualitative designs.

Despite the low methodologic quality and low level of evidence (i.e., primarily qualitative rather than quantitative research designs), the nurses believed the evidence supported the possibility of improved quality of life for parents who participated in peer support groups. The nurses believed parent participation in the support group would be low risk for harm. The nurses were encouraged by the APRNs and physicians to initiate a parent peer support group (*support*). The nurse researcher recommended a survey tool to measure parents' quality of life (QOL) before and after peer group participation (*information, support, resource*).

The APRNs helped the nurses contact a local psychologist to provide professional direction on setting up guidelines for peer support groups (*information, support*). The nurse researcher assisted with helping clinic nurses receive Institutional Review Board approval for studying QOL (*support*). The clinic manager secured private space in the clinic for the parent peer groups to meet (*support, resource*). The nurse researcher agreed to assist with data analysis related to the QOL survey (*support*). Physicians and APRNs agreed to refer parents to the support group (*support*).

The parent peer support group was implemented and met for 6 consecutive weeks. The QOL measurement demonstrated a statistically significant improvement in parents' perception of personal health. The clinic provided a time for the nurses to share their project and findings with all clinic staff (*opportunity*). In addition, the clinic paid the nurses' registration fees to attend the state Nurses' Association Convention where the nurses had a poster accepted about their parent peer support group EBP project (*opportunity*). The nurse researcher was intrigued with the gap in well-controlled studies about parent peer support groups and undertook an investigation to study the phenomenon. She agreed to acknowledge the clinic nurses in any subsequent manuscripts or presentations (*empowerment*).

The nurses were satisfied that parents of children with chronic heart conditions were receiving a valuable additional resource in ongoing parent peer support groups. In addition, the nurses believed they made an out-of-the-ordinary contribution to the well-being of the patients and families.

SUMMARY

Healthcare organizations need nurses who can take the initiative and respond creatively to the IOM mandate that 90% of clinical decisions be evidence based. Nurses who perceive a sense of empowerment are generally more committed and effective in meeting a healthcare organization's patient-centered goals. The link between an empowering work setting (i.e., access to information, resources, support, and opportunity) and desired organizational outcomes, such as EBP, are described in this chapter. Later chapters in this book discuss specific actions organizations and nurses can use to shape and strengthen a culture of EBP.

REFERENCES

Card, E., Tomes, C., Wood, J., Lee, C., Allen, L., Kellum, L., & Pandharipande, P. (2012). Implementation of delirium monitoring in the PACU. *Journal of PeriAnesthesia Nursing, 27*(3), e10. doi:10.1016/j.jopan.2012.04.056

Chandler, G. E. (1992). The source and process of empowerment. *Nursing Administration Quarterly, 16*(3), 65–71.

Christenbery, T., Williamson, A., Sandlin, V., & Wells, N. (2016). Immersion in evidence-based practice fellowship program. *Journal for Nurses in Professional Development, 32*(1), 15–20.

Clavelle, J. T., Porter O'Grady, T., Weston, M. J., & Verran, J. A. (2016). Evolution of structural empowerment: Moving from shared to professional governance. *Journal of Nursing Administration, 46*(6). 308–312. doi:10.1097/NNA.0000000000000350

Denton, T. (2015). Southern hospitality: How we changed the NPO practice in the emergency department. *Journal of Emergency Nursing, 41*(4), 317–322.

Dunning, T. (2013). Engaging clinicians in research: Issues to consider. *Journal of Nursing and Care, 2.* doi:10.4172/2167-1168.1000132

Fletcher, K. (2006). Beyond dualism: Leading out of oppression. *Nursing Forum, 41*(2), 50–59. doi:10.1111/j.1744-6198.2006.00039.x

Grassley, J. S., & Jones, J. (2014). Implementing skin-to-skin contact in the operating room following cesarean birth. *Worldviews on Evidence-Based Nursing, 11*(6), 414–416.

Hagen, J., & Walden, M. (2015). Development and evaluation of the barriers to nurses' participation in research questionnaire at a large academic pediatric hospital. *Clinical Nursing Research, 26,* 157–175. doi:10.1177/1054773815609889

Institute of Medicine. (2010). *The future of nursing: Leading change advancing health.* Washington, DC: National Academies Press.

Kanter, R. (1993). *Men and women of the corporation.* New York, NY: Basic Books.

Kuokkanen, L., & Leino-Kilpi, H. (2000). Power and empowerment in nursing: Three theoretical approaches. *Journal of Advanced Nursing, 31*(1), 235–241.

Laschinger, H. K., Almost, J., & Tuer-Hodes, D. (2003). Workplace empowerment and Magnet hospital characteristics: Making the link. *Journal of Nursing Administration, 33*(7–8), 410–422.

Laschinger, H. K., Finegan, J., & Shamian, J. (2001). The impact of workplace empowerment, organizational trust on staff nurses' work satisfaction and organizational commitment. *Health Care Management Review, 26*(3), 7–23.

Laschinger, H. K., Finegan, J. Shamian, & Wilk, P. (2001). Impact of structural and psychological empowerment on job strain in nursing work settings: Expanding Kanter's model. *Journal of Nursing Administration, 31*(5), 260–272.

Laschinger, H. K., & Havens, D. S. (1996). Staff nurse work empowerment and perceived control over nursing practice: Conditions for work effectiveness. *Journal of Nursing Administration, 26*(9), 27–35.

Manojlovich, M. (2007). Power and empowerment in nursing: Looking backward to inform the future. *Online Journal of Issus in Nursing, 12*(1), Manuscript 1. doi:10.3912/OJIN.Vol12No01Man01

McClellan, M. B., McGinnis, J. M., Nabel, E. G., & Olsen, L. A. M. (2008). *Evidence-based medicine and the changing nature of health care: 2007 IOM annual meeting summary.* Washington, DC: National Academies Press.

Melnyk, B. M. (2012). Achieving a high-reliability organization through implementation of the ARCC model for system wide sustainability of evidence-based practice. *Nursing Administration Quarterly, 36*(2), 127–135. doi:10.1097/NAQ.obo13e318249fb6a

Melnyk, B. M., Fineout-Overholt, E., Gallagher-Ford, L., & Kaplan, L. (2012). The state of evidence-based practice in US nurses: Critical implications for nurse leaders and educators. *Journal of Nursing Administration, 42*(9), 410–417.

Orgambidez-Ramos, A., & Borrego-Ales, Y. (2014). Empowering employees: Structural empowerment as antecedent of job satisfaction in university settings. *Psychological Thought, 7*(1), 28–36. doi:10.5964/psyct.v7i1.88

Patrick, A., & Laschinger, H. K. S. (2006). The effect of structural empowerment and perceived organizational support on middle level nurse managers role satisfaction. *Journal of Nursing Management, 14,* 13–22.

Rodwell, C. M. (1996). An analysis of the concept of empowerment. *Journal of Advanced Nursing, 22,* 305–313.

Ryles, S. M. (1999). A concept analysis of empowerment: Its relationship to mental health nursing. *Journal of Advanced Nursing, 29,* 600–607.

Scala, E., Price, C., & Day, D. (2016). An integrative review of engaging clinical nurses in nursing research. *Journal of Nursing Scholarship, 48*(4), 423–430.

Wilson, M., Sleutel, M., Newcomb, P., Behan, D., Walsh, J., Wells, J. N., & Baldwin, K. M. (2015). Empowering nurses with evidence-based practice environments: Surveying Magnet®, Pathway to Excellence®, and non-Magnet facilities in one healthcare system. *Worldviews in Evidence-Based Nursing, 12*(1), 12–21.

CHAPTER 16

Nursing Leadership: The Fulcrum of Evidence-Based Practice Culture

Thomas L. Christenbery

Objectives

After reading this chapter, learners should be able to:

1. Identify characteristics of formal and informal leaders
2. Describe ways nursing leaders encourage an organizational spirit of patient-centered inquiry
3. Outline a plan for implementing an evidence-based practice (EBP) healthcare culture

EVIDENCE-BASED PRACTICE (EBP) SCENARIOS

Scenario 1

A clinical nurse leader (CNL) mentioned to the chief nurse executive (CNE) that direct care nurses on the oncology unit were beginning an EBP project related to the management of intractable pain. The CNL inquired about available support for the direct care nurses in implementing the EBP project. The CNE noted that if schools of nursing were doing their job then the hospital would not have to absorb an additional educational cost. The CNE related that direct care nurses perhaps were moving too hastily on this project and mentioned physicians have used research for years; therefore, she did not want the nurses to seem to be underprepared. She asked the CNL to have the nurses wait until a thorough assessment of their EBP knowledge was conducted.

Scenario 2

A CNL mentioned to the CNE that direct care nurses on the oncology unit were beginning an EBP project related to management of intractable pain. The CNL inquired about available support for the direct care nurses in implementing the EBP project. The CNE stated, "I see the nurses are concerned about our current standard of care. That's the starting point for EBP success. Let the nurses know I am sending an announcement out this week with a list of the hospital's EBP resources. Let them know a faculty member from the university's school of nursing will be coming to the hospital to present a special series on the use of EBP. I am meeting with the chief of oncology medical practice tomorrow and will let her know we are initiating this project on the oncology unit."

Discussion

Clearly, the CNE in Scenario 1 placed blame on another entity for what she perceived to be a problem. In this scenario, direct care nurses were unrecognized for their spirit of inquiry and were discouraged from pursuing an EBP project about a critical patient care issue. The CNE mistook the use of research evidence as the working definition of EBP and may have inadvertently set up unhealthy competition between physicians and direct care nurses. The EBP project was in peril before it was formally started.

The CNE in Scenario 2 honored the nurses' commitment to begin the EBP project. The CNE understood that training in EBP is necessary but developing EBP skills and knowledge is an ongoing process. The CNE used her influence to endorse, support, and enlist collaborative backing in implementing an organizational EBP culture.

NURSING LEADERSHIP IN DEVELOPING AN EBP CULTURE

Making EBP a reality that is central to patient care is often a challenging endeavor for leaders in healthcare organizations (Stetler, Ritchie, Rycroft-Malone, & Charns, 2014). For more than two decades, studies have cited organizational barriers to successful implementation of EBP (Funk, Champagne, Tornquist, & Wiese, 1995). Organizational barriers that hinder direct care nurses from implementing EBP include perceived absence of authority, inadequate support, lack of resources, and few role models (Brown, Wickline, Ecoff, & Glaser, 2009; Kocaman et al., 2010; Koehn & Lehmen, 2008). In addition to organizational barriers, participant barriers also can impede implementation of an EBP culture. For example, EBP requires important changes in the way nurses think about patient concerns and the mental processes used to manage or resolve those concerns.

Facilitating a supportive EBP culture requires both decreasing organizational barriers to implementing EBP and promoting nurse readiness and preparedness for engagement in EBP. Research has repeatedly recognized *nursing leadership* as a necessary constituent of successful formation of an EBP culture. In fact, two of the most salient factors influencing the use of EBP are solid leadership support and EBP skill mastery (Hutchinson & Johnston, 2006; Moser, DeLuca, Bond, & Rollins, 2004). As discussed in this chapter, EBP skill mastery for direct care nurses is positively associated with nursing leadership advocacy for EBP. Not surprisingly, studies found leadership resistance to EBP and insufficient support from nursing leaders have an adverse effect on EPB implementation (Hutchinson & Johnston, 2006; Parahoo & McCaughan, 2001).

Nursing leadership is defined as the use of interpersonal skills to influence others to achieve specific goals (Sullivan & Garland, 2010). In healthcare organizations, nursing leadership is often designated as *formal* or *informal*. Formal leaders are officially assigned leadership status within a group or organization. Examples of formal leaders are chief nurse executive, nurse manager, and director of nursing research. In contrast, informal leaders are those who do not have official status but who are able to induce and inspire organizational participants to engage in or refrain from engaging in specific behaviors, such as EBP.

This chapter addresses the roles of formal and informal leaders in developing and sustaining an organizational culture of EBP. An organizational culture consists of beliefs, customs, and assumptions that guide participant behavior (O'Reilly, Chatman, & Caldwell, 1991). Healthcare settings with an embedded EBP culture demonstrate the EBP process as normative and expected behavior of nurses' everyday work life. Several healthcare organizations, especially those with Magnet® recognition, exemplify thriving EBP cultures (Fitzsimons & Cooper, 2012).

Much of the work concerning nursing leadership and its importance in cultivating a culture of EBP has been focused on formal leaders (Damschroder et al., 2009; Gifford, Davies, Edwards, & Graham, 2006; Sandstrom, Borglin, Nilsson, & Willman, 2011; Stetler et al., 2014). This may be related, in part, to the wider organizational role formal leaders have in envisioning, planning, articulating, implementing, and sustaining the formation of an EBP culture for an organization or significant areas within an organization. In addition, formal leaders are often extremely influential in helping produce conditions that influence adoption of EBP behaviors by direct care nurses (Weston, 2010). Successful formal leadership behaviors, associated with embedded EBP cultures, are often identified as *strategic leadership behaviors* (Stetler et al., 2014).

Strategic leadership behaviors identify overarching organizational goals and activate the means to achieve those goals as opposed to tactical leadership behaviors, which involve short-term actions to achieve a specific goal (Fulmer, Stumpf, & Bleak, 2009). Strategic leadership behaviors require clear goals, a timeline, and delineated lines of responsibility. Nursing leaders with a strategic focus for forming an organizational EBP culture must first conceptualize a vision of the culture, clearly articulate the importance of EBP, and plan for implementation and sustainment of EBP as a cultural norm. Effective strategic leaders understand that a realistic EBP culture is multifaceted and must be expressed explicitly and repeatedly to be recognized as a normative cultural behavior (Stetler et al., 2014).

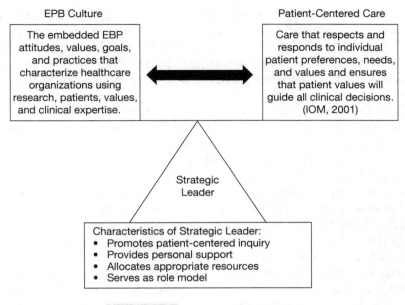

FIGURE 16.1 Leadership fulcrum

EBP, evidence-based practice.

Research has shown four recurrent formal nursing leadership behaviors that are used to begin and maintain the formation of an EBP culture (see Figure 16.1). The identified leadership behaviors are *promoting patient-centered inquiry, personal support, allocating recourses,* and *role modeling.* Each behavior, while often practical, is a critical component for developing a strategic plan to establish EBP as a cultural norm. Over time, the leadership behaviors contribute to making the EBP vision a reality for direct care nurses. Formal leadership behaviors, supportive of EBP, have been described in primary, secondary, and tertiary healthcare settings as well as Magnet- and non-Magnet-status healthcare organizations (Yoder et al., 2014).

Developing an EBP culture is a formidable endeavor. Learning and applying select strategic leadership behaviors help make an EBP culture an achievable goal. The following sections discuss the four strategic-based leadership behaviors for creating an EBP culture for healthcare organizations.

Patient-Centered Promoting Inquiry

Direct care nurses perceive leaders in healthcare organizations as placing higher priorities on nurses' achievement of organizational goals (e.g., patient morning hygiene completed on time) than on development of a spirit of inquiry (Pravikoff, Tanner, & Pierce, 2005; Vanhook, 2009). A spirit of inquiry fosters productive and creative mental skills that enable nurses to enlarge their capacities to question current clinical practice. As a result of direct care nurse inquiry about clinical care, the EBP process is put in motion and, accordingly, healthcare organizations often experience positive change.

All disciplines can claim *spirit of inquiry* as an essential component of their professional formation; however, each discipline defines and operationalizes spirit of inquiry in a way that specifically fits the discipline's philosophical perspective. In nursing, spirit of inquiry is considered a genuine sense of curiosity that initiates generation of information and knowledge to inform clinical practice. Consequently, spirit of inquiry in nursing ignites the flame of information literacy. The American Library Association (2016) defines *information literacy* as a set of abilities that enables individuals to recognize when knowledge is needed and the ability to locate, evaluate, and optimally use the needed knowledge. Information literacy is a valued EBP skillset in nursing (see Box 16.1). To summarize, *inquiry* refers to the effort on the part of a nurse to seek patient-centered truth, information, or knowledge. *Spirit* refers to a nurse's implicit sense of readiness to achieve a greater awareness and understanding of patient care.

A spirit of inquiry in nursing challenges the status quo related to patient care and is often a difficult step for nurses to make (Melnyk & Fineout-Overholt, 2015). Challenging the status quo is seen as a "risk taking" behavior that is often a difficult task for healthcare providers. Many healthcare providers prefer not to challenge the status quo because such a challenge may imply the possibility of an untoward consequence. Even when nurses are convinced of the effectiveness of EBP, they may avoid inquiry about standardized patient care because they do not believe they have the authority to initiate the EBP process (Yoder et al., 2014).

Research demonstrates that initiation of EBP is more likely to occur in organizations where nursing leaders inspire curiosity and inquisitiveness in others (Moser et al., 2004). Nursing leaders play an important role in inspiring and motivating direct care nurses to be inquisitive about the status quo of patient care. To initiate the first step in EBP, nursing leadership must encourage staff nurses to question current clinical practices such as usefulness of postdischarge telephone calls for patients with total hip replacement or effectiveness of a nursing care unit's surgical patient checklist. Encouraging inquiry is especially challenging when the target of inquiry may be a deeply held custom, belief, or institutional mandate related to patient care (e.g., all patients need vital signs checked every 4 hours).

For direct care nurses to engage fully in patient-centered practice, nursing leaders must demonstrate they value the curiosity and inquiry inherently associated with EBP. Direct care nurses view leaders with drive, enthusiasm, and credibility toward EBP as significantly influential in determining their initial steps for engaging in practice-related empirical inquiry (Rycroft-Malone et al., 2004). Questioning standards of practice to translate research findings into practice is

BOX 16.1 Information Literacy Competencies

- Determine the extent of information needed
- Efficiently and effectively access the needed information
- Evaluate information and its sources critically
- Incorporate selected information into one's knowledge base
- Use information effectively to accomplish a specific purpose
- Understand the economic, legal, and social issues surrounding the use of information, and the access and use of information ethically and legally

Source: American Library Association (2016).

still a recently new endeavor that many direct care nurses consider a form of risk-taking behavior. Nursing leaders who actively promote strong research values and demonstrate organizational acceptance of EBP demonstrate important characteristics that, in due course, encourage direct care nurse engagement in EBP (Gifford, Davies, Edwards, Griffin, & Lybanon, 2007). Nurse leaders who encourage direct care nurses to use evidence in practice help provide a means for nurses to improve patient care. Championing specific EBP-related behaviors is an effective way to help enhance a sense of staff accomplishment and empowerment (Christenbery, Williamson, Sandlin, & Wells, 2016).

Personal Support

Direct care nurses may be inexperienced and/or lack proficiency in EBP use. Nurses' unfamiliarity with EBP is a significant obstacle for nurse leaders who want to encourage EBP use in healthcare organizations. For direct care nurses to engage in EBP, they must value and recognize the significance of EBP; therefore, direct care nurses need ongoing support from nursing leadership about the importance of EBP and their direct care nursing roles in its implementation. Supportive EBP leadership is not focused on giving orders and managing details but rather is focused on providing nurses with the encouragement and support required to engage effectively in EBP. Informal relational behaviors, such as demonstrating an awareness of a staff member's EBP activities, promotes motivation to continue EBP activities. Leaders who recognize staff engaged in EBP by providing positive feedback are viewed as both inspirational and trustworthy, characteristics strongly associated with transformational leadership (Atkinson, 2011). Nursing leaders who personally and publicly appreciate and acknowledge the efforts of direct care nurses engaged in EBP are seen as leaders who stimulate sustainment of EBP within the organization (Gifford et al., 2006). Overt recognition of EBP performance publicly honors staff behaviors associated with EBP and, therefore, tends to reinforce those behaviors.

Effective communication is an essential component of support used by nursing leaders to promote the process of EBP. When asked what they require to successfully implement EBP, direct care nurses responded they need a leader who is available and uses good communication skills to provide necessary information about EBP (Gifford et al., 2006). Engagement with nurses and feedback about their use of EBP from nurse leaders has been found to be important in both the implementation and dissemination of EBP findings in clinical practice (Nilsson Kajermo, Nordstrom, Krusenbrant, & Lutzen, 2001).

Allocation of Time and Resources

Resource allocation is both a process and strategy in which organizational leaders decide where scarce resources could best be used to create desired organizational outcomes (Joiner, Castellanos, & Wartman, 2011). Optimizing resource allocation is essential in establishing an EBP culture. Nursing leaders have significant influence in shaping an EBP culture because they allocate time and human, material, and capital resources to create an environment supportive of EBP.

Developing an infrastructure amenable to EBP implementation is a key nursing leadership function. Research consistently cites the importance of nursing leadership in affording access to library resources and research experts and the provision of time for direct care nurses to efficiently and effectively assume EBP projects (Cummings, Estabrooks, Midodzi, Wallin, & Hayduk, 2007; Gifford et al., 2006; Miejers et al., 2006). Creating a modern culture in which EBP can develop requires state-of-the-art electronic resources such as subscriptions to electronic journals and access to computers and the Internet. An EBP culture does not flourish on a minimized budget.

Although the dedication of highly qualified CNEs and nurse researchers is essential for the implementation of EBP, such endeavors rarely occur without the allocation of substantial resources. EBP implementation depends on a nursing leader's influence in creating a context for EBP implementation to thrive (Newhouse, Dearholt, Poe, Pugh, & White, 2007; Rycroft-Malone, 2004). Providing real and tangible support, such as EBP fellowships and ongoing EBP education, is valued by staff and seen as support from nursing leadership to engage in EBP activities. Allocation of educational resources is critical to the success of EBP, and educational methods, whether interactive and learner driven or in the form of a traditional classroom lecture, need financial backing.

Intentionally embedding EBP policies (i.e., adoption of an EBP model) into the organization helps establish an EBP code of conduct for staff. Use of discretionary funds to sponsor staff attendance at EBP conferences is an important investment for engaging staff in external EBP-related activities. Direct care nurses who engage in external EBP conferences and workshops often return to the home organization with an enriched understanding of EBP and are willing to share the EBP-related knowledge they have gained. Scheduling a series of internal intensives or workshops is important for direct care nurses interested in learning about research and EBP and is also a way to invite nurses external to the organization to participate in EBP learning and sharing. Another method nursing leaders can use to influence the establishment of an EBP culture is assuring that organizational resources such as policies and documentation forms reflect nursing practice that is aligned with EBP.

Importantly, nurse leaders can employ a nurse researcher who supports the formation of an EBP council and EBP fellowship program to work closely with direct care nurses on developing their EBP projects. Healthcare organizations that cannot afford a full-time nurse researcher can partner with a school of nursing to engage a part-time nurse researcher faculty through a joint appointment arrangement. Such arrangements are seen as mutually beneficial to the healthcare organization and the school of nursing because synergistic engagement of nursing staff, research faculty, and students inspires deeper understandings of EBP and commitment to the EBP process. It is important for nursing leaders who control budgets to be cognizant of the potential financial savings associated with EBP. A culturally embedded EBP allows for provision of optimal patient-centered care, which in turn may lead to considerable long-term cost savings (National Institute for Health and Clinical Excellence, 2017). Estimated financial savings are up to eight times the return on initial financial investments for EBP projects (Bunting, Lee, Knowles, Lee, & Allen, 2011).

Role Modeling

Role modeling by nursing leadership conveys expected organizational norms. Nursing leaders who role model the use of EBP help build a capacity to normalize EBP throughout the organization. In fact, direct care nurses are more likely to engage in EBP if they notice their nursing leaders are actively engaged in EBP (Sredl et al., 2011). If nurse leaders, as role models, are not engaged in EBP, it is understandable that direct care nurses may refrain from implementing EBP activities. Seeing leaders actively involved in an EBP project and using evidence to solve organizational problems help persuade nurses as well as other healthcare organization participants to use EBP.

Formal interactions, such as coaching sessions or EBP committee involvement, are ways to mentor informal leaders who in turn can influence organizational understanding of EBP and reinforce behaviors related to EBP. An important aspect of EBP role modeling is the ability for nurse leaders to "talk the talk." For example, the use of EBP language (i.e., *best evidence, evaluating practice change*) is a form of role modeling in daily communication and conversations that leaders may use to reflect an organizational focus on the importance of EBP. Clearly, one of the most critical resources in the EBP process is support provided from role models who have expertise in the EBP process. CNEs, nurse managers, and APRNs are those most often cited as leaders who provide effective EBP role modeling (Stetler et al., 2014).

A significant form of role modeling is through the use of education. CNEs, nurse managers, and APRNs are often seen as the most effective EBP educators because they understand the EBP process. They generally have experience in implementing EBP projects and seeing projects through to completion (Fitzsimons & Cooper, 2012). Formal education endeavors, such as teaching a literature synthesis and integration course series to direct care nurses, demonstrate effective educational role modeling. Educational EBP role modeling by leaders helps increase and sustain nurses' mindfulness, knowledge, and skills related to EBP.

Summary of Formal Leadership Behaviors

The key to a well-developed EBP culture is nursing leadership with a strategic plan for building the EBP structure and using wise allocation of both human and material resources. Leadership behavior that is supportive of EBP is not an abstraction but rather a very real way to demonstrate implementation and maintenance of an EBP culture. A confluence of observable and concrete behaviors, over time, transforms traditional ways of implementing practice change into focusing the practice change on best available evidence consisting of research, patient values, and clinical expertise.

INFORMAL LEADERS

The EBP process provides a pathway to excellent clinical care. Direct care nurses can be closely involved in the process of initiating and implementing EBP changes. Favorable patient outcomes are frequently achieved when direct care nurses implement the EBP process and ultimately translate evidence into practice. Positive outcomes related to direct care nurse use of EBP include increased ability to provide safe care (Barnsteiner, 2011), enhanced patient quality of life (Wells, Pesaro, & McCaffery, 2008), cost-effective care (Sedwick, Lance-Smith, Reeder, & Nardi, 2012), and patient-specific clinical interventions (Scott & McSherry, 2008). Participation in EBP helps direct care nurses develop a professional sense of empowerment, related, in part, to their involvement and ownership of important patient care changes (Christenbery et al., 2016). Involvement in EBP also provides a means to enrich direct care nurses' critical thinking skills and enhance *informal leadership* abilities.

Very little is written about the direct care giver's informal leadership role in implementing EBP. The majority of literature discussing the leadership role and EBP is, understandably, focused on healthcare administrators. Without specific and strategic endorsement of healthcare administrators it is unlikely there would be an EBP culture. Nonetheless, direct care nurses have critical informal leadership roles to play in EBP implementation. This section of the chapter discusses aspects of informal roles.

An abundance of relevant research is easily accessible and applicable to patient care; however, the knowledge generated by healthcare research is insufficiently used by direct care nurses (Yoder et al., 2014). If research is used by direct care nurses, the research is often applied in an organizational top-down hierarchical approach, which indicates direct care nurses may be far removed from the analysis, interpretation, and decision to use current research findings (Reavy & Tavernier, 2008). Regardless, EBP is an expected core competency of all nurses (IOM, 2010). Direct care nurses, who are identified as informal leaders on their clinical units, may be an excellent informal leadership resource to encourage and teach other nurses how to effectively engage in the EBP process.

Encouraging a Spirit of Inquiry

Informal nurse leaders, skilled in the use of EBP, can help other nurses develop a spirit of intellectual curiosity about patient care. Helping nurses think beyond obvious or commonsense explanations regarding patient conditions and consider alternative explanations is one method to inspire intellectual curiosity. For example, a nurse may indicate that hyperkalemia in a patient with congestive heart failure was solely related to potassium supplement use. An EBP informal leader may encourage the nurse to consider alternative and/or additional explanations for the hyperkalemia, such as the patient is receiving an angiotensin-converting enzyme inhibitor or has a vaginal yeast infection. Encouraging nurses, with limited EBP experience, to consider additional or even competing hypotheses about patient conditions endorses a spirit of inquiry as the foundation for EBP.

Developing a Clinical Question

EBP informal leaders have an important role teaching other nurses how to formulate clinical questions using the PICOT format (see Chapter 6). The PICOT format helps nurses identify and clarify key concepts and variables related to their topic of inquiry. Identifying the topic's key concepts will help make the electronic search for best research evidence an easily surmountable task.

Searching for Best Evidence

A new nurse may understand he needs additional empirical evidence to enable him to provide the best pain management interventions for a patient with Stevens-Johnson syndrome, a condition he has not seen before. However, navigating the world of evidence surrounding a condition such as Stevens-Johnson syndrome can be a daunting and time-intensive endeavor. Informal EBP leaders can role model how to effectively access and search for the best empirical evidence. For example, role modeling skills and strategies to identify and use credible databases such as PubMed or National Institutes of Health Consensus statements is an invaluable step in learning to use EBP. Findings gathered from the empirical search about pain management for Stevens-Johnson syndrome enable the new nurse and the EBP informal leader to jointly articulate an evidence-based plan of care for promoting patient-centered pain management.

Critically Appraising the Evidence

Critically appraising scientific evidence is a vigorous intellectual effort for members of all disciplines. Even nurses with advanced practice degrees appreciate the support of colleagues when conducting a critical appraisal of relevant research literature. Direct care nurses who have limited experience in literature appraisal need the support and guidance provided by an EBP informal leader to successfully assess the merit of scientific evidence. Critical appraisal of research literature requires a rigorous and systematic method to adequately determine the quality, level, credibility, and usefulness of evidence. Critical appraisal of the literature is often a time-consuming process. For inexperienced nurses who are conducting a literature appraisal, consultation and discussion with an EBP informal leader may help assure the literature is being appraised efficiently and effectively. EBP informal leaders may want to suggest the use of online critical appraisal tools such as the Duke University Critical Appraisal Worksheet (Duke University Medical Center Library and Archives, 2016). In addition, nursing units sometimes have a standard critical analysis tool. Findings gleaned from the literature appraisal can be shared with the EBP informal leader and other staff nurses to promote discussion about the possibility of establishing a new innovative practice guideline for their nursing unit.

Integrating Evidence Into Practice

EBP informal leaders have a critical role to play in helping nurses integrate evidence, nurse expertise, and patient values into clinical practice. Change of shift report is an excellent opportunity for EBP informal leaders to encourage staff to discuss and compare best current evidence with actual practice on the nursing unit. For example, nurses on a chronic respiratory unit may believe sputum color is an indication of either viral or bacterial infection. An EBP informal leader and direct care nurse may review literature related to this topic. In evaluating the literature, they may discover there is not a credible correlation between sputum color and source of infection. Sharing this finding would be an excellent example of integrating best evidence into practice when discussed at change of shift report.

Evaluation of Outcomes

EBP informal leaders can serve as excellent role models for monitoring, evaluating, and reporting findings related to new evidence integrated into practice. Evaluating evidence to determine whether an intervention had the desired clinical effect and whether it was valued by the patient is a critical component of EBP. If the intervention did not have the desired effect or lacked patient value, the EPB informal leader can begin the discussion with other nurses on the unit regarding the unexpected outcomes, possible causes for the outcomes, and what alterations may need to be considered with regard to the intervention.

Teaching and encouraging the use of EBP skills does not occur in an isolated computer screen vacuum but rather occurs as a very real part of the nurse's and patient's environment. EBP informal leaders have multiple opportunities on their units to teach and inspire other nurses to become skillful in the use of EBP. Teaching nurses to question, access, appraise, integrate, and evaluate evidence related to clinical practice is to give them an essential skillset for nursing in the 21st century.

Direct care nurses who embrace EBP can influence patient care outcomes. EBP provides direct care nurses a methodical process to become responsibly involved with developing optimal solutions to patient care concerns. Involvement may be termed *ownership*. Ownership implies an obligation and responsibility to resolve patient care concerns instead of passing concerns to another discipline that may be less qualified to address direct patient care issues. Ownership of practice allows direct care nurses to have a clearer voice and immediate influence over the care and subsequent outcomes delivered to patients.

Summary of Informal Leadership Behaviors

Informal leaders, in relation to EBP implementation, are participants within a specific area of an organization who are perceived by peers as having EBP knowledge and expertise and are therefore worthy of emulating. Direct care nurses' ability to be informal leaders, in regard to EBP, rests on their abilities to inspire respect, confidence, and trust in other nurses. Direct care nurses who are EBP informal leaders are valuable to the healthcare organization in establishing a culture of EBP. In addition, EBP informal leaders are key support for formal leaders in implementing the vision and agenda to embed EBP as an organizational value and expected nursing activity.

SUMMARY

Effective nurse leaders understand the organization's overall purpose and goals for establishing an EBP culture. They develop strategies to achieve and maintain an EBP culture. Nurse leaders are clear about the needs of the organization's participants to help EBP grow and thrive as a means of delivering high-quality patient care. This chapter highlights ongoing strategies that effective nurse leaders use to attain and uphold an EBP culture. In addition, the chapter explores the underreported, yet vitally important, role that informal leaders have in fostering an EBP culture.

REFERENCES

American Library Association. (2016). Information literacy competency standards for higher education. Retrieved from http://www.ala.org/acrl/standards/information literacycompetency

Atkinson, S. M. (2011). Are you a transformational leader? *Nursing Management, 42*(9), 44–50.

Barnsteiner, J. (2011). Teaching the culture of safety. *The Online Journal of Issues in Nursing, 16*(3). doi:10.3912/OJIN.Vol16No03Man05

Brown, C. E., Wickline, M. A., Ecoff, L., & Glaser, D. (2009). Nursing practice knowledge attitudes and perceived barriers to evidence-based practice at an academic medical center. *Journal of Nursing, 65*(2), 371–381.

Bunting, B. A., Lee, G., Knowles, G., Lee, C., & Allen, P. (2011). The Hickory project: Controlling healthcare costs and improving outcomes for diabetes using the Asheville project model. *American Health and Drug Benefits, 4*(6), 343–350.

Christenbery, T., Williamson, A., Sandlin, V., & Wells, N. (2016). Immersion in evidence-based practice fellowship program. *Journal for Nurses in Professional Development, 32*(1), 15–20.

Cummings, G., Estabrooks, C., Midodzi, W., Wallin, L., & Hayduk, L. (2007). Influence of organizational characteristics and contact on research utilization. *Nursing Research, 56*(4), 24–39.

Damschroder, L. J., Aron, D. C., Keith, R. E., Kirsh, S. R., Alexander, J. A., & Lowery, J. C. (2009). Fostering implementation of health services research findings into practice: A consolidated framework for advancing implementation science. *Implementation Science, 4*, 50. doi:10:1186/1748-5908-4-50

Duke University Medical Center Library and Archives. (2016). Evidence-based practice: Appraise. Retrieved from http://guides .mclibrary.duke.edu/ebm/appraise

Fitzsimons, E., & Cooper, J. (2012). Embedding a culture of evidence-based practice. *Nursing Management, 19*(7), 14–19.

Fulmer, R., Stumpf, S., & Bleak, J. (2009). The strategic development of high potential leaders. *Strategy and Leadership, 37*(3), 17–22.

Funk, S. G., Champagne, M. T., Tornquist, E. M., & Wiese, R. A. (1995). Administrators views on barriers to research utilization. *Applied Nursing Research, 8*(1), 44–49.

Gifford, W. A., Davies, B., Edwards, N., & Graham, I. D. (2006). Leadership strategies to influence the use of clinical practice guidelines. *Nursing Leadership, 19*(4), 72–88.

Gifford, W. A., Davies, B., Edwards, N., Griffin, P., & Lybanon, V. (2007). Managerial leadership for nurses' use of research evidence: An integrative review of the literature. *Worldviews on Evidence-Based Nursing, 3*, 126–145.

Hutchinson, A. M., & Johnston, L. (2006). Beyond the BARRIERS scale: Commonly reported barriers to research use. *Journal of Nursing Administration, 36*(4), 189–199.

Institute of Medicine. (2010). *The future of nursing: Leading change advancing health*. Washington, DC: National Academies Press.

Joiner, K. A., Castellanos, N., & Wartman, S. A. (2011). Resource allocation in academic health centers: Creating common metrics. *Academic Medicine, 86*(9), 1084–1092. doi:10.1097/ACM .0b013e318226b18b

Kocaman, G., Seren, S., Lash, A. A., Kurt, S., Bengu, N., & Yurumezoglu, H. A. (2010). Barriers to research utilization by staff nurses in a university hospital. *Journal of Advanced Nursing, 19*(13–14), 1908–1918.

Koehn, M. I., & Lehmen, K. (2008). Nurses' perceptions of evidence-based practice. *Journal of Advanced Nursing, 62*(2), 209–215.

Melnyk, B. M., & Fineout-Overholt, E. (2015). *Evidence-based practice in nursing and healthcare: A guide to best practice.* Philadelphia, PA: Wolters Kluwer.

Miejers, J., Janssen, M., Cummings, G., Wallin, L., Estabrooks, C., & Halfens, R. (2006). Assessing the relationship between contextual factors and research utilization in nursing: A systematic literature review. *Journal of Advanced Nursing, 55*(5), 622–635.

Moser, L., DeLuca, N., Bond, G., & Rollins, A. (2004). Implementing evidence-based psychosocial practices: Lessons learned from statewide implementation of two practices. *The International Journal of Neuropsychiatric Medicine, 9*(12), 926–936.

National Institute for Health and Care Excellence. (2017). Clinical guidelines. Retrieved from https://www.ncbi.nlm.nih.gov/books/NBK11822

Newhouse, R. P., Dearholt, S., Poe, S., Pugh, L. C., & White, M. K. (2007). Organizational change strategies for evidence-based practice. *Journal of Nursing Administration, 37*(12), 552–557.

Nilsson Kajermo, K., Nordstrom, G., Krusenbrant, A., & Lutzen, K. (2001). Nurses' experiences of research utilization within the framework of an educational programme. *Journal of Clinical Nursing, 10,* 671–681.

O'Reilly, C. A., Chatman, J., & Caldwell, D. F. (1991). People and organizational culture: A profile comparison approach to assessing person-organization fit. *Academy of Management Journal, 34*(3), 487–516.

Parahoo, K., & McCaughan, E. M. (2001). Research utilization among medical and surgical nurses: A comparison of their self-reports and perception of barriers and facilitators. *Journal of Nursing Management, 9,* 21–30.

Pravikoff, D. S., Tanner, A. B., & Pierce, S. T. (2005). Readiness of U.S. nurses for evidence-based practice. *American Journal of Nursing, 105*(9), 40–47.

Reavy, K., & Tavernier, S. (2008). Nurses reclaiming ownership of their practice: Implementation of an evidence-based practice model and process. *Journal of Continuing Education in Nursing, 39*(4), 166–172.

Rycroft-Malone, J. (2004). The PARIHS Framework: A framework for guiding the implementation of evidence-based practice. *Journal of Nurse Care Quality, 16,* 297–304.

Rycroft-Malone, J., Harvey, G., Seers, K., Kitson, A., McCormack, B., & Titchen, A. (2004). An exploration of the factors that influence the implementation of evidence into practice. *Journal of Clinical Nursing, 13,* 913–924.

Sandstrom, B., Borglin, G., Nilsson, R., & Willman, A. (2011). Promoting the implementation of evidence-based practice: A literature review focusing on the role of nursing leadership. *Worldviews on Evidence-Based Nursing, 8*(4), 212–223. doi:10.1111/j.1741-6787.2011.00216.x

Scott, K., & McSherry, R. (2008). Evidence-based nursing: Clarifying the concepts for nurses in practice. *Journal of Clinical Nursing, 18*(8), 1085–1095. doi:10.1111/j. 1365-2702.2008.02588.x

Sedwick, M. B., Lance-Smith, M., Reeder, S. J., & Nardi, J. (2012). Using evidence-based practice to prevent ventilator-associated pneumonia. *Critical Care Nurse, 32*(4), 41–51. doi:10.4037/ccn2012964

Sredl, D., Melnyk, B. M., Hsueh, K-H, Jenkins, R., Ding, C. D., & Durham, J. (2011). Health care in crisis! Can nurse executives' beliefs about and implementation of evidence-based practice be key solutions in health care reform? *Teaching and Learning in Nursing, 6*(2). 73–79.

Stetler, C. B., Ritchie, J. A., Rycroft-Malone, J., & Charns, M. P. (2014). Leadership for evidence-based practice: Strategic and functional behaviors for institutionalizing EBP. *Worldviews on Evidence-Based Nursing, 11*(4), 219–226.

Sullivan, E. J., & Garland, G. (2010). *Practical leadership and management in nursing.* London, UK: Pearson Education.

Vanhook, P. M. (2009). Overcoming barriers to EBP. *Nursing Management, 40*(8), 9–11.

Wells, N., Pesaro, C., & McCaffery, M. (2008). Improving the quality of care through pain assessment and management. In R. G. Hughes (Ed.), *Patient and safety quality: An evidence-based handbook for nurses.* Rockville, MD: Agency for Healthcare Research and Quality.

Weston, M. J. (2010). Strategies for enhancing autonomy and control over nursing practice. *The Online Journal of Issues in Nursing, 15*(1). doi:10.3912/OJIN.Vol15No01Man01

Yoder, L. H., Kirkley, D., McFall, D. C., Kirksey, K. M., StalBaum, A. L., & Sellers, D. (2014). Staff nurses' use of research to facilitate evidence-based practice. *American Journal of Nursing, 114*(9), 26–37.

CHAPTER 17

A Prosperous Evidence-Based Culture: Nourishing Resources

Thomas L. Christenbery

Objectives

After reading this chapter, learners should be able to:

1. Differentiate evidence-based culture and infrastructure
2. Identify key components of an effective evidence-based practice (EBP) infrastructure
3. Assess benefits of a sound evidence-based infrastructure

EVIDENCE-BASED PRACTICE (EBP) SCENARIOS

Scenario 1

Bob, a nurse with several years of medical intensive care unit (MICU) experience, transferred to an MICU in a different state. At his former place of employment, Bob was accustomed to a bedside nursing report at shift change instead of the nurse-to-nurse report format used at his current medical center. Believing that the bedside nursing report enhanced patient safety, Bob decided to try to implement the bedside nursing change-of-shift report. He met with the nurse manager about this proposed change. The nurse manager was very supportive of the idea and told Bob to initiate the change. When Bob attempted the change, he met with resistance from other direct care nurses and the house staff expressed concern about this method of reporting. Being completely discouraged by the response, Bob relinquished the idea of the bedside nursing report and the traditional method of nurse-to-nurse report continued.

Scenario 2

David, a nurse with several years of MICU experience, transferred to an MICU in a different state. At his former place of employment, David was accustomed to a bedside nursing report at shift change instead of the nurse-to-nurse report format used at his current medical center. Believing that the bedside nursing report enhanced patient safety, David decided to try to implement the bedside nursing change of shift report. He met with the nurse manager about his proposed change. The nurse manager thought his idea had merit and arranged for David to work with another direct care nurse who was an EBP mentor for the medical center. The mentor helped David develop a PICOT (patient population, intervention, comparison, outcome, and time frame) question and showed him how to retrieve the most current evidence about change of shift report. She also helped David evaluate the level and quality of evidence. Once they amassed evidence to support the idea, the EBP mentor demonstrated how to implement change effectively on the unit by engaging key stakeholders in the decision and implementation processes. Six months later the EBP mentor and David evaluated the change and discovered that other nurses and house staff believed the new method of reporting enhanced patient safety, provided greater role satisfaction for nurses, and fostered patient-centered care.

Discussion

In Scenario 1, Bob had an idea that could possibly be of benefit to both patient care and nursing practice. Even though the idea was generated by an experienced nurse and supported by management, the implementation was met with skepticism and resistance that could not be overcome. In Scenario 2, an EBP mentor became a key central mechanism for implementing and sustaining the proposed EBP change. Adherence to the EBP steps was important for the change to be successful. Of equal importance was the role of mentor in assisting with implementing change by engaging key stakeholders in the decision-implementation process.

INFRASTRUCTURE AND EBP

The Institute of Medicine (2001) has charged healthcare organizations with creating an *infrastructure* to support EBP, thereby helping provide optimal patient care within a healthcare environment of rapidly expanding knowledge and change. Successful implementation of EBP in healthcare organizations requires a sound EBP infrastructure (Newhouse, 2007). *Infrastructure* is defined as the organizational structure and facilities (e.g., technology, resources) required for the operation of an enterprise, such as EBP. Organizational infrastructure differs from organizational culture in that a culture represents the cumulative attitudes, beliefs, and behaviors of an organization, whereas an infrastructure is the basic physical plant and systems that make up the organization (Tylor, 1974).

Several studies have found direct care nurses and advanced practice nurses need infrastructural support to augment their EBP cultural attitudes, beliefs, and behaviors (Melnyk, Fineout-Overholt, Gallagher-Ford, & Kaplan, 2012; Pravikoff, Tanner, & Pierce, 2005). Many nursing school graduates entering the workforce have excellent academic preparation related to EBP. Nevertheless, new graduate nurses care for patients with complex health issues and must learn numerous skills while being required to integrate EBP into patient care (National Council of State Boards of Nursing, 2013). New graduates require a sound organizational infrastructure to support implementation and further development of the EBP knowledge they learned while in school. Absence of an EBP organizational infrastructure jeopardizes new graduates' professional role satisfaction and compliance with best nursing practice standards (Newhouse, 2007).

In healthcare, infrastructure is the primary foundation that supports patient-centered clinical care (Foxcroft, Cole, Fulbrook, Johnston, & Stevens, 2000). As noted in Chapter 16, nurse leaders are the driving force in establishing an EBP culture because they have the responsibility for allocating needed resources to create an EBP infrastructure. In addition, nurse leaders are ultimately responsible for providing infrastructure to disseminate research findings and support the integration of those findings within respective healthcare organizations (American Nurses Association, 2004).

Healthcare organizations are at a critical juncture in terms of EBP. Nurses indicate they have positive attitudes toward EBP and are willing to engage in EBP (Melnyk et al., 2012). Yet they report the lack of adequate infrastructure as one of the primary impediments to full participation in EBP (LaPierre, Ritchey, & Newhouse, 2004; Melnyk et al., 2012). Nurses tend to implement EBP when they are internally motivated and have the support of an organizational infrastructure. Organizations with active EBP nursing endeavors are organizations with noticeable pledges of leadership support and dedicated commitment to supplying EBP infrastructure. Healthcare organizations must supply the necessary infrastructure for EBP to exist and flourish. The material and human resources that have been found to support an EBP infrastructure are discussed in the following sections (Christenbery, Williamson, Sandlin, & Wells, 2016; Melnyk et al., 2012; Pravikoff et al., 2005).

PERSONNEL

Designated personnel assigned to EBP operations are an essential, and costly, resource for EBP programs to be effective. Evidence-based practice personnel consist of both nursing professionals, who ideally have education and work-related experience related to research and EBP, and ancillary personnel. The number of EBP personnel required is generally dependent on the size of the healthcare organization. Large multisite medical centers may require an EBP department with several EBP personnel, whereas for smaller community healthcare organizations, one or two personnel may be adequate.

Nurse researchers are often a logical choice to lead EBP programs. Nurse researchers are committed to advancing quality and excellence in healthcare and, importantly, they base professional nursing practice on science (American Association of Colleges of Nursing, 2006). Direct care nurses report critical barriers to implementation of EBP. These include (a) lack of research mentors and

(b) personal inadequate understandings of research. It is therefore important that EBP programs employ nurse researchers who have both requisite EBP and research skills and knowledge to mentor nurses through an EBP trajectory. The EBP trajectory is composed of elements that nurse researchers have been well educated to address including question development, literature search, evidence appraisal, implementation design, evaluation, and professional dissemination of EBP project outcomes.

If a doctoral-educated nurse researcher is not available to oversee the EBP program, other appropriate supervisory personnel may be considered. Other EBP program supervisory personnel may include advanced practice nurses, clinical nurse leaders, and clinical nurse specialists. These nurses, usually educated at the master's degree level, must have commensurate EBP experience to match EBP leadership requirements.

EBP programs require additional support of ancillary personnel who are key participants in supporting the EBP goals and objectives of the nursing department (Siedlecki, 2016). The number of ancillary personnel is dependent on the scope of the EBP program and the annual number and type of EBP projects. For small EBP programs, minimal full-time supportive help is needed. Examples of EBP ancillary team members may include administrative assistant, librarian, statistician, and graphic designer.

EBP Mentors

One-third of nurses listed absence of an EBP mentor as one of the top three impediments to effective engagement in EBP (Fink, Thompson, & Bonnes, 2005). Evidence-based practice mentors are necessary for guiding other nurses in the development and use of EBP skills (Melnyk et al., 2004). Identified mentors for EBP endeavors include director of nursing research, advanced practice nurses, nurse graduates of EBP fellowship programs, and faculty linked to academic partnerships at schools of nursing (Kelly, Turner, Speroni, McLaughlin, & Guzzetta, 2013). EBP mentors provide EBP-specific knowledge, wisdom, encouragement, and one-on-one coaching. Mentors help both individuals and teams generate PICOT questions, assist in locating and evaluating the best available evidence, provide support in developing the EBP implementation plan, and offer guidance in designing a dissemination plan for key EBP project findings and outcomes. It is critical to have adequate numbers of EBP mentors to prevent delays in meeting with potential mentees. Delays in meeting with EBP mentees can easily lead to loss of EBP interest and, as a consequence, loss of potential answers to important EBP questions.

EBP/RESEARCH COUNCILS

Healthcare organizations with progressive EBP programs generally have active EBP/nursing research councils. Traditionally, healthcare organizations have relied on nursing policy and procedure committees to review and approve nursing care policies. Often the policy review committees relied little, if at all, on quality research and evidence-based literature to inform nursing practice (O'May &

BOX 17.1   Key Features of Evidence-Based Practice/Research Councils

---

- Identifies clinical practice issues requiring EBP solutions

- Provides important and immediate access to EBP mentors

- Provides a venue for sharing innovative clinical practice insight

- Allows for teamwork related to computer use, evidence searches, and critique of poster and podium presentations

- Serves as a venue for consulting and collaboration with other EBP healthcare institutions and professional organizations

- Provides important access to mentors

EBP, evidence-based practice.

Buchan, 1999; Porter-O'Grady, 1994). Evidence-based practice/research councils enable nurses to engage in the review of research and best evidence to better align nursing practice, policies, and procedures with the best available scientific knowledge (Becker et al., 2012).

Through an Evidence-Based Practice/Nursing Research Council, direct care nurses are afforded the foundation and infrastructure to systematically engage in and implement EBP and research endeavors. Councils are responsible for several important EBP activities; examples are that they may:

- Honor and promote scientific, evidence-based approaches to problem solving in the delivery of patient-centered care
- Support programs that promote direct care nurses in the implementation and integration of EBP projects
- Provide direction in the development of nursing EBP projects and nursing research proposals
- Develop, review, and disseminate nursing practice guidelines and practice alerts centered on the best available evidence
- Help determine the best methods and venues for dissemination of EBP project outcomes and research project findings (Becker et al., 2012; Brody, Barnes, Ruble, & Sakowski, 2012; see Box 17.1)

Councils can be unit-based or organization-wide endeavors and may focus on EBP function and/or role (Kramer et al., 2008). Composition of councils include direct care nurses, director of EBP and research, unit nurse managers, health science librarian, advanced practice nurses, clinical specialists, clinical nursing leaders, and faculty of associated schools of nursing. Councils generally meet once a month and direct care nurses must be given release time to attend council meetings.

EBP FELLOWSHIP

Nurses are the largest healthcare workforce targeted with meeting the Institute of Medicine (2009; Committee on the Robert Wood Johnson Foundation Initiative on the Future of Nursing, 2011) goal of integrating evidence into practice.

Yet nurses are faced with infrastructural obstacles regarding the translation of science into usable evidence for application to patient care decisions. Nurses repeatedly attribute both lack of knowledge and confidence in their critical appraisal skills of research reports as a consistent obstacle to implementing EBP (Melnyk et al., 2012; Profetto-McGrath, 2005; Wallis, 2012). Educating and empowering nurses to develop a spirit of inquiry and implement best EBP into patient-centered care is essential to both nursing and patient outcomes (Jackson, 2016). Evidence-based practice fellowship programs are an infrastructural support that has demonstrated effectiveness in helping nurses to become confident and skilled at appraising scientific evidence and integrating evidence into practice.

Evidence-based practice fellowships are a series of didactic and experiential workshops designed to enable clinicians, primarily direct care nurses, to develop, implement, evaluate, and disseminate EBP projects. The EBP projects focus specifically on issues in clinicians' work areas with the aim of improving practices to become efficient and effective in fostering positive patient-centered outcomes. Fellows are either systematically recruited by nurse managers or self-selected to enter the EBP program. Depending on the healthcare organization, fellowships generally meet once a month for 8 hours and extend for a period from 6 months to a year. During this time, the fellows blend their clinical knowledge and expertise with didactic instruction about research methodology, appraisal of levels and quality of evidence, guideline development, and change process theories, as discussed in Chapter 7.

During the course of the fellowship, the fellows work with a trained EBP coach to engage in innovative thinking about EBP behaviors, skills, and practices. Trained coaches are characteristically advanced practice nurses, nurse managers, clinical nurse educators, school of nursing faculty, or graduates of the EBP fellowship. The fellowships require intensive mentorships that involve four key players: fellows, coaches, nurse managers, and the director of the EBP program (see Box 17.2).

THE INTERNET AND INTRANET EVIDENCE-BASED INFRASTRUCTURE

It may be challenging to consider the Internet as infrastructure because no single organization owns the Internet. The Internet is a global collection of small and large networks that interconnect in multiple ways to form a single network entity. Even though a single organization does not own the Internet, healthcare organizations are responsible for monitoring and maintaining their Internet system; therefore, the Internet is an established part of an organization's infrastructure. To successfully implement EBP, nurses need research resources that may be efficiently retrieved through the Internet.

A well-developed internal website, known as an *intranet*, is also important for effective nurse implementation of EBP. An intranet is a network, created using World Wide Web software, with restricted access within an organization. The primary purpose of an EBP intranet is to share organization-specific EBP information between an organization's nurses. Intranet service also facilitates EBP working groups and teleconferences. EBP intranet users are generally novices in the world of EBP and research; therefore, intranet information needs to be organized and labeled so that nurses can easily and intuitively find information.

BOX 17.2   Evidence-Based Practice Roles

Director of EBP Program

- Provides leadership and direction in the development and implementation of the EBP program
- Ensures that strategic goals (e.g., safety, quality of life) of the healthcare organization are being addressed by the fellowship projects
- Optimizes the overall success of the mentor/fellow dyad
- Serves as research/EBP resource for mentor/fellow when questions arise
- Serves as liaison with EBP fellows and faculty
- Provides direction and mentorship to EBP coaches

Nurse managers

- Meet with mentors and fellows to monitor EBP project development
- Assess for potential needed resources related to EBP projects
- Foster accepting and positive environment for change on the clinical unit
- Provide needed time allotment to EBP fellows for participation in fellowship and completion of EBP projects

Mentors

- Share in-depth knowledge and skills in EBP as well as organizational change
- Convey positive beliefs and values about EBP
- Foster confidence in mentees to implement EBP projects
- Assist mentees in overcoming barriers to EBP
- Role model interdisciplinary collaboration to implement EBP projects

Fellows

- Identify clinical practice issues
- Implement EBP projects
- Disseminate projects at institution's designated EBP days

EBP, evidence-based practice.

Having a section devoted to dissemination of EBP projects or EBP results is also a key element of an EBP intranet.

LIBRARY RESOURCES

Many healthcare organizations, but not all, have access to some type of library resources. As noted in Chapter 3, health science librarians and libraries facilitate EBP by providing efficient access to research literature and are invaluable guides in appraising the research literature. If resources are not available within the healthcare organization, arrangements are sometimes made with local colleges and universities to provide access to them.

SUMMARY

This chapter differentiates EBP culture and EBP infrastructure. Benefits of an EBP infrastructure to nurses and patients are identified. Several examples of EBP resources and materials are described and the important roles each has in supporting full implementation of EBP are discussed.

REFERENCES

American Association of Colleges of Nursing. (2006). AACN position statement on nursing research. Retrieved from http://www.aacnnursing.org/Portals/42/News/Position -Statements/Nursing-Research.pdf

American Nurses Association. (2004). *Scope and standards for nurse administrators*. Washington, DC: Nursebooks.

Becker, E., Dee, V., Gawlinski, A., Kirkpatrick, T., Lawanson-Nichols, M., Lee, B., ... Zanotti, J. (2012). Clinical nurse specialists shaping policies and procedures via an evidence-based clinical practice council. *Clinical Nurse Specialist, 26*(2), 74–86. doi:10.1097/ NUR.0b013e3182467292

Brody, A. A., Barnes, K., Ruble, C., & Sakowski, J. (2012). Evidence-based practice councils: Potential path to staff nurse empowerment and leadership growth. *Journal of Nursing Administration, 42*(1), 28–33.

Christenbery, T., Williamson, A., Sandlin, V., & Wells, N. (2016). Immersion in evidence-based practice fellowship program. *Journal for Nurses in Professional Development, 32*(1), 15–20.

Committee on the Robert Wood Johnson Foundation Initiative on the Future of Nursing. (2011). *The future of nursing: Leading change, advancing health* Washington, DC: National Academies Press.

Fink, R., Thompson, C. J., & Bonnes, D. (2005). Overcoming barriers and promoting the use of research in practice. *Journal of Nursing Administration, 35*(3), 121–129.

Foxcroft, D. R., Cole, N., Fulbrook, P., Johnston, L., & Stevens, K. (2000). Organizational infrastructures to promote evidence based nursing practice. *Cochrane Database of Systematic Reviews, 3*. doi:10:1002/14651858.CD002212

Institute of Medicine. (2001). *Crossing the quality chasm: A new health system for the 21st century*. Washington, DC: National Academies Press.

Jackson, N. (2016). Incorporating evidence-based practice learning into a nurse residency program: Are new graduates ready to apply evidence at the bedside? *Journal of Nursing Administration, 46*(5), 278–283.

Kelly, K. P., Turner, A., Speroni, K. G., McLaughlin, M. K., & Guzzetta, C. E. (2013). National survey of hospital nursing research part 2. *Journal of Nursing Administration, 43*(1), 18–23. doi:10.1097/NNA.0b013e3182786029

Kramer, M., Schmalenberg, C., Maguire, P., Brewer, B. B., Burke, R., Chmielewski, L., ... Waldo, M. (2008). Structures and practices enabling staff nurses to control their practice. *Western Journal of Nursing Research, 30*(5), 539–559.

LaPierre, E., Ritchey, K., & Newhouse, R. (2004). Barriers to research use in the PACU. *Journal of PeriAnesthesia Nursing, 19*(2), 78–83.

Melnyk, B. M., Fineout-Overholt, E., Feinstein, N. F., Li, H., Wilcox, L., & Kraus, R. (2004). Nurses' perceived knowledge, beliefs, skills, and needs regarding evidence-based practice: Implications for accelerating the paradigm shift. *Worldviews on Evidence-Based Nursing, 1*, 185–193.

Melnyk, B. M., Fineout-Overholt, E., Gallagher-Ford, L., & Kaplan, L. (2012). The state of evidence-based practice in US nurses: Critical implications for nurse leaders and educators. *Journal of Nursing Administration, 42*(9), 410–417.

National Council of State Boards of Nursing. (2013). Transition to practice. Retrieved from https://www.ncsbn.org/transition-to-practice.htm

Newhouse, R. P. (2007). Creating infrastructure supportive of evidence-based nursing practice: Leadership strategies. *Worldviews on Evidence-Based Nursing, 4*(1), 21–29.

O'May, F., & Buchan, J. (1999). Shared governance: A literature review. *International Journal of Nursing Studies, 36,* 281–300.

Porter-O'Grady, T. (1994). Whole systems shared governance: Creating the seamless organization. *Nursing Economic$, 12*(4), 187–195.

Pravikoff, D. S., Tanner, A. B., & Pierce, S. T. (2005). Readiness of U.S. nurses for evidence-based practice. *American Journal of Nursing, 105*(9), 40–47.

Profetto-McGrath, J. (2005). Critical thinking and evidence-based practice. *Journal of Professional Nursing, 21*(3), 64–71.

Siedlecki, S. L. (2016). Building blocks for a strong nursing research program. In N. M. Albert (Ed.), *Building and sustaining a hospital-based nursing research program* (pp. 43–60). New York, NY: Springer Publishing.

Tylor, E. B. (1974). *Primitive culture: Researches into the development of mythology, philosophy, religion, art, and custom.* New York, NY: Gordon Press.

Wallis, L. (2012). Barriers to implementing evidence-based practice remain high for U.S. nurses. Getting past: "We've always done it this way" is crucial. *American Journal of Nursing, 112*(12), 15.

CHAPTER 18

Advancing Evidence-Based Practice Through Mentoring and Interprofessional Collaboration

Elaine Kauschinger

Objectives

After reading this chapter, learners should be able to:

1. Differentiate between *mentorship* and *preceptorship*
2. Describe the role of mentoring within the context of evidence-based practice (EBP)
3. Identify components of successful mentorship
4. Define *interprofessional collaboration*
5. Implement interprofessional collaborative EBP experiences

EVIDENCE-BASED PRACTICE (EBP) SCENARIOS

Scenario 1

Darrell was in his first month of employment as a nurse in the colonoscopy lab. He was delighted when he learned that Sheila had been assigned his mentor as part of a new hospital-wide "mentoring program." Darrell was perplexed that Sheila worked an opposite shift in the endoscopy lab. As Darrell's mentor, Sheila assigned him several research articles to read about management of upper GI endoscopy nausea so he could contribute to the creation of a poster abstract for a national conference. Using information he retained from an undergraduate research course, Darrell dutifully read and analyzed the articles. Sheila told him that he would need to attend several meetings to help her and other nurses develop ideas for the poster and help make the poster. Even though these meetings were not convenient for Darrell, he tried to attend. He grew frustrated in trying to be present for all the meetings and discuss a topic that was not of particular interest to him. Eventually, Darrell became uninterested and "dropped out" of the mentorship program. Sheila told her supervisor she was no longer mentoring Darrell because of his "lack of interest."

Scenario 2

Maria, a novice nurse, was in the first month of orientation on an oncology unit. She met many supportive direct care nurses on the unit but there was an experienced nurse, Ed, who shared Maria's deep interest in palliative care. Maria asked Ed to show her "the ropes" of how palliative care is integrated into oncology unit care. Ed taught her how to request a palliative care consult and support palliative care endeavors on the unit. Ed invited her to join a group of like-minded nurses who meet monthly at a local school of nursing to discuss palliative care issues. Ed also encouraged Maria to join a national palliative care society. During her first year on the oncology unit, Maria became interested in how to best manage palliative care patients' opioid tolerance. Ed suggested to Maria that opioid tolerance in palliative care would be an excellent EBP project that would be of interest to other nurses. Ed helped Maria develop a PICOT (patient population, intervention, comparison, outcome, and time frame) question, search for relevant research literature, appraise the literature, and develop a practice guideline for managing opioid tolerance in palliative care patients. Ed encouraged Maria to submit a poster abstract on managing opioid tolerance to a national palliative care society's annual meeting. Maria's poster won first prize. When Ed found out, he was ecstatic.

Discussion

Mentoring is a powerful experience that influences nursing careers and impacts patient care outcomes. The presence of a knowledgeable and committed EBP mentor enhances learning the art and science of EBP for the mentee (Christenbery, Williamson, Sandlin, & Wells, 2016; Fineout-Overholt, Levin, & Melnyk, 2004/2005). Scenarios 1 and 2 depict several positive and negative attempts at EBP mentoring. This chapter explores nurses working together in both individual mentoring experiences and as members of interprofessional collaborative teams to further the implementation of EBP.

PROFESSIONAL FORMATION

A profession is composed of individuals who possess specialized knowledge and skills, and who adhere to ethical and discipline-specific standards (Cruess, Johnston, & Cruess, 2004). Professional development is a means by which nurses maintain, advance, and broaden their nursing knowledge and enhance personal and professional qualities throughout their careers (Nursing and Midwifery Board of Australia, 2010). Because nursing attempts to preserve values associated with the profession (e.g., caring, integrity, diversity), professional development is an enduring behavior for nurses (Shaw & Fulton, 2015). Beyond traditional classroom environments, nurses seek opportunities to augment their professional development. Professional opportunities, such as *mentorship* and *interprofessional collaboration*, assist nurses in professional development by increasing nursing knowledge, skills, and values in important areas such as EBP, quality improvement, and research.

MENTORSHIP

Mentorship, as a concept, originated in the literature of ancient Greece. Mentorship was described more than 3,000 years ago in Homer's epic *The Odyssey* (Homer, 1990). Odysseus left home to fight in the Trojan War. While at war he entrusted the care of his household to Mentor, who served as a teacher and guide for Odysseus's young son, Telemachus.

Traditionally, *mentor* has been defined as a trusted counselor or guide (Fagenson-Eland, Marks, & Amendola, 1997). However, the meaning of the word *mentor* has evolved to include *teacher, sage, trusted advisor, friend*, and *expert*. Effective mentors provide direction, engender self-efficacy, and reinforce values (Wensel, 2006). History offers many examples of notable mentoring relationships, such as Socrates and Plato, Fonteyn and Nureyev, and Angelou and Winfrey. Each of these relationships provided unique opportunities to assist the mentee to learn, develop, and achieve professional fulfillment (Monsen & Cameron, 2004). Key components or characteristics of an effective mentoring relationship include (a) open communication and accessibility, (b) goals and challenges, (c) passion and inspiration, (d) caring personal relationship, (e) mutual respect and trust, (f) exchange of knowledge, (g) independence and collaboration, and (h) role modeling (Eller, Lev, & Feurer, 2014; see Figure 18.1).

Misunderstanding exists about the conceptualization of *mentor* and *preceptor* (Wensel, 2006). Sometimes, the words *mentor* and *preceptor* are inappropriately used interchangeably (McClure & Black, 2013). A preceptorship is an assigned, time-limited commitment in which a preceptor provides predetermined clinical instruction to a novice practitioner. A preceptorship may evolve into a reciprocal teaching–learning relationship between learner and preceptor (Chism, 2010). The preceptorship model in nursing originated in the 1970s to assist in the transitioning of newly graduated nurses from school to a professional work environment. As a means to enhance clinical reasoning (i.e., processing information to better understand patient problems or situations), the preceptor role eventually expanded into undergraduate nursing education to seamlessly guide nursing students from the theory of nursing to the application of theory (Omansky, 2010). In contrast to a preceptor, a mentor voluntarily provides a mentee with support for professional development that extends beyond an immediate clinical experience and nurtures a more profound sense of professional engagement and commitment to nursing (Lennox, Skinner, & Foureur, 2008; see Table 18.1).

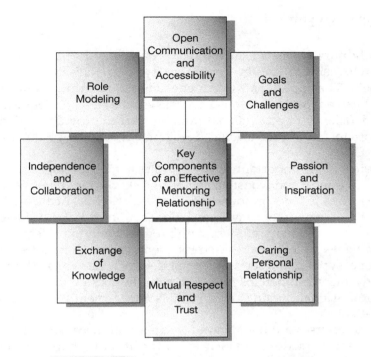

FIGURE 18.1   **Characteristics of a mentorship**

Source: From Eller, Lev, and Feurer (2014).

TABLE 18.1   **Differentiating Mentorship and Preceptorship**

Attribute	Mentorship	Preceptorship
Purpose	• Enables professional development • Supports professional development through new contexts and experiences	• Focus on developing clinical expertise • Assigned content to be learned
Origin	• Negotiated between mentor and mentee • Often initiated by mentee • May or may not be endorsed by employer	• Ascribed by employer
Duration	• Long-term commitment, often years • Dynamic, changes over time to meet mentee's needs	• Short-term commitment, limited to days or weeks
Setting	• Nonspecific	• Limited to clinical worksite
Termination	• Negotiated and mutually agreed upon between mentor and mentee	• When assigned term of preceptorship ends
Selection	• Mentee selects preceptor • Voluntary relationship	• Preceptor assigned by employer • Mandatory relationship
Goals	• Establish sense of place in profession • Improve problem-solving skills • Develop sense of professional autonomy	• Bridge theory-practice gap • Decrease work-related anxiety • Specific skill and knowledge acquisition

Source: Adapted from Lennox, Skinner, and Foureur (2008).

MENTORSHIP AND EBP

Traditionally, nurses were socialized into professional roles, including practice and research, using a master–apprentice system (Kalisch & Kalisch, 1986; Kohler, 2008). The apprentice system engendered a learning context in which nurses had few advocates in a hierarchical system. This problem was perpetuated by a deficiency of professional nursing staff to provide needed diversity and support to foster professional development for novice nurses (Andrist, 2006).

Mentoring is an important form of professional development for nurses. Receiving guidance and constructive feedback during mentorship enables direct care nurses to have profound learning experiences. Acquiring seemingly unmanageable amounts of new knowledge is a source of considerable stress for novice nurses and may interfere with progression into professional nursing roles. To mitigate professional role stress, mentors provide mentees with social and emotional support and serve as role models for achievement (Johnson, 2015). Additionally, mentorship helps nurses to gain the confidence needed to transition into professional nursing roles, such as engagement in EBP (Eller, Lev, & Feurer, 2014).

Direct care nurses are not always prepared with necessary knowledge and skills to base their practice on evidence. Many direct care nurses are educated at the associate degree or diploma level and have not had the benefit of a research course. Even with a bachelor of science in nursing (BSN) degree, direct care nurses may not have the expertise to rigorously and critically appraise research reports. Contemporary healthcare organizations use a variety of didactic and experiential approaches to educate the developing professional nursing workforce about the use of EBP. One of the most effective approaches for learning about EBP is through a mentoring relationship (Dearholt, White, Newhouse, Pugh, & Poe, 2008; Fineout-Overholt et al., 2004/2005; Roe & Whyte-Marshall, 2012). Using clinical experiences, EBP mentors capitalize on real-world opportunities to adapt EBP learning activities to meet the specific learning needs of mentees. EBP mentors are often effective because they act on EBP learning opportunities while favorable conditions exist in clinical areas.

Research demonstrates that engagement in EBP leads to significant improvements in patient outcomes and reduces the extensive time gap from generation of research to translation into patient care (Balas & Boren, 2000). Having an EBP mentorship is important, in part, because nurses are eager to see positive patient outcomes and nurses tend to be receptive to using the best and most current evidence (Melnyk, Fineout-Overholt, Gallagher-Ford, & Kaplan, 2012). Furthermore, nurses who use research to guide patient care tend to be more satisfied in their professional roles (Christenbery et al., 2016; Maljanina, Caramanica, Taylor, MacRae, & Beland, 2002; Retsas, 2000).

EBP mentorship targeted for direct care nurses has been identified repeatedly as a key element for successful implementation of EBP (Christenbery et al., 2016; Melnyk et al., 2012; Roe & Whyte-Marshall, 2012). Effective EBP mentorship for nurses has the potential to influence their convictions about EBP usefulness and can engender a lifelong commitment to the study and implementation of EBP. Multiple EBP implementation models (e.g., Johns Hopkins Nursing EPB

Model, Iowa Model) are available and depict key mentorship elements that are highly applicable to EBP mentoring relationships. For example, EBP mentoring must include the following:

- Helping nurses assess a healthcare organization's readiness for acceptance and sustainability of EBP
- Helping nurses identify key elements of an EBP culture (e.g., administrative support)
- Role modeling EBP (e.g., identifying a patient or population care problem, developing a PICOT question, appraising research literature, evaluating EBP outcome)
- Demonstrating interprofessional collaboration on implementing EBP projects
- Helping nurses identify internal (e.g., supplies, staffing) and external (e.g., accreditation, legislation) factors that impact the use of EBP
- Disseminating EBP outcomes

Many healthcare organizations employ advanced practice registered nurses (APRNs), clinical nurse specialists, and graduates from EBP fellowship programs. These nurses have often received both requisite and advanced EBP knowledge and experience to be effective EBP mentors. EBP mentors need to be able to support direct care nurses anywhere along the EPB continuum: from idea to outcome. EBP mentors have an especially important role in helping nurses to understand and apply the fundamentals of EBP.

The mentoring literature identifies several characteristics associated with effective mentors. Salient characteristics of effective mentors include approachability, effective interpersonal skills, positivity, supportive supervisory techniques, and professional development ability (Andrews & Wallis, 1999). In addition to these characteristics, EBP mentors must be able to be flexible with time and structure (Fineout-Overholt et al., 2004/2005). Direct care nurses are often pressed for time and cannot fit an inflexible EBP mentoring schedule into their lives. EBP mentors must be able to embrace teachable moments, which make achievements of succeeding in EBP possible for mentees. To be present for teachable moments means an EBP mentor must be accessible in the direct care nurse's work environment. Physical presence of an EBP mentor demonstrates an interest in the area in which the EBP project will occur. Being physically present provides the EBP mentor an opportunity to be attentive to topics that direct care nurses find important and might be interested in pursuing as unit-based EBP projects.

Nurses must recognize that mentorship is an ongoing, dynamic process that advances professional development of the novice nurse or of a professional nurse to a more advanced level. There are both benefits and challenges for the mentor and mentee in establishing a successful mentoring relationship. For the mentor, giving back to the profession is an enormous benefit, while availability of time and developing a successful mentoring experience can be challenging. Setting aside time for mentorship as well as finding an appropriate mentor can be challenging for the mentee.

Expertise has been characterized as having a vision of what is possible (Benner, 1982). Mentoring implies there is a level of expert knowledge that is being shared with the mentee. Using the Dreyfus Model of Skill Acquisition (Dreyfus & Dreyfus, 1980), nurses typically advance through five development stages: novice, advanced beginner, competent, proficient, and expert. To facilitate advancing skills, nurses receive substantial benefit from an EBP mentor who guides them from novice to expert in EBP engagement (see Table 18.2). Based on mutual interest, EBP mentorships are enduring, individualized partnerships that have a positive influence on providing scientifically sound patient-centered care.

TABLE 18.2   Novice to Expert

Stage		Characteristics of Mentee	Expected Level of Mentee Autonomy
1	Novice	• Adheres to established EBP rules and guidelines • Has minimal contextual perception • No discretionary judgment	• Needs explicit instruction and guidance about fundamental concepts of EBP (e.g., identify patient problems, write PICOT questions, correctly identify levels of evidence, access best available evidence)
2	Advanced Beginner	• Contextual perception still limited • All aspects of clinical situations given equal importance	• Straightforward tasks (e.g., assess basic patient problems and develop PICOT question) are likely achievable but supervision is still needed, especially in helping mentee see relationships among EBP tasks
3	Competent	• Copes with multiple tasks • Sees actions partly in terms of goals • Performs standardized and routine procedures	• Using own judgment, mentee is able to complete most fundamental EBP tasks
4	Proficient	• Sees what is most important in clinical situations • Perceives deviations from expected patterns	• Assumes full responsibility for identifying patient problems and patterns that deviate from the norm. Able to independently develop PICOT question, locate appropriate research literature, evaluate merits of research, synthesize research findings, and implement EBP plan
5	Expert	• No longer relies on rules, guidelines, or maxims • Grasp of situations and decision making intuitive • Vision of what is possible	• Is able to work independently with healthcare organization staff and lead interprofessional collaborative teams to address patient needs and implement standards of EBP

EBP, evidence-based practice; PICOT, patient population, intervention, comparison, outcome, time frame.
Source: Adapted from Dreyfus and Dreyfus, 1980.

COLLABORATION

In the current healthcare environment, patients are dependent on multiple providers from various disciplines for the provision of healthcare. For patient care to be safe, logically delivered, and of the highest quality, healthcare providers must practice as interprofessional collaborative teams (Sullivan, Kiovsky, Mason, Hill, & Dukes, 2015). Interprofessional collaboration has been defined as multiple healthcare workers from different disciplinary backgrounds (e.g., nursing, medicine, social work, pharmacology, neuroscience) working together with patients, families, caregivers, and communities to deliver optimal quality care (World Health Organization, 2010). Interprofessional collaboration is a primary factor in initiatives designed to influence the effectiveness of patient care, such as EBP (D'Amour, Ferrada-Videla, Rodriguez, & Beaulieu, 2005).

The Institute of Medicine (IOM) (2000) report *To Err Is Human* is unequivocal in its depiction of the breakdown or absence of communication among healthcare providers, especially between nurses and physicians. Communication collapse among healthcare providers leads to significant disruption and destabilization of healthcare environments, which, in due course, has a regrettable impact on patient care (Rabol et al., 2016). To promote healthier communication and interprofessional collaboration, egalitarian systems of healthcare delivery are replacing physician-centric healthcare environments. Healthcare environments are moving to a point at which input from all team members (e.g., patients, nurses, physicians, chaplains) is valued (Newhouse & Spring, 2010).

Ineffective or insufficient communication among healthcare professionals is a primary cause of patient harm (Leonard, Graham, & Bonacum, 2004; Woolf, Kuzel, & Dovey, 2004). In addition to adverse patient events, healthcare organizations report that communication issues among practitioners result in increased patient length of stay, resource waste, health provider dissatisfaction, and unwarranted attrition (Fisher & Peterson, 1993; Sexton, 2002; Zwarenstein & Reeves, 2002). Inadequate interprofessional communication in intensive care units among nurses and physicians contributes a minimum of a 1.8-fold increase in both patient mortality and patient length of stay (Baggs et al., 1999; Shortell et al., 1994).

Effective interprofessional collaboration and communication among healthcare providers is a challenging endeavor related, in part, to several interconnecting factors:

- Healthcare delivery is complex and constantly changing.
- Healthcare is delivered by providers from multiple disciplines with discipline-specific views of health and illness.
- Healthcare organizations are often hierarchical with noticeable power gaps between physicians and other members of the healthcare team, which may lead to inhibition of communication.
- Between and within the various healthcare professions are multiple levels of education and expertise that challenge communication.
- The educational background of some disciplines may not emphasize teamwork and communication (Zwarenstein & Reeves, 2002).

INTERPROFESSIONAL COLLABORATION AND EBP

For almost 20 years, the IOM has strongly emphasized interprofessional collaboration and communication among healthcare providers as a means to foster safe exchange of patient information and straightforward coordination of patient care (IOM, 2000). In 2003, the IOM issued a report that identified five competencies: *patient-centered care, quality improvement, EBP, informatics,* and *interprofessional teams.* The five competencies serve as a common vision to engender a commitment among healthcare professionals to meet patients' needs. The IOM report indicated healthcare provider education should prepare healthcare students to work together in interprofessional collaborative practice teams to provide the highest quality and safest possible patient care.

In 2011, the Interprofessional Education Collaborative (IPEC) identified four competency domains: (a) Values/Ethics, (b) Roles/Responsibilities, (c) Interprofessional Communication, and (d) Team and Teamwork. Each domain contains a set of specific and related competency statements to establish a framework for interprofessional education (see Box 18.1). The four domains conceptualize the interprofessional goals of six health education disciplines:

- American Association of Colleges of Nursing
- American Association of Colleges of Orthopaedic Medicine
- Association of Schools and Programs of Public Health
- American Association of Colleges of Pharmacy
- American Dental Education Association
- Association of American Medical Colleges

BOX 18.1   Four Competencies of Interprofessional Collaborative Practice

Competency 1

General Competency Statement: Work with individuals of other professions to maintain a climate of mutual respect and shared values. (Values/Ethics for Interprofessional Practice)
  Values/Ethics for Interprofessional Practice Subcompetencies:

1. Place interests of patients and populations at center of interprofessional healthcare delivery and population health programs and policies, with the goal of promoting health and health equity across the life span.

2. Respect the dignity and privacy of patients while maintaining confidentiality in the delivery of team-based care.

3. Embrace the cultural diversity and individual differences that characterize patients, populations, and the health team.

4. Respect the unique cultures, values, roles/responsibilities, and expertise of other health professions and the impact these factors can have on health outcomes.

5. Work in cooperation with those who receive care, those who provide care, and others who contribute to or support the delivery of prevention and health services and programs.

6. Develop a trusting relationship with patients, families, and other team members.

(continued)

BOX 18.1   **Four Competencies of Interprofessional Collaborative Practice** *(continued)*

---

7. Demonstrate high standards of ethical conduct and quality of care in one's contributions to team-based care.

8. Manage ethical dilemmas specific to interprofessional patient/population-centered care situations.

9. Act with honesty and integrity in relationships with patients, families, and other team members.

10. Maintain competence in one's own profession appropriate to scope of practice.

Competency 2

General Competency Statement: Use the knowledge of one's own role and those of other professions to appropriately assess and address the healthcare needs of patients and to promote and advance the health of populations. (Roles/Responsibilities)
Roles/Responsibilities Subcompetencies:

1. Communicate one's roles and responsibilities clearly to patients, families, community members, and other professionals.

2. Recognize one's limitations in skills, knowledge, and abilities.

3. Engage diverse professionals who complement one's own professional expertise, as well as associated resources, to develop strategies to meet specific health and healthcare needs of patients and populations.

4. Explain the roles and responsibilities of other care providers and how the team works together to provide care, promote health, and prevent disease.

5. Use the full scope of knowledge, skills, and abilities of professionals from health and other fields to provide care that is safe, timely, efficient, effective, and equitable.

6. Communicate with team members to clarify each member's responsibility in executing components of a treatment plan or public health intervention.

7. Forge interdependent relationships with other professions within and outside of the health system to improve care and advance learning.

8. Engage in continuous professional and interprofessional development to enhance team performance and collaboration.

9. Use unique and complementary abilities of all members of the team to optimize health and patient care.

10. Describe how professionals in health and other fields can collaborate and integrate clinical care and public health interventions to optimize population health.

Competency 3

General Competency Statement: Communicate with patients, families, communities, and professionals in health and other fields in a responsive and responsible manner that supports a team approach to the promotion and maintenance of health and the treatment of disease. (Interprofessional Communication)
Interprofessional Communication Subcompetencies:

1. Choose effective communication tools and techniques, including information systems and communication technologies, to facilitate discussions and interactions that enhance team function.

2. Communicate information with patients, families, community members, and health team members in a form that is understandable, avoiding discipline-specific terminology when possible.

(continued)

BOX 18.1   **Four Competencies of Interprofessional Collaborative Practice** (*continued*)

3. Express one's knowledge and opinions to team members involved in patient care and population health improvement with confidence, clarity, and respect, working to ensure common understanding of information and treatment and care decisions, as well as population health programs and policies.

4. Listen actively, and encourage ideas and opinions of other team members.

5. Give timely, sensitive, instructive feedback to others about their performance on the team, responding respectfully as a team member to feedback from others.

6. Use respectful language appropriate for a given difficult situation, crucial conversation, or interprofessional conflict.

7. Recognize how one's own uniqueness, including experience level, expertise, culture, power, and hierarchy within the health team, contributes to effective communication, conflict resolution, and positive interprofessional working relationships.

8. Communicate consistently the importance of teamwork in patient-centered care and population health programs and policies.

Competency 4

General Competency Statement: Apply relationship-building values and the principles of team dynamics to perform effectively in different team roles to plan, deliver, and evaluate patient/population-centered care and population health programs and policies that are safe, timely, efficient, effective, and equitable. (Teams and Teamwork)

Team and Teamwork Subcompetencies:

1. Describe the process of team development and the roles and practices of effective teams.

2. Develop consensus on the ethical principles to guide all aspects of patient care and teamwork.

3. Engage health and other professionals in shared patient-centered and population-focused problem solving.

4. Integrate the knowledge and experience of health and other professions to inform health and care decisions, while respecting patient and community values and priorities/preferences for care.

5. Apply leadership practices that support collaborative practice and team effectiveness.

6. Engage self and others to constructively manage disagreements about values, roles, goals, and actions that arise among healthcare and other professionals and with patients, families, and community members.

7. Share accountability with other professions, patients, and communities for outcomes relevant to prevention and healthcare.

8. Reflect on individual and team performance for individual, as well as team, performance improvement.

9. Use process improvement strategies to increase the effectiveness of interprofessional teamwork and team-based services, programs, and policies.

10. Use available evidence to inform effective teamwork and team-based practices.

11. Perform effectively on teams and in different team roles in a variety of settings.

Source: Interprofessional Education Collaborative (2016).

NURSING, INTERPROFESSIONAL COLLABORATION, AND EBP

Nurses must be leaders in the design, implementation, and evaluation of EBP. Nursing's role as a *full partner* with other healthcare disciplines underscores nursing's accountability in leading EBP initiatives. Nurses have important roles in advancing EBP as part of interprofessional collaboration. Whether nurses are *educators, clinicians, researchers,* or *administrators,* they have critical responsibilities in contributing to interprofessional collaboration and EBP responsibilities. The nursing workforce in each of these areas needs to use leadership skills and competencies to act as full EBP partners with other disciplines.

Nurse Educators

Nursing faculty members are responsible for developing nursing curricula that includes the nurse's role in interprofessional collaboration and EBP. Faculty members have a responsibility to integrate simulated interprofessional and EBP activities in the curriculum. Evaluation of educational outcomes and learner satisfaction about interprofessional collaboration and EBP projects is a faculty role. Evaluation of interprofessional collaboration and EBP activities should take place at the end of the nursing program. Evaluation also should be conducted 1 year postgraduation to evaluate whether alumni were academically prepared to integrate EBP and interprofessional collaboration into real-world work settings. Faculty must be alert for opportunities to enrich interprofessional EBP endeavors in the curriculum. Faculty must also evaluate their own members to determine whether their EBP knowledge, skills, and values are current and whether they can role model the practice of engaging in interprofessional collaboration and EBP activities (Newhouse & Spring, 2010).

Nurse Clinicians

Direct care nurses and other clinicians may have the most important roles in implementing interprofessional EBP in healthcare settings. As the largest workforce component of most healthcare settings, clinicians need to develop EBP knowledge and skills to efficiently and effectively disseminate EBP throughout the healthcare setting. Because of their proximity to patients and depth of patient care knowledge, clinicians need to be present on all interprofessional EBP committees and task forces. Clinicians are in an excellent position to provide healthcare organization administrators with input about facilitators and barriers to interprofessional collaboration and EBP. Because of their clinical expertise, clinicians are generally excellent at finding solutions and therefore should have positions at the "table" to help strategize removal of barriers to EBP. Clinicians need to be abstract reviewers and poster judges for in-house EBP poster events. Finally, clinicians who are EBP savvy and understand how to work in interprofessional activities and relationships can lead in promoting the translation of current and best evidence into practice (Newhouse & Spring, 2010).

Nurse Researchers

Nurse researchers have an important role in recommending EBP interprofessional models (e.g., Colorado Patient-Centered Interprofessional EBP Model, Johns Hopkins Nursing EBP Model). In addition, nurse researchers are able to test and measure the effectiveness of EBP models and make recommendations for use in designated healthcare settings. Healthcare organizations that implement interprofessional collaboration and EBP will need rigorous and systematic program evaluation activities to evaluate for desired outcomes, staff and patient satisfaction, and cost benefits. These program evaluation activities benefit from the planning and implementation skills of nurse researchers (Newhouse & Spring, 2010).

Nurse Administrators

Interprofessional collaboration and EBP are not the "normal way" of doing business in healthcare settings. Interprofessional collaboration EBP endeavors are new to many healthcare settings and therefore require demonstrable support and commitment from nurse administrators in these settings. Nurse administrators need to work closely with nurse clinicians and nurse researchers to detect positives and negatives about interprofessional collaboration and EBP and make required immediate adjustments. Nurse administrators need to work closely with schools of nursing administrators and faculty to keep both groups apprised of required knowledge and skills that nursing students need for working in environments that use interprofessional collaborative EBP. Clinicians will need the support and assurance from nurse administrators that they are supported as full participants in the implementation and dissemination of EBP.

SUMMARY

This chapter addresses the essential elements of mentorship and interprofessional collaboration for professional nursing development. Mentoring and interprofessional collaboration are discussed as opportunities for nurses to have key leadership roles in the implementation and dissemination of EBP. Methods to support successful EBP mentoring and interprofessional collaboration are presented.

REFERENCES

Andrews, M., & Wallis, M. (1999). Mentorship in nursing: A literature review. *Journal of Advanced Nursing, 29*(1), 201–207. doi:10.1046/j.1365-2648.1999.00884.x

Andrist, L. C. (2006). The history of the relationship between feminism and nursing. In L. C. Andrist, P. K. Nicholas, & K. A. Wolf (Eds.), *History of nursing ideas*. Boston, MA: Jones & Bartlett.

Baggs, J. G., Schmitt, M. H., Mushlin, A. I., Mitchell, P. H., Eldridge, D. H., Oakes, D., & Hutson, A. D. (1999). Association between nurse-physician collaboration and patient outcomes in three intensive care units. *Critical Care Medicine, 27,* 1991–1998.

Balas, E. A., & Boren, S. A. (2000). Managing clinical knowledge for health care improvement. *Yearbook of Medical Informatics, 1,* 65–70.

Benner, P. (1982). From novice to expert: Excellence and power in clinical nursing practice. Menlo Park, CA: Addison-Wesley.

Chism, L. A. (2010). The DNP graduate as expert clinician. In L. A. Chism (Ed.), *The doctor of nursing practice: A guidebook for role development and professional issues* (pp. 61–96). Burlington, MA: Jones & Bartlett.

Christenbery, T., Williamson, A., Sandlin, V., & Wells, N. (2016). Immersion in evidence-based practice fellowship program. *Journal for Nurses in Professional Development, 32*(1), 15–20.

Cruess, S. R., Johnston, S., & Cruess, R. L. (2004). Profession: A working definition for medical educators. *Teaching and Learning in Medicine, 16*(1), 74–76.

D'Amour, D., Ferrada-Videla, M., Rodriguez, L. S. M., & Beaulieu, M. D. (2005). The conceptual basis for interprofessional collaboration: Core concepts and theoretical frameworks. *Journal of Interprofessional Care, S1,* 116–131.

Dearholt, S. L., White, K. M., Newhouse, R., Pugh, L. C., & Poe, S. (2008). Educational strategies to develop evidence-based practice mentors. *Journal for Nurses in Staff Development, 24*(2), 53–59.

Dreyfus, S., & Dreyfus, H. (1980). *A five stage model of the mental activities involved in directed skill acquisition.* Unpublished doctoral study supported by the Air Force Office of Scientific Research, USAF (contract F49620-79-C0063), University of California, Berkeley, CA.

Eller, L. S., Lev, E. L., & Feurer A. (2014). Key components of an effective mentoring relationship: A qualitative study. *Nurse Education Today, 34*(5), 815–820.

Fagenson-Eland, E. A., Marks, M. A., & Amendola, K. L. (1997). Perceptions of mentoring relationships. *Journal of Vocational Behavior, 51*(1), 29–42.

Fineout-Overholt, E., Levin, R. F., & Melnyk, B. M. (2004/2005). Strategies for advancing evidence-based practice in clinical settings. *Journal of the New York State Nurses Association, Fall/Winter, 35,* 28–31.

Fisher, B., & Peterson, C. (1993). She won't be dancing anyway: A study of surgeons, surgical nurses, and elder patients. *Qualitative Health Research, 3,* 165–183.

Homer. (1990). *The Odyssey* (R. Fagles, Trans.). New York, NY: Vintage Books.

Institute of Medicine. (2000). *To err is human* (L. T. Kohn, J. M. Corrigan, & M. S. Donaldson, Eds.). Washington, DC: National Academies Press.

Interprofessional Education Collaborative. (2016). *Core competencies for interprofessional collaborative practice: 2016 update.* Washington, DC: Author.

Johnson, W. B. (2015). *On being a mentor: A guide for higher education faculty* (2nd ed.). New York, NY: Routledge

Kalisch, P. A., & Kalisch, B. J. (1986). *The advance of American nursing* (2nd ed.). Boston, MA: Little, Brown.

Kohler, R. E. (2008). From farm to family to career naturalist: The apprenticeship of Vernon Baily. *Isis, 99,* 28–56.

Lennox, S., Skinner, J., & Foureur, M. (2008). Mentorship preceptorship and clinical supervision: Three key processes for supporting midwives. *New Zealand College of Midwives Journal, 39,* 7–12.

Leonard, M., Graham, S., & Bonacum, D. (2004). The critical importance of effective teamwork and communication in providing safe care. *Quality and Safety in Health Care, 13,* 85–90.

Maljanina, R., Caramanica, L., Taylor, S. K., MacRae, J. B., & Beland, D. K. (2002). Evidence-based nursing practice, Part 2: Building skills through research roundtables. *Journal of Nursing Administration, 32*(2), 85–90.

McClure, E., & Black, L. (2013). The role of the clinical preceptor: An integrative literature review. *Journal of Nursing Education, 52*(6), 335–341. doi:10.3928/01484834-20130430-02

Melnyk, B. M., Fineout-Overholt, E., Gallagher-Ford, L., & Kaplan, L. (2012). The state of evidence-based practice in US nurses: Critical implications for nurse leaders and educators. *Journal of Nursing Administration, 42*(9), 410–417.

Monsen, J., & Cameron, R. S. (2004). *Working with emotions: Responding to the challenge of difficult pupil behaviour in schools.* London, UK: RoutledgeFalmer.

Newhouse, R. P., & Spring, B. (2010). Interdisciplinary evidence-based practice: Moving from silos to synergy. *Nursing Outlook, 58*(6), 309–317.

Nursing and Midwifery Board of Australia. (2010). *Continuing professional development registration standards.* Retrieved from http://www.nursingmidwiferyboard.gov.au/Registration-Standards/Continuing-professional-development.aspx

Omansky, G. L. (2010). Staff nurses' experiences as preceptors and mentors: An integrative review. *Journal of Nursing Management, 18*, 697–703. doi:10.1111/j.1365-2834.2010.01145.x

Rabol, L. I., Anderson, M. L., Ostergaard, D., Bjorn, B., Lilja, L., & Mogensen, T. (2016). Descriptions of verbal communication errors between staff: An analysis of 84 root-cause analysis reports from Danish hospitals. *BMJ Quality and Safety, 20*(3), 268–274.

Retsas, A. (2000). Barriers to using research in nursing practice. *Journal of Advanced Nursing, 31*(3), 599–606.

Roe, E. A., & Whyte-Marshall, M. (2012). Mentoring for evidence-based practice: A collaborative approach. *Journal for Nurses in Staff Development, 28*(4), 177–181.

Sexton, J. (2002). Error stress and teamwork in medicine and aviation: Cross sectional surveys. *British Medical Journal, 320*, 745–749.

Shaw, M. D., & Fulton, J. (2015). *Mentorship in healthcare* (2nd ed.). Cumbria, UK: M & K Publishing.

Shortell, S. M., Zimmerman, J. E., Rousseau, D. M., Gillies, R. R., Wagner, D. P., Draper, E. A., . . . Duffy, J. (1994). The performance of intensive care units: Does good management make a difference? *Medical Care, 32*, 508–525.

Sullivan, M., Kiovsky, R. D., Mason, D. J., Hill, C. D., & Dukes, C. (2015). Interprofessional collaboration and education. *American Journal of Nursing, 115*(3), 47–54.

Wensel, T. M. (2006). Mentor and preceptor: What is the difference? *American Journal Health-System Pharmacy, 63*, 1597.

Woolf, S. H., Kuzel, A. J., & Dovey, S. M. (2004). A string of mistakes: The importance of cascade analysis in describing, counting, and preventing medical errors. *Annals of Family Medicine, 2*, 317–326.

World Health Organization. (2010). *Framework for action on interprofessional education and collaborative practice.* Retrieved from http://whqlibdoc.who.int/hq/2010/WHO_HRH_HPN_10.3_eng.pdf

Zwarenstein, M., & Reeves, S. (2002). Working together but apart: Barriers and routes to nurse-physician collaboration. *Joint Commission Journal on Quality Improvement, 28*, 242–247.

CHAPTER 19

Evidence-Based Practice: Sequential Layering of BSN, MSN, and DNP Competencies and Opportunities

Thomas L. Christenbery

Objectives

After reading this chapter, learners should be able to:

1. Differentiate the expected evidence-based practice (EBP) competencies for nurses educated at BSN, MSN, and DNP levels

2. Describe organizational opportunities that are appropriate in supporting EBP for nurses educated at BSN, MSN, and DNP levels

3. Identify expected EBP outcomes for nurses educated at BSN, MSN, and DNP levels

EVIDENCE-BASED PRACTICE (EBP) SCENARIOS

Scenario 1

Joan, a direct care nurse who graduated from a BSN program 6 months ago, works in a head and neck oncology clinic. The unit's nursing manager knew Joan had didactic EBP content in her BSN program. The manager asked Joan to lead an interdisciplinary and collaborative effort to initiate new practice guideline protocols for treatment of lymphedema. Joan was able to effectively search the research literature and find several Level I articles, of sound quality, about innovative treatments for lymphedema. Joan believed many of the new lymphedema treatment recommendations would be beneficial and well received by patients who are seen at the clinic. As for the next EBP steps, Joan had to tell her unit manager she did not know how to form an interdisciplinary team or even develop practice guidelines based on best evidence. Joan felt she was letting both her manager and, more important, the patients down.

Scenario 2

Sharam, an advanced practice registered nurse (APRN) who graduated from a DNP program 6 months ago, sees patients in a head and neck oncology clinic. The unit's leadership knew Sharam completed a practice change project on the unit as part of her scholarly work requirement for the DNP degree. The DNP practice change project was evaluated as being successful for both patients and staff. Unit leadership asked Sharam if she would design, direct, and evaluate an interdisciplinary and collaborative project to implement new protocols for the treatment of lymphedema. Building on her experiences and knowledge from the DNP program, Sharam was able to coordinate an interprofessional team to design, implement, and evaluate new lymphedema protocols for the unit. Sharam was grateful for the opportunity to involve members from other disciplines in a nursing-led initiative to improve patient care.

Discussion

In Scenario 1, the unit manager had excellent intentions of involving a new nurse in an EBP endeavor. However, the EBP endeavor exceeded the nurse's knowledge and skillset. Involving the nurse as a member of a team that would initiate protocol guidelines for change would have been an appropriate request. The nurse would likely have achieved success and felt a sense of accomplishment in her abilities to contribute to an EBP endeavor. In Scenario 2, unit leadership selected a nurse who was prepared to lead a multilayered EBP project that required extensive EBP knowledge and skills. The results of this selection were beneficial to the nurse, leadership, team members, and patients.

PROVIDING OPPORTUNITY FOR EBP

Implicitly, nurses do not mean much to healthcare organizations unless they have the *opportunity* to develop and advance within the organization. Opportunity within an organization refers to a chance to increase work-related knowledge and skills and subsequently experience professional growth. Organizational opportunity is important to nurses because it allows them to show out-of-the-ordinary capabilities and be seen as successful and promotable (Kanter, 1993). Opportunities to use knowledge and skills to implement EBP gives nurses a means to provide quality patient-centered care and achieve expected organizational goals and, as a consequence, receive recognition.

Each academic discipline (e.g., medicine, engineering) has distinct inquiry-based applications that are characteristic of that discipline (Cohen & Lloyd, 2014). Evidence-based practice is an inquiry-based application to practice that is central to nursing. To provide optimal patient care in the current dynamic healthcare environment, education for nurses must include development of EBP knowledge and skills. Strong influences impact the EBP role of nurses and include the following:

- *Scientific advances*, such as pharmacogenomics, targeted cancer therapies, and treatments for drug-resistant bacteria
- *Shifting patient population demographics*, notably in age, race, ethnicity, and culture
- *Healthcare technologies*, such as telemedicine, wearable medical devices, and portal technology

These and other important influences require nurses to provide unique and sophisticated ways of thinking about and implementing EBP that is commensurate with their practice degree level in nursing (i.e., bachelor of science in nursing [BSN], master of science in nursing [MSN], doctor of nursing practice [DNP]).

The American Association of Colleges of Nursing (AACN), as the collective voice for baccalaureate and graduate nursing education (MSN, DNP), works to establish quality standards for nursing education and, thereby, influences the nursing profession to improve healthcare (AACN, 2016). The AACN Essentials Series outlines the necessary curriculum content and expected *competencies* of graduates from BSN (AACN, 2008), MSN (AACN, 2001), and DNP (AACN, 2006) programs (see Table 19.1). Each degree level has a specific AACN Essential that addresses expected EBP competencies of nurses:

- BSN: Essential III—Scholarship for Evidence-Based Practice
  - Professional nursing practice is grounded in the translation of current evidence into one's practice
- MSN: Essential IV—Translating and Integrating Scholarship Into Practice
- DNP: Essential III—Clinical Scholarship and Analytical Methods for Evidence-Based Practice

Sequentially, each EBP Essential provides a foundation that builds necessary knowledge and skills from entry-level practice (BSN) to terminal practice degree (DNP). Achievement of essential EBP knowledge and skills at each degree level prepares nurses to fully engage in AACN-designated EBP capacities (see Table 19.1). The Institute of Medicine (IOM) and other authoritative groups have directed healthcare professionals to build a safer healthcare system for the 21st century (American Hospital Association, 2002; IOM, 2000, 2001, 2004, 2010). To achieve this goal, healthcare organizations need to provide opportunities for nurses, educated at each degree level, to engage in appropriate and expected levels of EBP competencies.

Nurses, whether educated at the BSN, MSN, or DNP degree level, are members of the professional healthcare team. The term *professional* indicates the formation of a professional identity as the foundation for professional functioning at each degree level (Adams, Hean, Sturgis, & Macleod-Clark, 2006). As professionals, nurses are knowledge workers who use clinical knowledge and skills that encompass substantial breadth and depth. Professional nurses use EBP to foster critical reasoning, sound clinical judgment, and effective communication to

TABLE 19.1   American Association of Colleges of Nursing EBP Essentials Crosswalk

Baccalaureate Level Essential III: Scholarship for Evidence-Based Practice	Master's Level Essential IV: Translating and Integrating Scholarship Into Practice	Doctor of Nursing Practice Level Essential III: Clinical Scholarship and Analytical Methods for Evidence-Based Practice (EBP)
1. Explain the interrelationships between theory, practice, and research.	1. Integrate theory, evidence, clinical judgment, research, and interprofessional perspectives using translational processes to improve practice and associated health outcomes for patient aggregates.	1. Use analytical methods to critically appraise existing literature and other evidence to determine and implement the best evidence for practice.
2. Demonstrate an understanding of the basic elements of the research process and models for applying evidence to clinical practice.	2. Advocate for the ethical conduct of research and translational scholarship with particular attention to the protection of the patient as a research participant.	2. Design and implement processes to evaluate outcomes of practice, practice patterns, and systems of care within a practice setting, healthcare organization, or community against national benchmarks to determine variances in practice outcomes and population trends.
3. Advocate for the protection of human subjects in the conduct of research.	3. Articulate to a variety of audiences the evidence base for practice decisions, including the credibility of sources of information and the relevance of the practice problem confronted.	3. Design, direct, and evaluate quality improvement methodologies to promote safe, timely, effective, efficient, equitable, and patient-centered care.
4. Evaluate the credibility of sources of information, including but not limited to databases and Internet resources.	4. Participate, leading when appropriate, in collaborative teams to improve care outcomes and support policy changes through knowledge generation, knowledge dissemination and planning, and evaluating knowledge implementation.	4. Apply relevant findings to develop practice guidelines and improve practice and the practice environment.
5. Participate in the process of retrieval, appraisal, and synthesis of evidence in collaboration with other members of the healthcare team to improve patient outcomes.	5. Apply practice guidelines to improve practice and the care environment.	5. Use information technology and research methods appropriately to: ● Collect appropriate and accurate data to generate evidence for nursing practice

(continued)

TABLE 19.1   American Association of Colleges of Nursing EBP Essentials
Crosswalk *(continued)*

Baccalaureate Level Essential III: Scholarship for Evidence-Based Practice	Master's Level Essential IV: Translating and Integrating Scholarship Into Practice	Doctor of Nursing Practice Level Essential III: Clinical Scholarship and Analytical Methods for Evidence-Based Practice (EBP)
		⬤ Inform and guide the design of databases that generate meaningful evidence for nursing practice ⬤ Analyze data from practice ⬤ Design evidence-based interventions ⬤ Predict and analyze outcomes ⬤ Examine patterns of behavior and outcomes ⬤ Identify gaps in evidence for practice
6. Integrate evidence, clinical judgment, interprofessional perspectives, and patient preferences in planning, implementing, and evaluating outcomes of care.	6. Perform rigorous critique of evidence derived from databases to generate meaningful evidence for nursing practice.	6. Function as a practice specialist/consultant in collaborative knowledge-generating research.
7. Collaborate in the collection, documentation, and dissemination of evidence.		7. Disseminate findings from evidence-based practice and research to improve healthcare outcomes.
8. Acquire an understanding of the process for how nursing and related healthcare quality and safety measures are developed, validated, and endorsed.		
9. Describe mechanisms to resolve identified practice discrepancies between identified standards and practice that may adversely impact patient outcomes.		

Source: American Association of Colleges of Nursing (2006, 2008, 2011).

deliver impactful patient-centered care (Melnyk & Fineout-Overholt, 2015). The following sections identify the required AACN EBP Essentials from BSN to DNP and describe the knowledge and skills required for achieving EBP competencies for each degree level.

NURSING ROLES IN EBP

Bachelor of Science in Nursing

In today's multifaceted healthcare environment, baccalaureate education is the minimum degree required for entry into professional nursing practice (AACN, 2008; American Nurses Association, 1965). BSN graduates are educated to practice with patients, families, communities, and populations across the human life span and the continuum of healthcare environments (AACN, 2008). Baccalaureate *EBP education is the foundation upon which MSN and DNP evidence-based practice nursing education builds.*

Nurses educated at the BSN level engage in patient-centered care that assesses, respects, and addresses patients' values, preferences, and expressed needs (Grenier & Knebel, 2003). Patient-centered care involves the coordination of patient care, listening to and communicating with patients, and educating patients and their families about health, prevention, and disease management (IOM, 2001). BSN graduates are an indispensable human link for translating a plan of care to patients and families (AACN, 2008). A sound EBP skillset is required to provide the best possible evidence to inform critical fundamental nursing actions. Engagement in EBP enables BSN-level nurses to design, coordinate, and manage optimal patient-centered care across healthcare environments.

The current healthcare environment actively involves nurses in clinical decision making and, therefore, has made it necessary for healthcare organizations to hire a larger proportion of nurses who have earned a BSN degree (AACN, 2015). Within the current dynamic and complex healthcare environment, BSN-level nurses provide patient care centered on EBP. BSN graduates use research and other forms of relevant evidence to implement care that is patient specific, high quality, and cost effective (AACN, 2008). Understanding advances in science and the influence scientific advances can bring to patient care is essential knowledge for baccalaureate-educated nurses. It is equally critical for BSN-level nurses to understand patient values and preferences brought to the healthcare setting.

The translation of current evidence into practice is a cornerstone of professional nursing (White, Dudley-Brown, & Terhaar, 2016). The AACN Essentials (2008) identify specific elements of EBP scholarship necessary for BSN-level nurses to begin the translation of relevant evidence into practice. Evidence-based practice scholarship for BSN graduates includes (a) identification of a practice or system issue and/or problem, (b) critical appraisal and integration of evidence, and (c) evaluation of EBP outcomes. BSN-educated practitioners generally fulfill the important role of providing nursing care at the patient's point of care and are eminently qualified to monitor patient outcomes and identify practice concerns or problems (AACN, 2015). Several EBP models, as described in the Appendix, are useful in helping to guide BSN-level nurses in the evaluation and application of scientific evidence surrounding patient-centered clinical concerns.

At the BSN level, nurses are educated with a foundational understanding of how best evidence is developed. A basic understanding of evidence development includes appraisal of qualitative and quantitative research processes, clinical decision-making knowledge, awareness of interprofessional perspectives, and patient values as applied to clinical practice (AACN, 2008). To enhance sound clinical judgments and augment clinical decision-making processes, healthcare organizations must provide BSN-educated nurses opportunities to contribute to EBP endeavors for which they have been educated. These EBP endeavors include opportunities to:

- Identify a need for clinical information about the care of patients, communities, and/or populations
- Convert a clinical information need into an answerable question (i.e., PICOT) that focuses on prevention, prognosis, therapy, diagnosis, etiology, or meaning
- Acquire relevant information and evidence to answer a clinical question
- Critically appraise evidence, related to an identified need, for validity (closeness to truth), impact (size of the effect), and applicability (usefulness to clinical practice or setting)
- Integrate the appraised evidence with professional clinical expertise and the patient's unique biology, context, values, and preferences to develop patient-centered interventions
- Apply evidence-based interventions within the context of collaborative decision making with the recipients of care
- Evaluate the previous steps for efficiency and effectiveness to improve implementation for future use
- Assist in disseminating EBP results internally and externally to a healthcare organization

Healthcare organizations must be committed to providing opportunities for BSN graduates to engage in the previous EBP steps. The steps help BSN graduates understand the research process, think critically about patient care concerns, and develop information literacy skills that enable them to find and appraise credible evidence. Opportunities to engage in the steps empower BSN graduates to inform and transform their nursing practice and patient outcomes.

Master of Science in Nursing

Master's level education is the critical interlinkage of nursing's education trajectory. MSN graduates are educated with broad knowledge and practice expertise that builds and expands on BSN-level practice. For any advanced practice nursing role or nurse educator role, MSN education prepares nurses with a richer understanding of the discipline and engages them in higher-level practice and leadership in diverse healthcare settings (AACN, 2011). MSN graduates are prepared to address significant gaps in healthcare delivery.

The AACN Essentials for MSN education emphasize *advanced nursing knowledge* and *higher level leadership skills*, which have a significant impact on the delivery of EBP healthcare (AACN, 2011). Building on baccalaureate degree preparation, master's degree nurses are prepared with broad knowledge and leadership expertise to address the AACN Essential of *translating and integrating scholarship (i.e., evidence) into practice*. Complexities of health and illness and the dynamic healthcare environment of today make expanded EBP knowledge and advanced leadership skills a necessity in translation of best evidence into practice (Moseley, 2012).

Translation and integration of evidence into practice, policy, and population health improvement is defined as the adoption and dissemination of sound interventions that have a significant impact on health (Gonzales, Handley, Ackerman, & O'Sullivan, 2012). Effective translation of evidence into practice has been sluggish and inconsistent across U.S. healthcare organizations (Madon, Hofman, Kupfer, & Glass, 2007; Ogilvie, Craig, Griffin, Macintyre, & Wareham, 2009; Zerhouni, 2005). Clinical practice inconsistencies contribute greatly to the illogical variation and substandard delivery of healthcare (Avorn & Fischer, 2010; Davis & Taylor-Vaisey, 1997; Gonzales et al., 2012; Haynes, Hayward, & Lomas, 1995). Guidelines, used alone, for translation of evidence into practice rarely have a positive impact on practice change (Davis & Taylor-Vaisey, 1997).

Nurses educated at the master's degree level who understand the art and science of *implementation* and *dissemination* of best evidence are needed to fully facilitate the translation of evidence into practice (White et al., 2016). The National Institutes of Health defined *implementation* as the use of strategies to adopt and integrate interventions centered on best evidence to change practice patterns within select settings. *Dissemination* is defined as targeted distribution of knowledge and intervention materials to a specific population or clinical practice audience (National Institutes of Health, 2016).

Advanced technical and adaptive knowledge and skills are needed to effectively translate evidence into practice. Graduates of MSN programs have substantive understandings of healthcare technology and organizational and human behavior. Advanced technical and behavioral knowledge enables master's educated nurses to foster interdisciplinary EBP teams, thereby encouraging adoption of relevant evidence-based interventions into practice and ensuring an EBP collaborative culture within healthcare organizations (Septimus et al., 2014).

MSN-educated nurses assume increasing accountabilities, responsibilities, and leadership roles (AACN, 2011) to effectively translate and integrate evidence into practice. The following are key responsibilities of MSN-educated nurses in translating and integrating evidence into practice:

- Critically assess and challenge the status quo of practice, policy, and procedure to seek questions that can lead to improvement of patient care
- Advance clinical practice knowledge by collaboratively applying best evidence to disseminate outcomes within the local setting as well as larger venues
- Incorporate implementation science and improvement science to support effective EBP

- Mentor other nurses and health professionals (e.g., physicians, social workers) in implementation of EBP
- Engage in the cyclical process of identifying relevant clinical questions and searching for and *creating* the evidence for solutions and innovations
- Evaluate outcomes and identify important questions based on the outcome evaluation
- Lead healthcare teams in the implementation of EBP

MSN-educated nurses have a critical place in role modeling and leading healthcare teams in the translation and application of best evidence into practice at the point of care. Healthcare organizations are required to provide MSN-educated nurses opportunities to use their critical thinking skills to bring EBP to both individual patient care situations and to broader communities.

Doctor of Nursing Practice

DNP-educated nurses are prepared in specialized advanced nursing with a focus on practice that is innovative and evidence based (AACN, 2006). DNP education prepares nurses to develop EBP clinical scholarship and engage in analytical methods that augment EBP. Clinical scholarship is a purposeful and systematic endeavor that emphasizes inquiry, outcomes, and evidence to support nursing practice (Sigma Theta Tau International Clinical Scholarship Task Force, 1999).

Scholarship integration enables DNP graduates to use isolated facts to make important connections that provide new conceptualizations and meanings to nursing care interventions. To improve health outcomes, DNP graduates integrate evidence derived from diverse sources and multiple disciplines and apply relevant findings to clinical problems (AACN, 2006; Diers, 1995). DNP graduates use advanced administrative skills to provide leadership to teams of healthcare providers in the implementation of EBP. DePalma and McGuire (2005) noted that integrating clinical practice knowledge and leading EBP initiatives at the DNP level require the following:

- Advanced nursing competency in translation of research into practice
- Ability to strategize evaluation of clinical practice
- Aptitude for improving the reliability of healthcare outcomes
- Active participation in collaborative healthcare research

DNP graduates are prepared to generate clinical evidence through their practices and serve as leaders in guiding healthcare improvements (AACN, 2006; White et al., 2016). To accomplish clinical knowledge translation and master key leadership roles for EBP, DNP-level nurses:

- Use analytical methods and expert critical appraisal skills to determine the merit of scientific literature and other evidence as appropriate sources of best knowledge for clinical practice change
- Create and implement innovative processes to evaluate clinical practice, practice patterns, and systems of care outcomes against national benchmarks

- Design, lead, and evaluate quality improvement work
- Develop practice guidelines centered on relevant, evidence-based findings
- Use advanced technologies and research methods to:
  - Collect data to generate evidence
  - Design meaningful clinical databases
  - Analyze practice-based data
  - Design innovative evidence-based interventions
  - Predict the probability of select outcomes
  - Review data for patterns of human and organizational behavior
  - Identify gaps in evidence for practice
- Consult with individuals and healthcare teams in collaboration of knowledge-generating research efforts
- Mentor others in the art and science of disseminating EBP findings

DNP graduates are expected to critically appraise and apply evidence to achieve optimal patient outcomes (Pipe, Wellik, Buchda, Hansen, & Martyn, 2005). Beyond important foundational involvement with EBP, DNP graduates must be engaged in translating scientific findings into clinical practice, improve reliability of healthcare outcomes, and actively collaborate in healthcare research. DNP graduates use their advanced EBP practice skills and knowledge to generate new ideas to guide improvements in clinical practice.

SEQUENTIAL ADVANCEMENT OF EBP KNOWLEDGE AND SKILLS

Evidence-based practice competencies in nursing advance along the trajectory of BSN, MSN, and DNP degrees. Each degree assumes a certain level of EBP competency. In addition, each degree provides the foundation knowledge and skills to accomplish the next level of EBP competency until a terminal practice degree (i.e., DNP) is achieved. For example, at the BSN level nurses are expected to *explain* critical interrelationships between theory, practice, and research. Moving to the MSN level, nurses are expected to integrate theory, practice, and research for the purpose of translating findings into practice. At the terminal practice degree level, nurses apply the integrated findings of theory, practice, and research to create practice guidelines for groups of nurses and other healthcare professionals.

Another example of successive EBP steps through nursing's academic trajectory is focused on research. At the BSN level, nurses advocate for the protection of humans as research participants. The MSN level requires nurses to advocate for the ethical conduct of programs of research and translational scholarship. DNP nurses are also expected to protect participants in research but also must be active consultants/collaborators in knowledge-generating research.

Critical appraisal is another step-wise EBP example. At the BSN level, nurses evaluate sources of information to determine the level and quality of evidence. At the MSN level, nurses perform rigorous and systematic critiques of evidence, derived from data-driven research, to generate meaningful clinical practice evidence. At the DNP level, nurses use sophisticated analytic methods (e.g., meta-analysis, systematic review, meta-synthesis) to critically appraise research literature to determine the best evidence to generate into clinical practice.

As a closing example of advancing stages of EBP, BSN-level nurses integrate evidence, clinical experience, and patient reference to plan, implement, and evaluate outcomes of patient-centered care. MSN-level nurses, using best evidence, lead collaborative teams to improve care outcomes and support policy changes. At the DNP level, nurses design and implement innovative processes to evaluate outcomes of practice

SUMMARY

The role of the nurse in EBP has not always been clear. This chapter clarifies and delineates the roles and expectations of the nurse in EBP at each professional nursing degree level. In line with AACN Essentials and IOM mandates, the chapter underscores EBP activities for BSN, MSN, and DNP graduates that help ensure safe, effective, and efficient care. Evidence-based practice knowledge and skill requirements for each nursing degree level are reviewed. Organizational obligations to provide EBP opportunities for each level of degree preparation are emphasized.

REFERENCES

Adams, K., Hean, S., Sturgis, P., & Macleod-Clark, J. (2006). Investigating the factors influencing professional identity of first-year health and social care students. *Learning in Health and Social Care, 5*(2), 55–68.

American Association of Colleges of Nursing. (2006). *The essentials of doctoral education for advanced nursing practice*. Retrieved from http://www.aacnnursing.org/Portals/42/Publications/DNPEssentials.pdf

American Association of Colleges of Nursing. (2008). *The essentials of baccalaureate education for professional nursing*. Retrieved from http://www.aacnnursing.org/Portals/42/Publications/BaccEssentials08.pdf

American Association of Colleges of Nursing. (2011). *The essentials of master's education in nursing*. Retrieved from http://www.aacnnursing.org/Portals/42/Publications/MastersEssentials11.pdf

American Association of Colleges of Nursing. (2015). The impact of education on nursing practice. Retrieved from http://www.aacnnursing.org/News-Information/Fact-Sheets/Impact-of-Education

American Association of Colleges of Nursing. (2016). Vision and mission. Retrieved from http://www.aacnnursing.org/About-AACN/AACN-Governance/Vision-and-Mission

American Hospital Association. (2002). *In our hands: How hospital leaders can build a thriving workforce*. Washington, DC: Author.

American Nurses Association. (1965). *A position paper*. New York, NY: Author.

Avorn, J., & Fischer, M. (2010). Bench to behavior: Translating comparative effectiveness research into improved clinical practice. *Health Affairs, 29*(10), 1891–1900.

Cohen, E. B., & Lloyd, S. J. (2014). Disciplinary evolution and the rise of transdiscipline. *Informing Science: The International Journal of Transdiscipline, 17*, 189–215.

Davis, D. A., & Taylor-Vaisey, A. (1997). Translating guidelines into practice: A systematic review of theoretic concepts, practical experience, and research evidence in the adoption of clinical practice guidelines. *Canadian Medical Association Journal, 157*, 408–416.

DePalma, J. A., & McGuire, D. B. (2005). Research. In A. Hamric, J. Spross, & C. Hanson (Eds.), *Advanced practice nursing: An integrative approach* (3rd ed, pp. 257–300). Philadelphia, PA: Elsevier Saunders.

Diers, D. (1995). The discipline of nursing. *Journal of Professional Nursing, 11*(1), 24–30.

Gonzales, R., Handley, M. A., Ackerman, S., & O'Sullivan, P. S. (2012). Increasing the translation of evidence into practice policy and public health improvements: A framework for training health professionals in implementation and dissemination science. *Academic Medicine, 87*(3), 271–278. doi:10.1097/ACM.0b013e3182449d33

Grenier, A. C., & Knebel, E. (Eds.). (2003). *Health professions education: A bridge to quality.* Washington, DC: National Academies Press.

Haynes, R. B., Hayward, R. S., & Lomas, J. (1995). Bridges between health care research evidence and clinical practice. *Journal of the American Medical Informatics Association, 2*(6), 342–350.

Institute of Medicine. (2000). *To err is human* (L. T. Kohn, J. M. Corrigan, & M. S. Donaldson, Eds.). Washington, DC: National Academies Press.

Institute of Medicine. (2001). *Crossing the quality chasm: A new health system for the 21st century.* Washington, DC: National Academies Press.

Institute of Medicine. (2004). *Keeping patients safe: Transforming the work environment of nurses.* Washington, DC: National Academies Press.

Institute of Medicine. (2010). *The future of nursing: Leading change advancing health.* Washington, DC: National Academies Press.

Kanter, R. M. (1993). *Men and women of the corporation.* New York, NY: Basic Books.

Madon, T., Hofman, K. J., Kupfer, L., & Glass, R. I. (2007). Public health implementation science. *Science, 318*(5837), 1728–1729. doi:10.1016/j.cnur.201202.004

Melnyk, B. M., & Fineout-Overholt, E. (2015). *Evidence-based practice in nursing and healthcare: A guide to best practice.* Philadelphia, PA: Wolters Kluwer.

Moseley, M. J. (2012). The role of the advanced practice registered nurse in ensuring evidence-based practice. *Nursing Clinics of North America, 47,* 269–281.

National Institutes of Health. (2016). Dissemination and implementation research in health (RO1). Retrieved from https://grants.nih.gov/grants/guide/pa-files/PAR-16-238.html

Ogilvie, D., Craig, P., Griffin, S., Macintyre, S., & Wareham, N. J. (2009). A translational framework for public health research. *BioMed Central Public Health, 9,* 116.

Pipe, T. B., Wellik, K. E., Buchda, C. M., Hansen, C. M., & Martyn, D. R. (2005). Implementing evidence-based practice in nursing. *Urologic Nursing, 25*(5), 365–370.

Septimus, E., Yokoe, D. S., Weinstein, R. A., Perl, T. M., Maragakis, L. L., & Berenholtz, S. M. (2014). Maintaining the momentum for change: The role of the 2014 updates to the compendium in preventing healthcare associated infections. *Infection Control and Hospital Epidemiology, 35*(5), 460–463.

Sigma Theta Tau International Clinical Scholarship Task Force. (1999). Clinical scholarship resource paper. Retrieved from http://www.sigmanursing.org/docs/default-source/position-papers/clinical_scholarship_paper.pdf?sfvrsn=4

White, K. M., Dudley-Brown, S., & Terhaar, M. F. (2016). *Translation of evidence into nursing practice and health care* (2nd ed.). New York, NY: Springer Publishing.

Zerhouni, E. A. (2005). US biomedical research: Basic, translational, and clinical sciences. *Journal of the American Medical Association, 294*(11), 1352–1358.

CHAPTER 20

Evidence-Based Practice: Empowering Nurses

Thomas L. Christenbery

Objectives

After reading this chapter, learners should be able to:

1. Define *nurse empowerment*
2. Describe how empowerment supports evidence-based practice (EBP)
3. Identify aspects of a healthy work environment

EVIDENCE-BASED PRACTICE (EBP) SCENARIOS

Scenario 1

Direct care nurses on a postsurgical unit wanted to develop and initiate a clinical practice guideline (CPG) for patient fall reduction, specific to the postsurgical unit. The nurses understood that an EBP project would be a realistic approach to developing a CPG for fall reduction. The nurses met with their direct supervisor to discuss the possibility of the EBP project. The nurses thought it would be helpful to know the fall incidence rate for the unit and subsequently asked their direct supervisor for the patient fall data. The supervisor told the nurses that fall incident data constituted legal information and they could not have *access* to it. She also told the nurses that staffing was short and they should be using their time as a *resource* for direct patient care and not be concerned with developing new safety protocols. The supervisor told the nurses not to be disheartened because a hospital-wide fall reduction plan was being considered. She told them it seemed they missed their *opportunity* for an EBP project. The nurses acquiesced and wished they felt more *supported* by management.

Scenario 2

Direct care nurses on a postsurgical unit wanted to develop and initiate a CPG for patient fall reduction, specific to the postsurgical unit. The nurses understood that an EBP project would be a realistic approach to developing a CPG for fall reduction. The nurses met with their direct supervisor to discuss the possibility of the EBP project. The nurses thought it would be helpful to know the actual fall incidence for the unit and subsequently asked their direct supervisor for the data. The supervisor replied, "Of course you may have *access* to that information" because she received that information monthly from the hospital safety committee. The supervisor stated, "There is a great *opportunity* for one of you to be a member of the hospital safety committee and the committee could really use a direct care nurse as a member." The supervisor also told them of a nurse on the unit who was a DNP student and was very good at accessing electronic *resources* such as the Cochrane Database of Systematic Reviews and Ovid. She was certain the DNP student would be willing to help them find the most up-to-date *knowledge/information* on patient fall reduction in hospitals. The nurses felt *supported* in this endeavor and confidently began making plans to proceed with the EBP fall reduction project.

Discussion

In Scenarios 1 and 2, both groups of direct care nurses identified a legitimate practice concern that fell within the realm of nursing to address as an EBP project. In Scenario 1, the nurses' healthcare organization did not extend the fundamental elements of structural empowerment, which left the nurses disempowered and struggling to move forward with an EBP project. In Scenario 2, the nurses detected the four structural elements of empowerment and were able to plan for a successful EBP project.

EMPOWERMENT

Health implies more than the absence of disease (World Health Organization, 1948). Similarly, a healthy work environment infers more than the absence of organizational dysfunction. A healthy person who is active and contributing to the well-being of society is analogous to a healthy work environment in which employees are active participants who collectively achieve desired organizational goals. A healthy work environment creates a desirable place to work, in part, by providing structural elements that positively impact the effectiveness of the work (Weston, 2010). Authoritative bodies indicate that nurses who practice in healthy work environments tend to contribute to desired clinical outcomes, have constructive views of the nursing profession, and have positive self-images as practicing nurses (American Association of Critical-Care Nurses [AACN], 2005; Nursing Organizations Alliance, 2004).

In addition to authoritative bodies, research indicates that nurses who work in healthy environments lean toward a greater sense of empowerment that positively impacts role satisfaction, relationships with formal leadership, attrition, and commitment to a healthcare organization's goals (Cohen, Stuenkel, & Nquyen, 2009; Heath, Johanson, & Blake, 2004; McDonald, Tullai-McGuinness, Madigan, & Shively, 2010; Nedd, 2006). In nursing literature, empowerment is a central theme that describes the relationship between healthcare organization culture and nurse participation in achieving organizational goals (Knol & van Linge, 2009). Across scholarly literature, *empowerment* is defined as the ability to get things done (Irvine, Leatt, Evans, & Baker, 1999; Kanter, 1993; Knol & van Linge, 2009). Empowerment enables organizational participants to achieve work-related goals (Laschinger, 1996; Wilson & Laschinger, 1994).

According to Kanter (1993), empowerment arises from mobilizing four organizational structural components:

- *Support:* Having access to organizational support for work-related responsibilities and decision making
- *Resources:* Having access to resources that will be needed to perform work-related activities
- *Knowledge:* Having access to relevant organizational information to engage in work-related roles
- *Opportunity:* Having opportunities for organizational advancement and involvement in activities beyond an assigned job description

Healthcare organizations that manifest these four structural components empower nurses and other organizational participants to engage in satisfying and effective organizational-related behaviors. The elements of structural empowerment support shared governance. Shared governance is a model of nursing practice in which direct care nurses are entrusted with the power to influence institutional policies and decisions that have implications for delivery of patient-centered care (Porter-O'Grady, 2009). The conceptual foundations of shared governance are based in Kanter's Theory of Structural Empowerment (Kanter, 1993). Structural empowerment fosters transformational leadership (i.e., leadership approach that enhances participants' motivation, job performance, and morale by connecting their self-identity to the mission and philosophy of the organization), open communication, and collegial and empathetic professional relationships (Linnen & Rowley, 2014). Support, resources, knowledge, and opportunity are discussed in Chapters 16, 17, 18, and 19, respectively, as structural components necessary for successful implementation of EBP in healthcare settings. The degree of nurse empowerment associated with implementation of EBP is dependent, in part, on the presence of each structural component in the healthcare organization (Kanter, 1993). Nurses' work engagement becomes more effective and achievement of healthcare organizational goals improve when healthcare organizations provide opportunity and empowerment to all nurses across the organizational hierarchy (Kanter, 1993; Manoilovich, 2007). Nurses are academically prepared to work within the scope of their practice and are worthy of being members of an empowered workforce.

The elements of structural empowerment seem to cross international and healthcare cultural boundaries. Aiken and coworkers (2001) compared nurse staffing, work environments, and patient outcomes across five countries (i.e., the United States, England, Scotland, Canada, and Germany). These countries, with widely different systems of healthcare delivery, reported similarities among workplace structural empowerment.

EMPOWERMENT AND EBP

EBP is defined as the systematic evaluation and implementation of sound scientific research, integrated with clinical expertise and patient preferences that facilitate optimal health outcomes for patients (Lenz & Barnard, 2009; Melnyk et al., 2004; Neville & Horbatt, 2008; Pravikoff, Tanner, & Pierce, 2005; Sackett, Straus, Richardson, Rosenberg, & Haynes, 2000). Implementation of EBP fosters both innovative nursing care strategies and autonomy in clinical practice that stimulate workplace empowerment (Belden, Leafmen, Nehrenz, & Miller, 2012).

Nurses who engage in EBP report heightened motivation, autonomy, and clinical expertise (Belden et al., 2012). Important nursing care concepts, such as accountability, responsibility, and innovation, have a positive correlation to structural empowerment when centered on best evidence, clinical expertise, and patient values (Faulkner & Laschinger, 2008; Laschinger & Wong, 1999). Nurses who have access to the four components of structural empowerment to engage in EBP report higher productivity levels, greater sense of professional accomplishment, and involvement in innovative care processes. *Importantly, empowered nurses are more likely to share sources of power with those perceived to have less empowerment* (Knol & van Linge, 2009). Healthcare organizations that undergird the components of structural empowerment as a means to support EBP directly impact nurses' sense of empowerment in professional practice (Knol & van Linge, 2009; see Box 20.1).

BOX 20.1   Examples of Healthcare Organization Empowerment Behaviors

Organizations that encourage empowerment provide the following:

- Opportunities for professional growth and development
- Stimulating and challenging work
- Opportunities to gain new work-related knowledge and skills
- Access to resources to accomplish work
- Time allotted to complete work
- Encouragement to find meaningfulness in work
- Information to accomplish work
- Support from management to meet responsibilities and complete work activities
- Opportunities to work collaboratively with other departments and interprofessional teams
- Recognition for work well done
- Tangible recognition from organizational leadership for work well done

In addition to EBP, nurse access to opportunity, support, knowledge, and resources supports many other professional workplace engagements. Empowered nurses are able to strategize and foster many healthcare organization activities that support EBP. When nurses act in an empowered manner, healthcare organization phenomena such as healthy work environments, meaningfulness of work, vision and innovation, and community leadership are positively influenced and help create a broader supportive culture that is welcoming and conducive to EBP.

NURSE EMPOWERMENT AND HEALTHY WORK ENVIRONMENTS

Empowered nurses are generally employed in healthy work environments that provide organizational structure for participant empowerment. Healthy work environments manifest attributes of interprofessional collaboration, effective communication, accountability, shared clinical decision making, and visible, dependable organizational leadership (AACN, 2005; Brody, Barnes, Ruble, & Sakowski, 2012; Nursing Organizations Alliance, 2004). Nurses working in healthy organizations often report a greater sense of empowerment (Heath et al., 2004).

Engagement in EBP enhances workplace empowerment by providing nurses opportunities to change standards of practice and improve quality of care. Having direct evidence-based input into clinical decision making increases nurses' ownership of clinical practice and instills an additional sense of pride in their work and work setting (Christenbery, Williamson, Sandlin, & Wells, 2016; Heath et al., 2004). To meet healthcare organization and public expectations about EBP, nurses must feel empowered. For almost two decades, research and theory have supported structural empowerment (Kanter, 1993) and its application to enhancing work environments that empower nurses (Laschinger, 1996).

MEANINGFUL WORK ENVIRONMENT

Meaningful work is defined as work that provides essence to what organizational participants do and brings fulfillment to their lives (Chalofsky, 2003; Lieff, 2009). The opportunity to find meaning in daily work positively influences participants' commitment to work and work engagement (Laschinger, Finegan, & Wilk, 2009; May, Gilson, & Harter, 2004). Nursing research, specifically, indicates that nurses who use EBP and are employed in organizations supportive of EBP feel greater role satisfaction and a sense of empowerment (Melnyk, Fineout-Overholt, Giggleman, & Cruz, 2010; Melnyk, Fineout-Overholt, & Mays, 2008).

Nurses engaged in EBP report a heightened awareness about the impact of their EBP work. In other words, EBP provides a sense of meaning to their clinical work (Brody et al., 2012; Melnyk et al., 2010). Having additional control and responsibility in implementing practice change through EBP promotes leadership, knowledge, and skills. The meaningfulness of EBP encourages some nurses to become more involved in their healthcare organizations, such as assuming leadership roles on committees (e.g., EBP Council, Nursing Research Committee). Seeking and attaining leadership roles in healthcare organizations serve to enhance further a feeling of empowerment for nurses.

VISION AND INNOVATION

Visionary nurses view nursing care as an essential link between science and humanity (Hader, 2014). Visionary behavior includes planning for the future using innovation and insight. Nurses have a responsibility to be inventive in visualizing a healthy future for patients, the nursing profession, and the global community. Several health-related variables are converging and building a demand for visionary nurses: (a) aging population, (b) increased complexity of patient care, (c) expansion of knowledge that undergirds healthcare, (d) concerns about basic patient safety and quality of care, (e) need for higher levels of academic preparation for nurses, and (f) ongoing shortage of prepared nursing faculty. If healthcare is to be transformed to meet the rising needs of patients and communities, visionary nurses will be central to that transformation. EBP is one method used to prepare and encourage visionary nurses.

Nurses express a sense of empowerment through an expanded scope of organizational vision that EBP provides (Christenbery et al., 2016). The interprofessional collaboration that EBP fosters enables nurses to see beyond individual patients to the broader unit and the healthcare organization as a whole. EBP rouses a spirit of camaraderie and teamwork supporting a vision of optimal patient care and a best-practice environment between departments within healthcare organizations. EBP provides nurses with opportunities to engage in activities that broaden their visions of healthcare and healthcare systems. For example, work on EBP councils provides nurses with exposure to teamwork between departments while maintaining a focus on optimal patient care.

Visionary nurses engage in innovative behavior. In nursing, innovation is the process of translating a vision into a nursing service that a patient or community will value. In the current complex and dynamic healthcare environment, nursing innovative behavior is essential for optimal EBP (Knol & van Linge, 2009). Empowerment motivates employees to initiate and engage in innovative organizational behaviors (Spreitzer, 1995).

Nursing literature identifies two categories of innovation: (a) *reactive* and (b) *proactive*. Reactive innovation seems to be the default innovation as it is the most frequently observed category of innovation that nurses use (Tonuma & Winbolt, 2000). Less noted in nursing is the creativity associated with proactive innovation (Gilmartin, 1999). A primary aim of EBP is to encourage nurses to engage in proactive innovation. Innovation is a function of organizational context (Kanter, 1988) and is facilitated by structural components of empowerment (Spreitzer, 1995).

COMMUNITY LEADERSHIP

The experience of having autonomy and responsibility for implementing evidence-based change accelerates the growth of leadership skillsets for nurses (Brody et al., 2012). Often EBP leadership skills transcend the healthcare organization. Empowered nurses are often involved in EBP committees and task forces (e.g., EBP council) that impact change in healthcare organizations. The empowered nurses may also serve on community boards or in community leadership positions that focus on the nurses' EBP phenomenon of interest. For example, a nurse whose EBP project is recognized for enhancing parental bonding in the neonatal intensive care unit may be asked to serve on a March of Dimes-related committee. Hospital leaders who support such community involvement for direct care nurses are demonstrating the element of opportunity in structural empowerment and promoting a community-wide positive image of nursing.

To meet healthcare organization and public expectations about EBP, nurses must feel empowered. For almost two decades, research and theory have supported structural empowerment (Kanter, 1993) and its application to enhancing work environments that empower nurses (Laschinger, 1996).

SUMMARY

This chapter describes ways nurses are expected to act when empowered to solve patient care problems and promote positive healthcare decisions. The chapter reviews how empowered nurses birth new ideas and innovations and engage in EBP to contribute and utilize new knowledge for the advancement of patient care. The chapter emphasizes how nursing leadership and those who practice professional nursing are responsible for setting up cultures of care that empower nurses to engage in EBP.

REFERENCES

Aiken, L. H., Clarke, S. P., Sloane, D. M., Sochalski, J., Busse, R., & Clarke, H., . . . Shamian, J. (2001). Nurses' reports on hospital care in five countries. *Health Affairs, 20*(3), 43–53.

American Association of Critical-Care Nurses. (2005). Standards for establishing and sustaining healthy work environments: A journey to excellence. *American Journal of Critical Care, 14*(3), 187–197.

Belden, C. V., Leafmen, J., Nehrenz, G., & Miller, P. (2012). The effect of evidence-based practice on workplace empowerment of rural registered nurses. *Journal of Rural Nursing and Health Care, 12*(2), 64–76.

Brody, A. A., Barnes, K., Ruble, C., & Sakowski, J. (2012). Evidence-based practice councils: Potential paths to staff nurse empowerment and leadership growth. *Journal of Nursing Administration, 42*(1), 28–33.

Chalofsky, N. (2003). An emerging construct for meaningful work. *Human Resource Development International, 6*, 69–83.

Christenbery, T., Williamson, A., Sandlin, V., & Wells, N. (2016). Immersion in evidence-based practice fellowship program. *Journal for Nurses in Professional Development, 32*(1), 15–20.

Cohen, J., Stuenkel, D., & Nquyen, Q. (2009). Providing a healthy work environment for nurses: The influence on retention. *Journal of Nursing Care Quality, 24*(4), 308–315.

Faulkner, J., & Laschinger, H. (2008). The effects of structural and psychological empowerment on perceived respect in acute care nurses. *Journal of Nursing Management, 16*, 214–221.

Gilmartin, M. J. (1999). Creativity: The fuel of innovation. *Nursing Administrative Quarterly, 23*(21), 1–8.

Hader, R. (2014). Visionary leader. *Nursing Management, 45*(6), 28. doi:10.1097/01.NUMA .0000451077.33462.3a

Heath, J., Johanson, W., & Blake, N. (2004). Healthy work environments: A validation of the literature. *Journal of Nursing Administration, 34*(11), 524–530.

Irvine, D., Leatt, P., Evans, M. G., & Baker, R. G. (1999). Measurement of staff empowerment within health service organizations. *Journal of Nursing Measurement, 7*(1), 79–96.

Kanter, R. M. (1988). When a thousand flowers bloom: Structural collective and social conditions for innovation in organization. *Research and Organizational Behavior, 10*, 169–211.

Kanter, R. M. (1993). *Men and women of the corporation* (2nd ed.). New York, NY: Basic Books.

Knol, J., & van Linge, R. (2009). Innovative behavior: The effect of structural and psychological empowerment on nurses. *Journal of Advanced Nursing, 65*(2), 359–370.

Laschinger, H. S. (1996). A theoretical approach to studying work empowerment in nursing: A review of studies testing Kanter's theory of structural empowerment on nurses. *Nursing Administration Quarterly, 20*(2), 25–41.

Laschinger, H. S., Finegan, J., & Wilk, P. (2009). Context matters: The impact of unit leadership and empowerment on nurses' organizational commitment. *Journal of Nursing Administration, 39*, 228–235.

Laschinger, H. S., & Wong, C. (1999). Staff nurse empowerment and collective accountability: Effect on perceived and self-related work effectiveness. *Nursing Economic$, 17*, 308–316.

Lenz, B. K., & Barnard, P. (2009). Advancing evidence-based practice in rural nursing. *Journal for Nurses in Staff Development, 25*(1), E14–E19.

Lieff, S. J. (2009). The missing link in academic career planning and development: Pursuit of meaningful and aligned work. *Academic Medicine, 84*, 1383–1388.

Linnen, D., & Rowley, A. (2014). Encouraging clinical nurse empowerment. *Nursing Management, 45*(2), 44–47.

Manoilovich, M. (2007). Power and empowerment in nursing: Looking backward to inform the future. *Online Journal of Issues in Nursing, 12*(1), 1–10. doi:10.3912/OJIN.Vol12No01Man01

May, D., Gilson, R., & Harter, L. (2004). The psychological conditions of meaningfulness safety and availability and the engagement of the human spirit at work. *Journal of Occupational and Organizational Psychology, 77*, 11–37.

McDonald, S., Tullai-McGuinness, S., Madigan, E., & Shively, M. (2010). Relationship between staff nurse involvement in organizational structures and perception of empowerment. *Critical Care Nurse Quarterly, 33*(2), 148–162.

Melnyk, B. M., Fineout-Overholt, E., Feinstein, N. F., Li, H., Wilcox, L., & Kraus, R. (2004). Nurses' perceived knowledge, beliefs, skills, and needs regarding evidence-based practice: Implications for accelerating the paradigm shift. *Worldviews on Evidence-Based Nursing, 1*, 185–193.

Melnyk, B. M., Fineout-Overholt, E., Giggleman, M., & Cruz, R. (2010). Correlates among cognitive beliefs EBP implementation, organizational culture, cohesion and job satisfaction in evidence-based practice mentors from a community hospital system. *Nursing Outlook, 58*(6), 301–308.

Melnyk, B. M., Fineout-Overholt, E., & Mays, M. Z. (2008). The evidence-based practice beliefs and implementation scales: Psychometric properties of two new instruments. *Worldviews on Evidenced-Based Nursing, 5*(4), 208–216.

Nedd, N. (2006). Perceptions of empowerment and intent to stay. *Nursing Economic$, 24*(1), 13–18.

Neville, K., & Horbatt, S. (2008). Evidence-based practice: Creating a spirit of inquiry to solve clinical problems. *Orthopedic Nursing, 27*, 331–337.

Nursing Organizations Alliance. (2004). Principles and elements of a healthful practice/work environment. Retrieved from http://www.aone.org/resources/healthful-practice-work.pdf

Porter-O'Grady, T. (2009). *Interdisciplinary shared governance: Integrating practice transforming health care.* Sudbury, MA: Jones & Bartlett.

Pravikoff, D. S., Tanner, A. B., & Pierce, S. T. (2005). Readiness of U.S. nurses for evidence-based practice. *American Journal of Nursing, 105*(9), 40–47.

Sackett, D. L., Straus, S. E., Richardson, W. S., Rosenberg, W., & Haynes, R. B. (2000). *Evidence-based medicine: How to practice and teach EBM* (2nd ed.). New York, NY: Churchill Livingstone.

Spreitzer, G. M. (1995). Psychological empowerment in the workplace: Dimensions measurement and validation. *Management Journal, 38*(5), 1442–1465.

Tonuma, M., & Winbolt, M. (2000). From rituals to reason: Creating an environment that allows nurses to nurse. *International Journal of Nursing Practice, 6*(4), 214–218.

Weston, M. J. (2010). Strategies for enhancing autonomy and control over nursing practice. *ANA Online Journal of Issues in Nursing, 15*(1), Retrieved from http://www.nursingworld.org/MainMenuCategories/ANAMarketplace/ANAPeriodicals/OJIN/TableofContents/Vol152010/No1Jan2010/Enhancing-Autonomy-and-Control-and-Practice.aspx

Weston, M. J. (2010). Strategies for enhancing autonomy and control over nursing practice. *The Online Journal of Issues in Nursing, 15*(1). doi:10.3912/OJIN.Vol15No01Man01

Wilson, B., & Laschinger, H. S. (1994). Staff nurse perception of job empowerment and organizational commitment. *Journal of Nursing Administration, 24*(4S), 39–47.

World Health Organization. (1948). *Constitution of the World Health Organization*. Geneva, Switzerland: Author.

Evidence-Based Practice Models

Nurses and other healthcare professionals have developed several evidence-based practice (EBP) models that aid in the implementation of EBP. These models serve as organizing guides that integrate the most current research to create best patient care practices. In addition to helping nurses integrate credible evidence into practice, EBP models help assure complete implementation of EBP projects and optimize the use of nurses' time and healthcare resources. No single EBP model can meet the needs of every organization and every patient situation. Therefore, we are providing model definitions, essential steps, salient points, and information resources for the models to help readers identify the EBP model that best fits their current, specific EBP needs.

Model Definition	Essential Steps	Salient Points to Consider
Iowa Model of EBP (Titler et al., 2001). The Iowa Model focuses on the entire healthcare system (e.g., patient, practitioner, infrastructure) to implement and guide practice decisions based on best available research and evidence.	1. Identify either a "problem-focused trigger" or "knowledge-focused trigger" that will generate the need for a practice change. 2. Determine whether the "trigger" is a healthcare organization priority. 3. Reflect a team's topic of interest and include interested stakeholders. The team will search, appraise, and synthesize literature related to the topic. 4. Evaluate the availability and merit (e.g., level of evidence, quality of evidence) of evidence. If evidence availability and merit are lacking, conduct research. 5. If credible and reliable evidence is available, pilot the practice change. 6. Appraise pilot for level of success. If pilot is successful, disseminate findings within the organization and implement recommended change into practice.	• Recommended for use at organizational systems level • Uses pragmatic problem-solving approach to EBP implementation • Detailed flowchart (see Chapter 11) guides decision-making process • Clearly identified decision points and feedback loops throughout the model • Emphasizes necessity of pilot project before initiating system-wide project • Designed for interprofessional collaboration • Has sustained test of time

(continued)

Model Definition	Essential Steps	Salient Points to Consider
Stetler Model (Ciliska et al., 2011; Stetler, 2001). The Stetler Model enables practitioners to assess how research findings and other pertinent evidence are implemented in clinical practice. The model examines how to use evidence to create change that fosters patient-centered care.	Steps in this model are referred to as *phases*. Phase I. *Preparation:* Identify a priority need. Identify the purpose of the EBP project, context in which the project will occur, and relevant sources of evidence. Phase II. *Validation:* Assess sources of evidence for level and overall quality. Determine whether source has merit and goodness of fit and whether to accept or reject the evidence in relation to project purpose. Phase III. *Comparative Evaluation/ Decision Making:* Evidence findings are logically summarized and similarities and differences among sources of evidence are evaluated. Determine whether it is acceptable and feasible to apply summation of findings to practice. Phase IV. *Translation/Application:* Develop the "how to's" for implementation of summarized findings. Identify practice implications that justify application of findings for change. Phase V. *Evaluation:* Identify expected outcomes of the project and determine whether the goals of EBP were successfully achieved.	• Designed to encourage critical thinking about the integration of research findings • Promotes use of best evidence as an ongoing practice • Helps lessen errors in critical decision-making activity • Allows for categorization of evidence as external (e.g., research) or internal (e.g., organization outcome data) • Emphasizes use by single practitioner but may include groups of practitioners or other stakeholders
Ottawa Model of Research Use (Graham & Logan, 2004 Graham et al., 2006). The Ottawa Model is an interactive model that depicts research as a dynamic process of interconnected decisions made and actions taken by stakeholders.	The model is composed of three phases: (a) Assess barriers and supports. (b) Monitor intervention and extent of use. (c) Evaluate outcomes. Subsumed under the three phases are six designated primary elements that must be considered when integrating research into practice: I. **Assess barriers and supports:** 1. *Evidence-based innovation:* Clearly identify what the innovation is and what the implementation will involve. 2. *Potential adopters:* Identify potential adopters with characteristics that could influence the adoption of the innovation (see Rogers' Change Theory in Chapter 7).	• Patients are central to the model's process and their health outcomes are the primary focus. • The model focuses on the unit-level environment instead of the entire healthcare organization. • The prescriptive aim of the model is to assess, monitor, and evaluate.

(continued)

Model Definition	Essential Steps	Salient Points to Consider
	3. *The practice environment:* Identify leaders, formal and informal, who can inspire change. Assess environment for needed resources. II. **Monitor intervention and extent of use:** 4. *Implementation of intervention strategies:* Select appropriate strategies to increase awareness of implementation and provide necessary education and training for conducting the implementation. 5. *Adoption of innovation:* Determine the extent of adoption of implementation. III. **Evaluate outcomes:** 6. Evaluate the impact of innovation on patients, practitioners, stakeholders, and healthcare organization.	
Promoting Action on Research Implementation in Health Services (PARiHS) Framework (Rycroft-Malone, 2004). The PARiHS Framework provides a method to implement research into practice by *exploring the* interactions among three key elements: (a) evidence, (b) context, and (c) facilitation.	1. **Evidence:** Search for and identify the best available evidence from research, clinician experience, patient values, organization data, and information. 2. **Context:** This is the local environment where the practice change will occur. Adoption of practice change is dependent on contextual features such as organizational culture and level of acceptance, leadership investment, and evaluation of desired outcomes. 3. **Facilitation:** Organizational participants use their knowledge and skills to foster implementation of practice change.	• Explicitly uses facilitation as a factor impacting integration of research findings into practice • Does not address generation of new knowledge • Focus is on unit settings more than system-wide environment • Codified (e.g., research data) and noncodified (e.g., practitioner experience) sources of evidence used

(continued)

Model Definition	Essential Steps	Salient Points to Consider
ACE (Academic Center for Evidence-Based Practice) Star Model of Knowledge Transformation© (Kring, 2008; Stevens, 2004). As a framework, the ACE Star Model aids in systematically integrating best evidence into practice. The model has five major stages that depict forms of knowledge in relative sequence. Research moves through the cycles to combine with other forms of knowledge before integration into practice occurs.	**Five Stages:** 1. **Discovery:** This stage involves searching for new knowledge found in traditional quantitative and qualitative methodologies. 2. **Evidence Summary:** The primary task is to synthesize the body of research knowledge into a meaningful statement of evidence for a given topic. This is a knowledge-generating stage, which occurs simultaneously with new findings that may arise from the synthesis. 3. **Translation:** The aim of translation is to provide clinicians with a practice document (e.g., clinical practice guideline) derived from the synthesis and summation of research findings. 4. **Integration:** Practitioner and healthcare organization practices are changed through formal and informal channels. 5. **Evaluation:** An array of EBP outcomes are evaluated on impact, quality, and satisfaction.	• Focus on promoting use of EBP for direct care nurses • Includes use of qualitative evidence • Primary goal of model is knowledge transformation • Does not incorporate nonresearch evidence (patient values, practitioner's experience) • Identifies factors that impact adoption of innovation
Advancing Research and Clinical Practice Through Close Collaboration (ARCC) (Melnyk & Fineout-Overholt, 2015).	1. Assess the healthcare organization for readiness for change and implantation of EBP project. 2. Identify potential and actual barriers to and facilitators of EBP project. 3. Identify EBP champions to work with direct care nurses or specific clinical units. 4. Implement evidence into practice. 5. Evaluate EBP outcomes.	• Promotes use of EBP among advanced practice nurses and direct care nurses • Identifies a network of stakeholders who are supportive of the EBP project • Cognitive behavioral theory underpinnings • Emphasis on healthcare organizational readiness and identification of facilities and barriers • Encompasses research, patient values, and clinical expertise as evidence.

(continued)

Model Definition	Essential Steps	Salient Points to Consider
Johns Hopkins Nursing Evidence-Based Practice Model (JHNEBP) (Newhouse, Dearholt, Poe, Pugh, & White, 2007). The JHNEBP Model applies a problem-solving approach to clinical decision making. The model is designed to meet the EBP needs of direct care nurses using an uncomplicated three-step process referred to as PET: (a) Practice Question, (b) Evidence, and (c) Translation.	1. **Practice Question:** Using a team approach, the EBP question is identified. 2. **Evidence:** The team searches, appraises, rates the strength of evidence, describes quality of evidence, and makes a practice recommendation on the strength of evidence. 3. **Translation:** In this stage, feasibility is determined, an action plan is created, and change is implemented and evaluated. Findings are presented to the healthcare organization and broader nursing community.	• Emphasizes individual use • Well-developed tool kit that provides nurses with guide for question development, evidence-rating scale, and appraisal guide for various forms of evidence
Knowledge-to-Action (KTA) Process Framework (Graham et al., 2006). The KTA is a model of knowledge creation and knowledge integration.	**Phases:** 1. Identify problems that need to be addressed and begin searching for evidence and research about the identified problem. 2. Adapt the knowledge use to a local context. 3. Identify barriers to use of knowledge. 4. Select, adapt, and implement interventions. 5. Monitor the use of implanted knowledge. 6. Evaluate outcomes related to knowledge use. 7. Sustain appropriate knowledge use.	• Adapts well for use with individuals, teams, and healthcare organizations • Is grounded in planned action theory, which makes the model adaptable to a variety of settings • Breaks knowledge-to-action process into manageable sections.

REFERENCES

Ciliska D., DiCenso, A., Melynk, B. M., Fineout-Overholt, E., Stettler, C. B., Cullent, L., . . . Dang. D. (2011) Models to guide implementation of evidence-based practice. In B. M. Melnyk & E. Finout-Overholt (Eds.), *Evidence-based practice in nursing and healthcare: A guide to best practice* (2nd ed., pp. 241–275). Philadelphia, PA: Wolters-Kluwer.

Graham, I. D., & Logan, J. (2004). Innovations in knowledge transfer and continuity of care. *Canadian Journal of Nursing Research, 36*(2), 89–103.

Graham, I. D., Logan, J., Harrison, M., Straus, S., Tetroe, J., Caswell, W., & Robinson, N. (2006). Lost in knowledge translation: Time for a map? *Journal of Continuing Education in the Health Professions, 26*(1), 13–24. doi:10.1002/chp.47

Kring, D. L. (2008). Clinical nurse specialist practice domains and evidence-based practice competencies: A matrix of influence. *Clinical Nurse Specialist 22*(4), 179–183.

Melnyk, B. M., & Fineout-Overholt, E. (2015). *Evidence-based practice in nursing and healthcare: A guide to best practice*. Philadelphia, PA: Wolters Kluwer.

Newhouse, R. P., Dearholt, S. L., Poe, S. S., Pugh, L. C., & White, K. M. (2007). *Johns Hopkins nursing: Evidence-based practice model and guidelines*. Indianapolis, IN: Sigma Theta Tau International.

Rycroft-Malone, J. (2004). The PARIHS framework: A framework for guiding the implementation of evidence-based practice. *Journal of Nursing Care Quality, 19*(4), 297–304.

Stetler, C. B. (2001). Updating the Stetler Model of research utilization to facilitate evidence-based practice. *Nursing Outlook 49,* 272–279.

Stevens, K. R. (2012). Star Model of EBP: Knowledge transformation. Academic Center for Evidence-Based Practice, The University of Texas Health Science Center at San Antonio. Retrieved from http://www.acestar.uthscsa.edu.

Titler, M. G., Kleiber, C., Steelman, V. J., Rakel, B. A., Budreau, G., Everett, L. Q., . . . Goode, C. J. (2001). The Iowa model of evidence-based practice to promote quality care. *Critical Care Nursing Clinics of North America, 13*(4), 497–509.

Index

CPSIA information can be obtained
at www.ICGtesting.com
Printed in the USA
LVHW101639200820
663728LV00008B/752